Problem Solving in Endocrinology and Metabolism

To Rhona, Hannah, Douglas, Alice, Kathleen and Euan for being a great family, and especially to Fiona for her support during this and many other projects (LK)

To Indrani and Ishani (AB)

Problem Solving in
Endocrinology and Metabolism

Lee Kennedy
James Cook University, Queensland, Australia

Ansu Basu
City Hospital, Birmingham, UK

CLINICAL PUBLISHING
OXFORD

CLINICAL PUBLISHING
An imprint of Atlas Medical Publishing Ltd

Oxford Centre for Innovation
Mill Street, Oxford OX2 0JX, UK

T: +44 1865 811116
F: +44 1865 251550
W: www.clinicalpublishing.co.uk

Distributed in the USA and Canada by:
Clinical Publishing
30 Amberwood Parkway
Ashland OH 44805 USA

T: 800 247 6553 (toll free within U.S. and Canada)
F: 419 281 6883
E: order@bookmasters.com

Distributed in UK and Rest of World by:
Marston Book Services Ltd
PO Box 269, Abingdon
Oxon OX14 4YN, UK

T: +44 1235 465500
F: +44 1235 465555
E: trade.orders@marston.co.uk

First published 2007

A catalogue record for this book is available from the British Library

ISBN 1 904392 79 2
ISBN 978 1 904392 79 8

Project manager: Gavin Smith, GPS Publishing Solutions, Herts, UK
Series design by Pete Russell, Faringdon, Oxon, UK
Typeset by Mizpah Publishing Services Pvt Ltd, Chennai, India
Printed by TG Hostench S.A., Barcelona, Spain

Contents

Abbreviations

17-OHP 17-hydroxyprogesterone
ACTH adrenocorticotrophic hormone
ADH antidiuretic hormone
AECA anti-endothelial cell antibodies
AIDS acquired immune deficiency syndrome
AIT amiodarone-induced thyrotoxicosis
AITD autoimmune thyroid disease
ALD adrenoleukodystrophy
AMI acute myocardial infarction
AMP adenosine monophosphate
ANCA antineutrophil cytoplasmic antibody
anti-TPO antithyroid peroxidase
APA aldosterone-producing adenoma
APS autoimmune polyendocrine deficiency syndromes
autoimmune polyglandular syndromes
adrenergic postprandial syndrome
AQP2 aquaporin-2
ARR ratio of plasma aldosterone to plasma renin
ATP adenosine triphosphate
AVP arginine vasopressin
BAH bilateral adrenal hyperplasia
BMD bone mineral density
BMI body mass index
BMR basal metabolic rate
CAH congenital adrenal hyperplasia
CBZ carbimazole
CC clomiphene citrate
CEE conjugated equine oestrogen
CI confidence interval
CRH corticotrophin-releasing hormone
CT computed tomography
CTLA-4 cytotoxic T lymphocyte antigen
DA dopamine agonist
DDAVP 1-desamino-8-d-arginine vasopressin
DHEA dehydro-3-epiandrosterone
DHEAS DHEA sulphate
DI deiodinase
DIT diiodothyronine
DITPA 3, 5-diiodothyropropionic acid
DOC deoxycorticosterone
DST dexamethasone suppression test
ECG electrocardiogram
ED erectile dysfunction
EDTA ethylenediamintetraacetic acid
EPHESUS Eplerenone Neurohormonal Efficacy and Survival Study
FAI free androgen index
FNAC fine needle aspiration cytology
FSH follicle-stimulating hormone
GFR glomerular filtration rate
GH growth hormone
GLP glucagon-like peptide
GMP guanosine monophosphate
GnRH gonadotrophin-releasing hormone
GTP guanosine triphosphate
hCG human chorionic gonadotrophin
HIV human immunodeficiency virus
HLA human leucocyte antigen
HPA hypothalamic–pituitary–adrenal axis
HRT hormone replacement therapy
HU Hounsfield Unit
ICSI intracytoplasmic sperm injection
IGF insulin-like growth factor
IPSS inferior petrosal sinus sampling
ITU intensive therapy unit
JNC7 Joint National Committee 7
LH luteinizing hormone
LOD laparoscopic ovarian drilling
MDT multidisciplinary team
MEN multiple endocrine neoplasia
MIBG ^{123}I-metaiodobenzylguandine
MIVAT minimally invasive video-assisted thyroidectomy

MMAS Massachusetts Male Aging Study
MMI methimazole
MNG multinodular goitre
MORE Multiple Outcomes of Raloxifene Evaluation
MRI magnetic resonance imaging
NAION non-arteritic ischaemic optic neuropathy
NANC non-adrenergic non cholinergic [neurones]
NEFA non-esterified fatty acid
NHANES National Health and Nutrition Examination Study
NS non-significant
oGTT oral glucose tolerance test
OR odds ratio
PADAM partial androgen deficiency in ageing men
PCOS polycystic ovarian syndrome
PDE-5 phosphodiesterase-5 inhibitor
PKA protein kinase A
POF premature ovarian failure
PPAR-γ peroxisome proliferator-activated receptor-γ
PPTD post-partum thyroid disturbance
PSV peak systolic velocity
PTH parathyroid hormone
PTHrP parathyroid-related protein
PTU propylthiouracil
RALES Randomised Aldactone Evaluation Study
RR relative risk
SAGH subclinical autonomous glucocorticoid hypersecretion
SAME Syndrome of apparent mineralocorticoid excess
SCA silent corticotroph adenomas
SCC side chain cleavage
SERM selective oestrogen receptor modulator
SERPINA serine protease inhibitor superfamily member A7
SES sick euthyroid syndrome
SHBG sex hormone-binding globulin
SIADH syndrome of inappropriate ADH secretion
SMR standard mortality ratio
SPECT single photon emission computed tomography
SST Short synacthen test
T_3 triiodothryronine
T_4 thyroxine
TBG thyroxine-binding globulin
TBI traumatic brain injury
TBII TSH receptor antibodies (TSH binding inhibitory immunoglobulins)
TED thyroid eye disease
TNF tumour necrosis factor
TPO thyroid peroxidase
TRAB TSH receptor antibody
TRH thyrotrophin-releasing hormone
TSH thyroid-stimulating hormone
TTR transthyretin
UFC urine free cortisol
VLCFA very low chain fatty acids
VMA vanillylmandelic acid
WHI Women's Health Initiative

SECTION ONE

01

Thyroid

PROBLEM

01 Graves' Disease

Case History

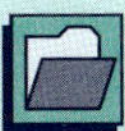

A previously fit 32-year-old woman notices tremor and heat intolerance. She has lost one and a half stones (9.5 kg) in weight over the past 6 months. You note signs of hyperthyroidism and a diffuse goitre. Her mother is treated for hypothyroidism. The patient smokes 20 cigarettes per day. She and her husband want to start a family in the foreseeable future.

How should she be investigated?

Does she require a thyroid scan?

What is the preferred first line of treatment?

If she has a child, how likely is the child to be affected by Graves' disease?

Background

Thyrotoxicosis occurs in 2% of women and 0.2% of men. In younger people, Graves' disease is by far the commonest diagnosis, with peak onset at 20–40 years. Treatment is with drugs, radioactive iodine or surgery. Thionamide drugs are generally the first line of therapy in young women.[1,2] They have been used for over 50 years. They are safe and well tolerated. Up to 10% of patients experience mild side effects including urticaria, skin rash, joint pain, altered taste and nausea. These do not usually necessitate stopping the drug. The most serious side effect is agranulocytosis which occurs in less than 0.4%. Patients should always be warned to report skin rash, sore throat or any other untoward side effect, and this warning should be recorded in their notes. If side effects are reported, full blood count and differential should be requested urgently and consideration should be given to stopping the drug.

There are three thionamide drugs—carbimazole (CBZ), methimazole (MMI), and propylthiouracil (PTU). They are similar in their clinical effect. There have been no substantial head-to-head studies comparing them. CBZ is the most commonly used drug in the UK, whereas MMI is used in the USA and in many European countries. PTU is usually used as second line treatment. It has a shorter duration of action and therefore is best given in divided doses. PTU may have free radical scavenging activity, and it is not the drug of first choice before or after radioactive iodine because it may diminish the effectiveness of the latter. Skin rashes may be commoner with MMI—reported rate in trials was 7% for CBZ compared with 12% for MMI.[2] PTU is the drug of choice in acute severe thyrotoxicosis as it decreases conversion of T_4 to T_3.

In practice, duration of antithyroid treatment does not appear to be critical. Endocrinologists have all encountered patients who stop taking their drugs after a few months and do not relapse and others who relapse even after prolonged treatment. There is consensus that patients should be treated for at least 6 months, and certainly until serum thyrotropin (TSH) is no longer suppressed and levels of TSH receptor antibodies (TBII) have decreased. Longer treatment may lead to decrease in goitre size, and thus lower risk of relapse. Evidence slightly favours longer than 6 months' treatment; common practice is between 12 and 18 months, and there is no evidence to favour longer treatment.

Most endocrinologists commence patients on high dose and gradually decrease to maintenance dose according to response. Block and replace regimens were based on the hypothesis that antithyroid drugs had immune-modulating and antioxidant properties, and thus may modify the natural history of the disease. Exposure to higher doses of the drug for longer necessitates concurrent thyroid hormone treatment. The two regimens have been compared in 12 studies involving a total of over 1700 patients. The compliance with follow-up varied in these studies. On an intention-to-treat basis, and with follow-up greater than 2 years, relapse rate is just over 50% with either regimen. Higher dose of drug increases risk of side effects. There was no difference in the incidence of agranulocytosis. However, skin rashes were more common in block and replace studies—10% for block and replace vs. 5% for titration (odds ratio [OR] 2.62; 95% confidence interval [CI] 1.20 to 5.75). More people withdrew because of side effects in the block and replace groups.

Treatment with thyroxine following antithyroid drugs was hypothesized to decrease autoantigen exposure and thus lower relapse rate. Three studies have combined thyroxine and low-dose antithyroid drug after initial stabilization with antithyroid drug. No difference in relapse rate was found. In three further studies, antithyroid drug was followed by a period of thyroxine treatment. In these studies relapse rate was 31% in the thyroxine-treated patients and 29% in those treated with placebo (not significant).

Thyrotoxicosis may temporarily worsen after ^{131}I because of a combination of radiation-induced thyroiditis and increased TBII. Severe exacerbation occurs in less than 1%. Antithyroid drugs are frequently used prior to ^{131}I to achieve more rapid symptom control. There is no real proof that pre-treatment with antithyroid drugs prevents exacerbation of thyrotoxicosis after treatment, but the increase in TBII is less marked, and exacerbations may thus be less severe.[3] Resumption of antithyroid drugs after radioactive iodine achieves symptom control but does not alter the outcome.[4] Antithyroid drugs are generally stopped 4–10 days before therapy and resumed 7 days after.

Genetics of Graves' disease

Graves' disease results from interaction between genetic and environmental factors. Up to 60% of patients have family history of autoimmune thyroid disease (AITD). About a third of first-degree relatives will develop, or have developed, AITD, and around half will be positive for autoantibodies. Concordance rates are higher for monozygotic twins than for dizygotic twins. Genetic influences are thought to account for up 80% of the susceptibility to Graves' disease.[5]

The human leucocyte antigen (HLA) complex located at chromosome 6p21 has three classes of antigen:

- class I—HLA-A, B and C
- class II—HLA DP, DQ and DR
- class III—complement, tumour necrosis factor (TNF)-α, heat shock protein-70 and other immune regulatory genes.

This is a highly polymorphic region of the genome, conferring susceptibility to a range of diseases. HLA-DR3 is the most useful marker. Among patients with Graves' disease 40–50% are HLA-DR3 positive, compared with 15–30% of the general population. Recent studies have identified associations with other HLA alleles, most notably DQA1*0501. HLA is probably important in all ethnic groups, but the precise associations in non-Caucasians differ from the above. Cytotoxic T lymphocyte antigen-4 (CTLA-4), located at chromosome 2q33, is a costimulatory molecule involved in interaction between T lymphocytes and antigen-presenting cells. At least four polymorphisms have been identified and confer susceptibility to autoimmune endocrine disease.[6] Together, HLA antigens and CTLA-4 confer around half the susceptibility to Graves'. Other candidate genes include immune regulatory genes, such as the vitamin D receptor, TSH receptor and thyroglobulin.

Recent Developments

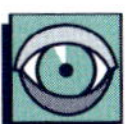

1. Wang *et al.*[7] have shown that the A/G polymorphism at position 40 in exon 1 of CTLA-4 may be a marker for relapse after antithyroid drug therapy. Early identification of patients liable to relapse may allow us to target definitive treatment early.
2. The Nurses' Health Study[8] followed 115 109 women aged 25–42 over 12 years. The incident diagnosis of Graves' was 4.6 per 1000. Smoking was a risk factor (hazard ratio

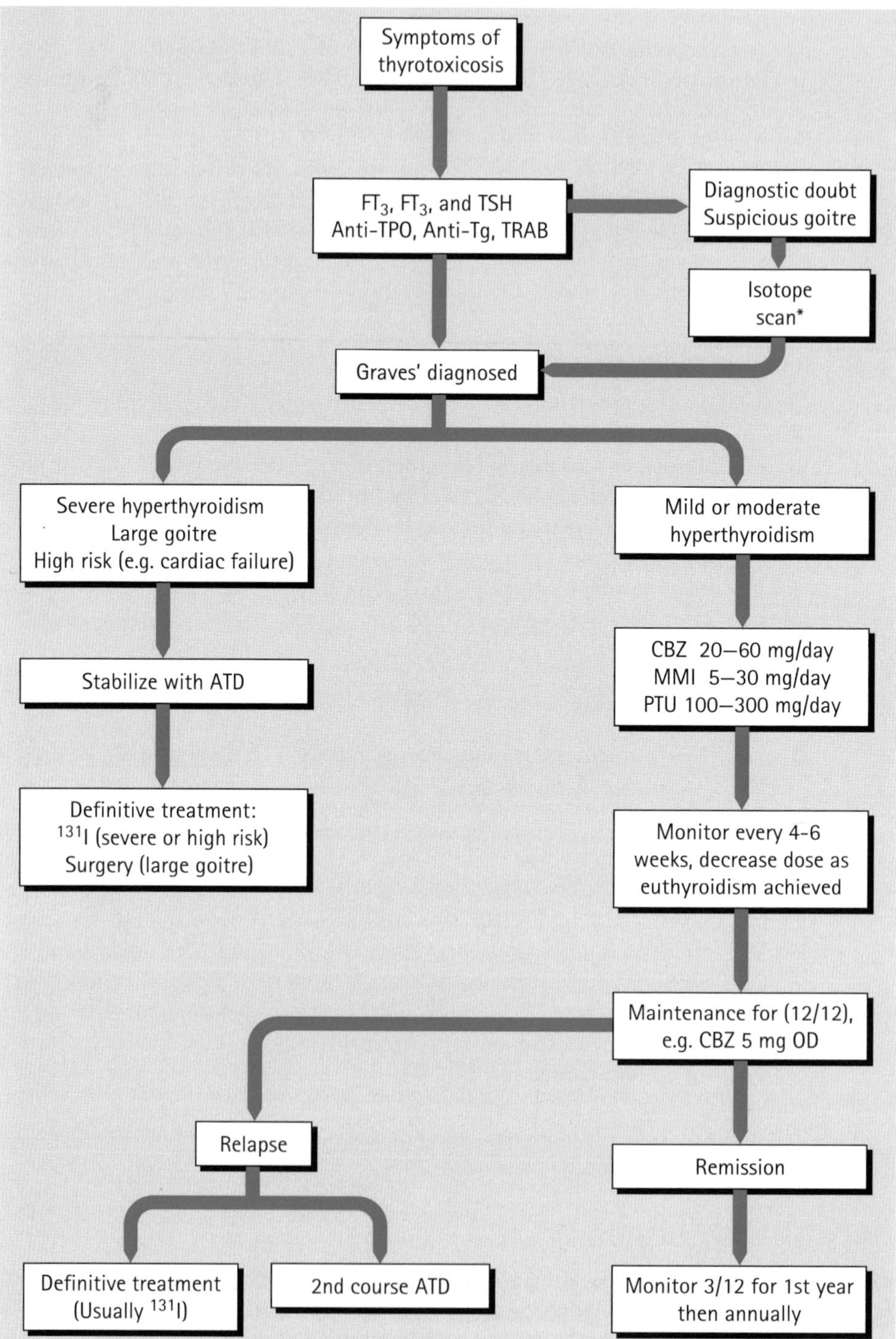

Fig. 1.1 Use of antithyroid drugs. *Scan with technetium-99m pertechnetate or iodide. ATD = antithyroid drugs; CBZ = carbimazole; MMI = methimazole; PTU = propylthiouracil; Tg = thyroglobulin; TPO = thyroid peroxidase; TRAB = TSH receptor antibodies.

1.93). Obesity was associated with lower risk of Graves'—hazard ratio for individuals with body mass index (BMI) greater than 30 kg/m^2 was 0.68 (95% CI 0.49 to 0.92).

3 Colour Doppler sonography may be useful in diagnosis of thyroid disorders. This is a safe, non-invasive technique to assess blood flow in the thyroid arteries. Results correlate highly with thyroid volume and function. In a preliminary study,[9] thyroid blood flow at baseline was highly correlated with outcome after 14 months of antithyroid drug therapy. Relapse could be predicted with a sensitivity of 71% and specificity of 100%.

Conclusions

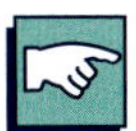

Initial investigations should include thyroid hormone, TSH and thyroid antibodies, including TBII. Full blood count and liver tests should be requested at baseline and at intervals in patients taking antithyroid drugs (Figure 1.1). Thyroid scanning is not routinely warranted unless there is doubt about the diagnosis. Antithyroid drug treatment is usually the first line treatment. Radioactive iodine has been increasingly used in recent years. There is no evidence of teratogenicity. Obviously, it is absolutely contraindicated during pregnancy and most endocrinologists would avoid its use within 6–12 months of conception. The above patient should not be overly concerned about the implications of the disease for her children although, if female, they will inherit a roughly one in three lifetime chance of developing AITD.

Further Reading

1 Cooper DS. Antithyroid drugs. *N Engl J Med* 2005; **352**: 905–17.

2 Abraham P, Avenell A, Watson WA, Park CM, Bevan JS. Antithyroid drug regimen for treating Graves' hyperthyroidism (Review). *Cochrane Library* 2005; **3**: 1–48.

3 Andrade VA, Gross JL, Maia AL. Serum thyrotropin-receptor autoantibody levels after ^{131}I therapy in Graves' patients: effect of pretreatment with methimazole evaluated in a prospective, randomized study. *Eur J Endocrinol* 2004; **151**: 467–74.

4 Bonnema SJ, Bennedbaek FN, Gram J, Veje A, Marving J, Hegedus L. Resumption of methimazole after ^{131}I therapy of hyperthyroid diseases: effect on thyroid function and volume evaluated by a randomised clinical trial. *Eur J Endocrinol* 2003; **149**: 485–92.

5 Tomer Y, Davies TF. Searching for the autoimmune thyroid disease susceptibility genes: from gene mapping to gene function. *Endocr Rev* 2003; **24**: 694–717.

6 Vaidya B, Pearce S. The emerging role of the CTLA-4 gene in autoimmune endocrinopathies. *Eur J Endocrinol* 2004; **150**: 619–26.

7 Wang PW, Liu RT, Juo SHH, *et al*. Cytotoxic T lymphocyte-associated molecule-4 polymorphism and relapse of Graves' hyperthyroidism after antithyroid withdrawal. *J Clin Endocrinol Metab* 2004; **89**: 169–73.

8 Holm I, Manson JE, Michels KB, Alexander EK, Willett WC, Utiger RD. Smoking and other lifestyle factors and the risk of Graves' hyperthyroidism. *Arch Intern Med* 2005; **165**: 1606–11.

9 Saleh A, Cohnen M, Fürst G, Mödder U, Feldkamp J. Prediction of relapse after antithyroid drug therapy of Graves' disease: value of color Doppler sonography. *Exp Clin Endocrinol Diabetes* 2004; **112**: 510–13.

PROBLEM

02 Hyperthyroidism – Multinodular Goitre

Case History

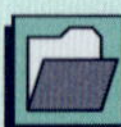

A 65-year-old man has noted a swelling in his neck, gradually increasing in size over the past 3 years. Although generally healthy, he has mild angina, which is stable at present. He is being treated with atenolol and isosorbide mononitrate, and uses sublingual nitrate only occasionally. Isotope scan shows 50 g goitre with patchy uptake. His thyrotropin (TSH) is undetectable but his free T_4 is only marginally elevated at 26 pmol/l (normal 12–25 pmol/l).

Should his hyperthyroidism be treated?

He is concerned about radioactive iodine therapy, can we reassure him?

Is long-term antithyroid drug treatment advisable?

If he opts for surgery, should he have a subtotal or total thyroidectomy?

Background

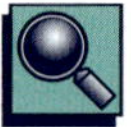

Goitre affects up to 15% of females and 4% of males in developed countries. It is commoner in areas of absolute or relative iodine deficiency. Up to 13% of the world population (i.e. 1.5 billion people) have goitre. Thyroid volume, and prevalence of goitre, increases with age. The differential diagnosis of goitre in elderly people is shown in Table 2.1.

Table 2.1 Goitre in elderly subjects

Diagnosis	Frequency (%)
Non-toxic multinodular	51
Toxic multinodular	24
Solitary nodule	10
Toxic adenoma	5
Graves' disease	4
Hashimoto's thyroiditis	4
Simple goitre	1
Other causes	1

Adapted from Diez.[1]

Autoimmune disease and simple goitre are much more common in younger people, whereas multinodular goitre (non-toxic and toxic) are much more common in elderly people.

Thyroid cancer should always be considered, especially in very young or elderly people with goitre. It accounts for less than 1% of all malignancies in the UK, and malignancy is only present in less than 10% of all excised cold thyroid lesions. The following features increase suspicion of malignancy—age (old or very young), male sex, recent onset and rapid enlargement, irregular shape, fixation to surrounding structures, and enlargement of regional lymph nodes.

Patients with goitre should always be asked about episodes of thyroid dysfunction, family history, and if there has been a history of neck irradiation (which predisposes to thyroid cancer). If hyperthyroid, ask about recent intake of iodine-containing compounds. The commonest obstructive symptoms are tracheal symptoms with dyspnoea and stridor, particularly on exertion; next come oesophageal, mainly dysphagia for solid food; recurrent laryngeal nerve palsy causing hoarseness and venous obstruction causing facial plethora are less common; sympathetic nerve compression with Horner's syndrome is uncommon.

Box 2.1 Pemberton's manoeuvre

Raise the arms above the head until they are touching the side of the head. Hold the posture for one minute. Development of facial plethora or inspiratory stridor indicates that the goitre is causing compression.

Fine needle aspiration biopsy, open biopsy, or thyroidectomy should be considered if there is suspicion of malignancy. Where there are compressive symptoms, a suggestion of retrosternal extension or in any large (>100 g) goitre, computed tomography (CT) or magnetic resonance imaging (MRI) should be carried out to delineate the size of the goitre prior to surgery (Figure 2.1). A general guide to estimating thyroid volume is suggested in Table 2.2.

Thyrotoxicosis occurs in 2% of women and in 0.2% of men, and 15% of episodes of clinically apparent thyrotoxicosis occur in people over the age of 60. In elderly people, thyrotoxicosis is most commonly due to multinodular goitre (45–50%), followed by Graves' (20%), iatrogenic (15%) and solitary adenoma (10%). In 5–10% there is no goitre and the aetiology is unclear.

Among the US population, 2.5% have thyrotropin (TSH) of <0.1 mIU/l, including patients treated with thyroxine. There has been considerable debate about the need to treat subclinical hyperthyroidism. Current opinion[2,3] favours treatment, but not for all patients. About 5% of patients progress to clinical thyrotoxicosis each year. Relative risk of developing atrial fibrillation is around 3.0. Overall, 15% of patients with new atrial fibrillation are hyperthyroid. Risk of peripheral embolism has been reported to be as high as 10%. Rate control and anticoagulation are important as indicated. Clinical thyrotoxicosis is a risk factor for osteoporosis. Subclinical thyrotoxicosis increases bone turnover. Some studies have demonstrated beneficial effects of treating subclinical thyrotoxicosis on bone mineral density (BMD). Post-menopausal women with subclinical hyperthyroidism may lose up to 2% BMD per year, with loss being most apparent from

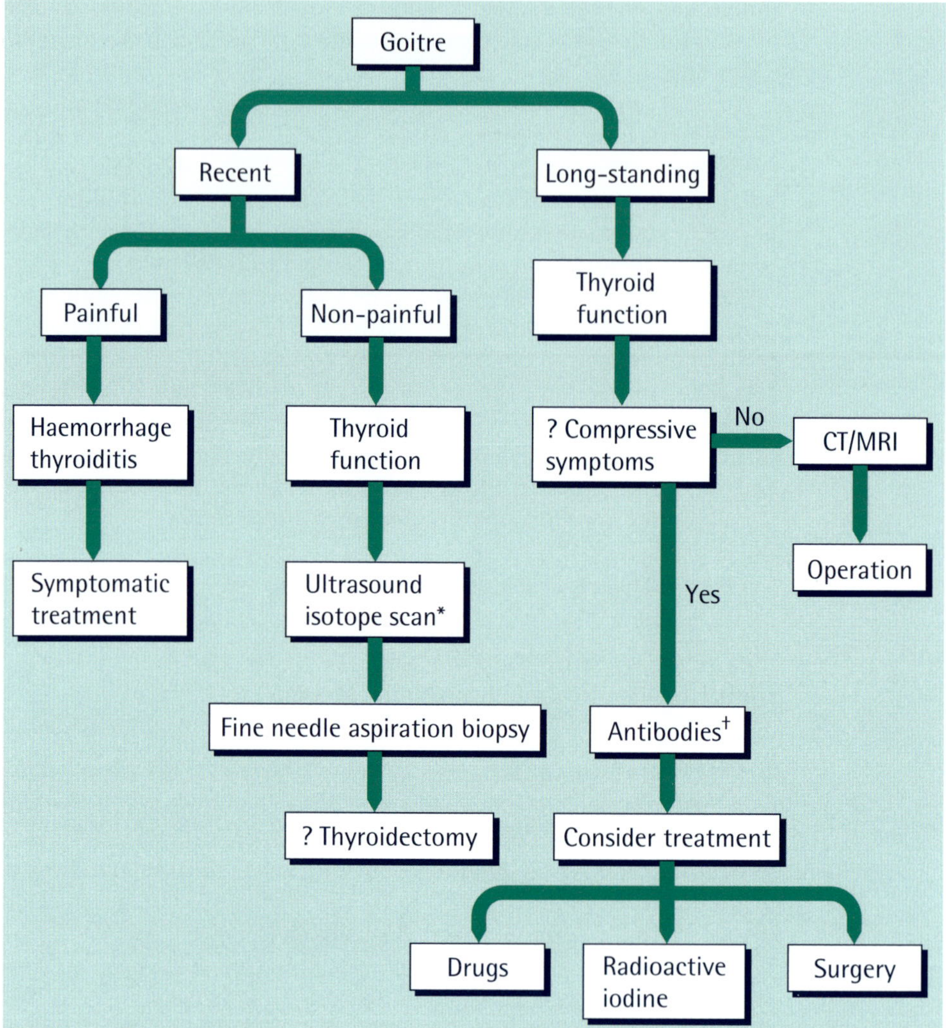

Fig. 2.1 Investigation of goitre in the elderly patient. *Isotope scan with technetium 99m pertechnetate or Iodine-123; †Antibodies, antithyroid peroxidase (TPO) and thyrotropin (thyroid-stimulating hormone [TSH]) receptor antibodies.

cortical bone. Observations that quality of life is impaired and risk of cognitive decline is increased need to be confirmed.

Choice of treatment depends on age, underlying diagnosis, and the presence of co-existent illnesses, and patient preference. Recent studies provide some reassurance about long-term drug treatment: Azizi and colleagues[4] showed that long-term methimazole was as safe and effective as radioactive iodine and there was no cost difference. Patients with hyperthyroidism require long-term follow-up whatever treatment they have. Pearce[5] has reviewed adverse events reported from over five million prescriptions of thionamide drugs in the UK between 1981 and 2003. Neutrophil dyscrasia (agranulocytosis or neutropaenia) was rare (0.1–0.5% of cases). It occurred mainly early in treatment (median

Table 2.2 Estimating the size of a goitre

Size (g)	Comparison	Compressive symptoms
<20	Normal thyroid	Not present
	Not visible or palpable	
40	Terminal phalanx of thumbs	Highly unlikely
	Large clove of garlic	
60	Apricot (small)	Unlikely
80	Hen's egg (small)	Possible if extends posteriorly or retrosternally
120	Lemon or orange (small)	Likely
200	Orange (large) or grapefruit	Probable

time 30 days) when the patient was likely to be on a high dose. It may be commoner with propylthiouracil, and is more frequently fatal in elderly people.

Many patients worry about potential risks from radioactive iodine therapy, particularly thyroid carcinoma, leukaemia and genetic damage. The treatment has been used for around 60 years now and long-term studies have confirmed that it is safe. Indeed, there is significantly greater risk from untreated, or undertreated, thyrotoxicosis. Hypothyroidism is much less likely with multinodular goitre compared with diffuse toxic goitre as the radioactive iodine is selectively taken up by the hyperfunctioning nodules. Rare side effects include transient thyrotoxicosis, sialadenitis and radiation thyroiditis—all usually seen with higher doses.

Most specialist centres now favour total rather than partial thyroidectomy for benign disease affecting both lobes of the gland. The major advantage is in avoiding the need for further operation should the gland re-grow or should thyroid cancer be discovered incidentally. Clearly, the patient would require thyroxine replacement following total thyroidectomy. In specialist hands, the rates of temporary vocal cord paralysis (1–2%) and hypoparathyroidism (5–10%) for a total thyroidectomy are comparable with permanent rates of 1% and 2% respectively for subtotal and total thyroidectomy.

Recent Developments

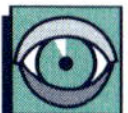

1. Uptake of radioactive iodine into multinodular goitres is often fairly low, meaning that many patients need repeated doses. Albino *et al.*[6] administered 0.1 mg of recombinant human TSH (rhTSH) 1 and 2 days prior to ^{131}I. Iodine uptake increased from 12% to 54%. The treatment was highly successful, and thyroid volume decreased within a few months. There was an appreciable incidence of transient thyrotoxicosis and painful thyroiditis with the treatment, and 65% of patients became hypothyroid.

2. Significant advances have been made in thyroid surgery, including use of thyroid artery embolization prior to surgery for large goitres, ablation of thyroid nodules using ethanol and thus avoiding the need for operation, and autotransplantation of cryopreserved thyroid tissue in patients developing postoperative hypothyroidism. Experience

is increasing with minimally invasive video-assisted thyroidectomy (MIVAT).[7] Although not suitable for large and invasive goitres, this technique has the advantages of not requiring general anaesthesia and short hospital stay, and low complication rate.

3 In a follow-up study of nearly 16 000 person years, Franklyn *et al.*[8] showed that patients treated with ^{131}I had a slight excess mortality (standard mortality ratio [SMR] 1.14, confidence interval 1.04 to1.24) compared with the background UK population. This was due to cardiovascular disease and was not apparent in patients rendered hypothyroid. These data confirm the safety of radioactive iodine and emphasize the need for effective treatment, even if hypothyroidism develops.

Conclusions

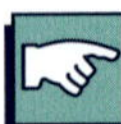

The above patient has three significant problems: goitre, subclinical hyperthyroidism and angina. Recent evidence leaves little doubt that the hyperthyroidism should be treated. Radioactive iodine would be the treatment of first choice in most centres. This is safe and effective, and will help to shrink the goitre, or at least stop it growing further. Available evidence suggests that long-term treatment with thionamide drugs is a safe alternative. The patient will need ongoing follow-up for his thyroid disease whatever option he chooses. He may be more likely to be followed up by an endocrinologist if he remains on drug treatment. Surgery is relatively contraindicated because of his angina. In specialist centres, total or near-total thyroidectomy would be preferred to avoid the possibility of a second operation.

Further Reading

1 Diez JJ. Goiter in adult patients aged 55 years and older: etiology and clinical features in 634 patients. *J Gerontol A Biol Sci Med Sci* 2005; **60**: 920–3.

2 Hoogendoorn EH, den Heijer M, van Dijk APJ, Hermus AR. Subclinical hyperthyroidism: to treat or not to treat? *Postgrad Med J* 2004; **80**: 394–8.

3 Biondi B, Palmieri EA, Klain M, Schlumberger M, Filetti S, Lombardi G. Subclinical hyperthyroidism: clinical features and treatment options. *Eur J Endocrinol* 2005; **152**: 1–9.

4 Azizi F, Ataie L, Hedayati M, Mehrabi Y, Sheikholeslami F. Effect of long-term continuous methimazole treatment of hyperthyroidism: comparison with radioiodine. *Eur J Endocrinol* 2005; **152**: 695–701.

5 Pearce SHS. Spontaneous reporting of adverse reactions to carbimazole and propylthiouracil in the UK. *Clin Endocrinol* 2004; **61**: 589–94.

6 Albino CC, Mesa CR, Olandoski M, *et al.* Recombinant human thyrotropin as adjuvant in the treatment of multinodular goiters with radioiodine. *J Clin Endocrinol Metab* 2005; **90**: 775–80.

7 Ruggieri M, Straniero A, Mascaro A, *et al.* The minimally invasive open video-assisted approach in surgical thyroid diseases. *BMC Surg* 2005; **5**: 9–14.

8 Franklyn JA, Sheppard MC, Maisonneuve P. Thyroid function and mortality in patients treated for hyperthyroidism. *JAMA* 2005; **294**: 71–80.

PROBLEM

03 Thyroid Nodule

Case History

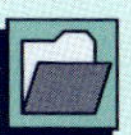

JC is a 48-year-old man who has developed a swelling in the right side of his neck over the past 3 months. It is not painful, and he has no compressive symptoms. His health is generally good. You note a 2 cm diameter swelling in relation to the right lobe of the thyroid. He is clinically euthyroid and thyroid function is normal.

What is your differential diagnosis?

How would you investigate the swelling further?

He would like to know what the chances are that the lump is malignant.

He is afraid of surgery and asks if it is safe to follow him up medically.

Background

Thyroid nodules are extremely common. Around 5% of the US population has a thyroid nodule, and most of these are greater than 2 cm in their maximum diameter.[1] The vast majority (>95%) are benign. With ultrasound detection, the prevalence of thyroid nodules is even higher—up to 50% in women over the age of 60 years, a finding borne out by autopsy studies. Prevalence of thyroid nodules is also considerably higher in areas of relative iodine deficiency. Lesions less than 1 cm in diameter are called 'micronodules'.

Expert assessment is essential to detect cancerous lesions, and to decrease likelihood of the patient having unnecessary surgery.[2] Widespread use of fine needle biopsy has decreased the proportion of patients requiring surgery while increasing the proportion of excised glands that have significant pathology. A proposed schema for investigation and management of thyroid nodules is shown in Figure 3.1. Initial assessment should include history and careful examination (look for irregularity of the nodule, size, fixation to surrounding tissues, regional lymph node enlargement and hoarseness), thyroid function tests, autoantibodies (antithyroid peroxidase (anti-TPO) and anti-thyroglobulin), fine needle aspiration cytology (FNAC) with or without ultrasound guidance, and inspection of the vocal cords if surgery is likely. Additional investigations include ultrasound, computed tomography (CT) or magnetic resonance imaging (MRI), plasma calcitonin measurement, flow-volume loop if there are respiratory symptoms, chest X-ray, and isotope scan of the thyroid. Thyroglobulin is useful for postoperative surveillance of patients with thyroid tumours but its measurement at presentation is not of diagnostic benefit.

FNAC is the cornerstone of investigation in the endocrine clinic.[3] However, it does not always yield diagnostic information. Around 10% are non-diagnostic, 75% are benign, and 5% show papillary, anaplastic or medullary cell carcinomas. The remaining 10% are follicular

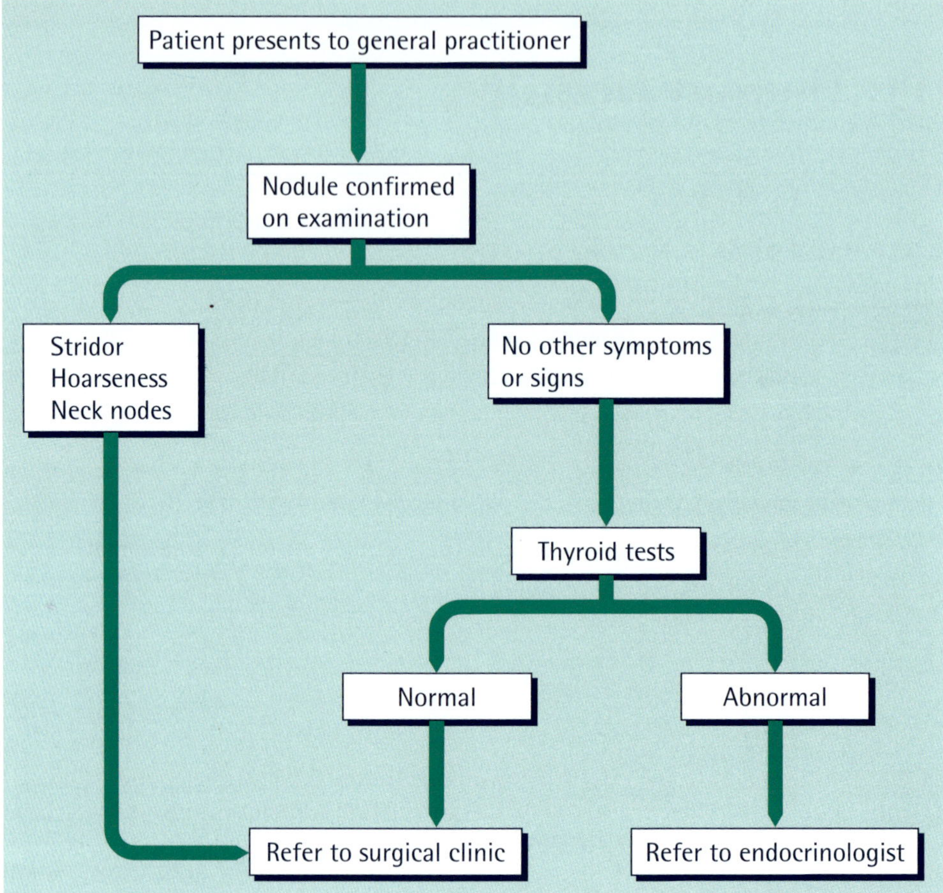

Fig. 3.1 Evaluation of a thyroid nodule. Adapted from Utiger[1]—patients with suspicious lesions should be referred to a combined or surgical clinic within 2 weeks of presentation.

lesions of which 20% are carcinomas. In these, carcinoma can only be distinguished from adenoma on the basis of invasion of the capsule, blood vessels or lymphatics. This distinction cannot be made on FNAC, and these lesions are therefore usually referred for surgery. Different diagnostic categories of FNAC are now recognized and routinely used (Table 3.1).

Differential diagnosis for the above patient is set out in Figure 3.2. Papillary carcinoma is the most common malignancy of endocrine glands. Its incidence is increasing throughout the world, particularly in young women. Some of this apparent increase may be due to increased detection of early and occult lesions. Incidence of papillary cancer is 2.3 per 100 000 women per year and 0.9 per 100 000 men. Each year in England and Wales, 900 new cases are diagnosed and 250 deaths from the condition. With optimal management, the overall outlook is very good with up to 90% of those diagnosed in middle life surviving 10 years. The adequacy of surgical management, postoperative thyroid ablation with radioactive iodine, and careful monitoring for recurrences are all important determinants of prognosis.

Table 3.1 Diagnostic categories from fine needle aspiration cytology

Category	Description
Thy 1	*Non-diagnostic* Action: Repeat (? with ultrasound guidance)
Thy 2	*Non-neoplastic* Action: Repeat at 3–6 months*
Thy 3	*All follicular lesions* Action: Discuss with MDT, thyroid lobectomy†
Thy 4	*Abnormal, suspicious of malignancy* Action: Discuss with MDT, thyroid lobectomy†
Thy 5	*Diagnostic of malignancy* Action: Management by surgeon and oncologist

*Two non-neoplastic biopsies are required to exclude malignancy. †With completion thyroidectomy depending on intra-operative and histological findings. MDT = multidisciplinary team.

The following recommendations should be considered:

- Patients with suspected or proven thyroid cancer should be managed by an endocrine surgeon or by a surgeon with appropriate experience in endocrine surgery.
- Proven cancer should be managed in a centre with appropriate cytology, pathology, endocrinology, nuclear medicine, genetics and oncology.
- Differentiated thyroid cancer (papillary and follicular) should be managed by total lobectomy as a minimum procedure. Total or 'completion' thyroidectomy may be needed depending on intra-operative and pathological findings.
- Radioactive iodine ablation should be considered in patients who have undergone total thyroidectomy. This will improve detection of recurrence and is associated with improved survival.
- Patients with differentiated cancer should be treated with titrated doses of thyroxine to achieve complete thyrotropin (TSH) suppression (<0.1 mIU/l). TSH and thyroglobulin should be monitored at regular intervals. Increased thyroglobulin suggests recurrent tumour.
- Management and regular review should be undertaken by a multidisciplinary team.
- Rare forms of thyroid cancer including medullary carcinoma, anaplastic lesions, and lymphoma should be managed in a specialist centre.

Thyroid cancer is best managed by a specialist team. Prognosis of localized disease is excellent (Table 3.2). Following total thyroidectomy and radioactive iodine ablation, the patient is started on suppressive doses of thyroxine. Follow-up iodine scanning is carried out at 4–6 months and thereafter annually. Thyroxine is stopped 6 weeks prior to each scan and the patient is started on triiodothyronine (20 μg three times daily). This is stopped 2 weeks prior to radioactive iodine ablation. Increased TSH is necessary to ensure that a high proportion of radioactive iodine is taken up. Use of recombinant human TSH (rhTSH)

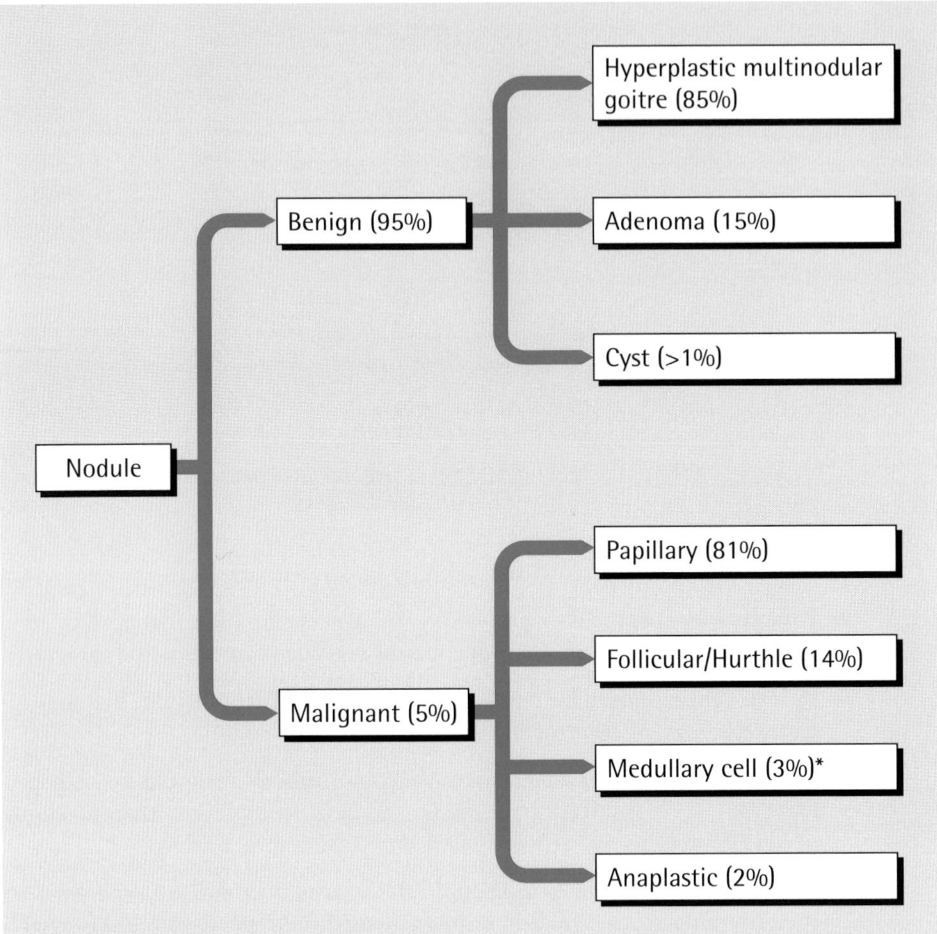

Fig. 3.2 Differential diagnosis of a 2 cm thyroid nodule. *75% of medullary cell cancers are sporadic, 25% are familial—mostly associated with multiple endocrine neoplasia type 2 (MEN2). Hurthle (oxyphilic) cells are large follicular cells with abundant pink-staining material. The tumours can be benign and are often slow growing. Prognosis and treatment is similar to other follicular lesions.

Table 3.2 Prognosis from papillary thyroid cancer

Stage	Description	Mortality (%)*
I	<45 years, tumour <1 cm, no metastases T1 N0 M0	1.7
II	>45 years, any size metastases Any T, any N, M1	15.8
III	>45 years, local invasion T4, N0, M0 or any T, N1, M0	30.0
IV	>45 years with metastases Any T, any N, M1	60.9

*Mortality is 10-year cancer specific mortality.

shortens the period during which the patient is hypothyroid. Thyroglobulin is most useful as a marker for recurrence when TSH is not suppressed and should thus be checked at the time of follow-up scan—if the thyroid has been successfully ablated, thyroglobulin should be negative. TSH suppression is also useful in some cases of benign thyroid disease—TSH is a growth factor for both benign and malignant thyroid cells.

Recent Developments

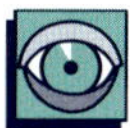

1. Papillary cancers are often present in multiple foci within the thyroid. This may arise from metastatic primary tumour or independent development of multiple tumours. Shattuck *et al.*[4] have recently investigated the clonal origin of multifocal papillary cancers in women by studying polymorphisms of the androgen receptor gene on the X chromosome. They confirmed that multifocal papillary cancers, in many cases, may develop as independent primary tumours.
2. Nodules greater than 2 cm in diameter generally trigger intervention. The natural history of smaller lesions and occult thyroid carcinomas is largely unknown. Indeed, many of them are never diagnosed. Papillary cancers have a higher chance of being multifocal and of local spread, whereas papillary and follicular lesions are equally likely to spread distantly. A recent study from Germany has suggested that intervention before tumours grow to 2 cm is highly beneficial for prognosis.[5]
3. FNAC has been invaluable in risk stratification of lesions. There is considerable interest in minimally invasive surgery for low-risk thyroid lesions. Ultrasound-guided laser photocoagulation is useful for treatment of benign lesions[6] and has good cosmetic results with low risk of side effects.

Conclusions

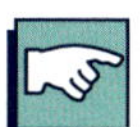

The above patient is over 45 years of age and has a swelling of recent onset which is greater than 2 cm in diameter. Investigations with a view to considering surgery are definitely indicated. However, it is most likely that this is a benign nodule—either a dominant hyperplastic nodule in a multinodular goitre or, thinking of his age, a benign adenoma. Thyroid function tests, autoantibody measurements, ultrasound and isotope scanning should all be considered but the major investigation is FNAC. If the lesion is low risk, it is safe to defer surgery and carry out further biopsy at 3–6 months, as treatment of papillary and follicular cancers with surgery, radioactive iodine ablation and suppressive thyroxine therapy is highly effective. Early treatment of all high-risk lesions is recommended.

Further Reading

1. Utiger RD. The multiplicity of thyroid nodules and carcinomas. *N Engl J Med* 2005; **352**: 2376–8.
2. Pacini F, Burron L, Ciuoli C, Di Cairano G, Guarino E. Management of thyroid nodules: a clinicopathological, evidence-based approach. *Eur J Nucl Med Mol Imaging* 2004; **31**: 1443–9.
3. Nguyen GK, Lee MW, Ginsberg J, Wragg T, Bilodeau D. Fine-needle aspiration of the thyroid: an overview. *Cytojournal* 2005; **2**: 12–24.

4 Shattuck TM, Westra WH, Ladenson PW, Arnold A. Independent clonal origins of distinct tumour foci in multifocal papillary thyroid carcinoma. *N Engl J Med* 2005; **352**: 2406–12.

5 Machens A, Holzhausen HJ, Dralle H. The prognostic value of primary tumor size in papillary and follicular thyroid carcinoma. *Cancer* 2005; **103**: 2269–73.

6 Døssing H, Bennedbaek F, Hegedüs L. Effect of ultrasound-guided interstitial laser photocoagulation on benign solitary solid cold thyroid nodules—a randomised study. *Eur J Endocrinol* 2005; **152**: 341–5.

PROBLEM

04 Sick Euthyroid Syndrome

Case History

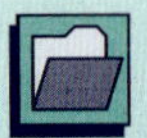

A 56-year-old man presents with an acute myocardial infarction. Examination reveals mild cardiac failure. He has been feeling quite tired and experiencing chest pains with only minimal exertion. His thyroid tests reveal a low free T_4 at 10 pmol/l (normal 12–25 pmol/l) and thyrotropin (thyroid-stimulating hormone [TSH]) at the lower end of the reference range (0.6 mIU/l, normal 0.15–3.5 mIU/l).

Could his thyroid test results have a bearing on his reported state of health?

How would you investigate this further?

Does he require thyroid replacement therapy?

Background

Modern thyroid tests with free hormone measurements and high-sensitivity thyrotropin (TSH) assays have made it easier to diagnose thyroid dysfunction. Sick euthyroid syndrome refers to the physiological changes that occur in patients with non-thyroidal illness in the absence of thyroid disease. Clinicians are often advised not to check thyroid tests during a severe intercurrent illness as thyroid disease. However, we now recognize that the changes that occur in thyroid function in patients with sepsis, myocardial infarction, cardiac failure, and other critical illnesses are of prognostic importance. The physiological basis for these changes is now becoming understood. Thyroid hormone measurements in these circumstances can be helpful and the possibility that interventions to correct the thyroid changes in these circumstances may improve prognosis has been entertained.

The common patterns of abnormality are:

- Low T_3—the commonest abnormality due to impaired peripheral conversion of T_4 to T_3 and accompanied by increased reverse T_3.
- Low T_3 and T_4—due to decreased thyroid production and changes in binding proteins.
- Low T_3, T_4 and TSH—alteration in the hypothalamic pituitary axis in patients who are very ill.

Only 0.3% of triiodothyronine (T_3) and 0.03% of thyroxine (T_4) in the circulation is free, and therefore metabolically active. Thyroid hormone in the plasma is transported as follows:

- 70–80%—thyroxine-binding globulin (TBG)
- 10–15%—transthyretin (TTR)
- 10–15%—albumin

There is a considerable body of knowledge about how these thyroid hormone transport proteins change in non-thyroidal illness. In steady state, the changes will be in total but not free hormone levels. However, in the short term, as in the context of an acute illness, rapid alteration in transport protein levels may shift the equilibrium between bound and free hormone, and thus affect levels of the latter. Furthermore, binding inhibitors associated with the non-esterified fatty acid (NEFA) fraction of plasma are increased in acute illness.

TBG is the major transport protein. The 46.3 kDa protein is a member of the serine protease inhibitor superfamily (SERPINA7), and is homologous with other anti-proteases including α_1-antichymotrypsin and α_1-antitrypsin. The gene is located on the X chromosome (Xq22.2) and mutations can cause either increased or decreased expression. Conditions associated with changes in TBG are summarized in Table 4.1. The autosomal dominant form of TBG deficiency may be due to changes in a regulator gene as TBG can be increased by oestrogen treatment in this condition.

Transthyretin (TTR) was formerly known as thyroxine-binding pre-albumin because of its electrophoretic mobility. The protein transports both thyroid hormones and

Table 4.1 Conditions associated with altered levels of thyroxine-binding globulin

Excess	Deficiency
Pregnancy	Androgen treatment
Oestrogen treatment	Corticosteroids (high dose)
Newborn	Nephrotic syndrome
Porphyria	Acromegaly
Active hepatitis	Genetic (X-linked recessive and autosomal dominant)

Increased TBG increases total thyroid hormone levels and *vice versa*.

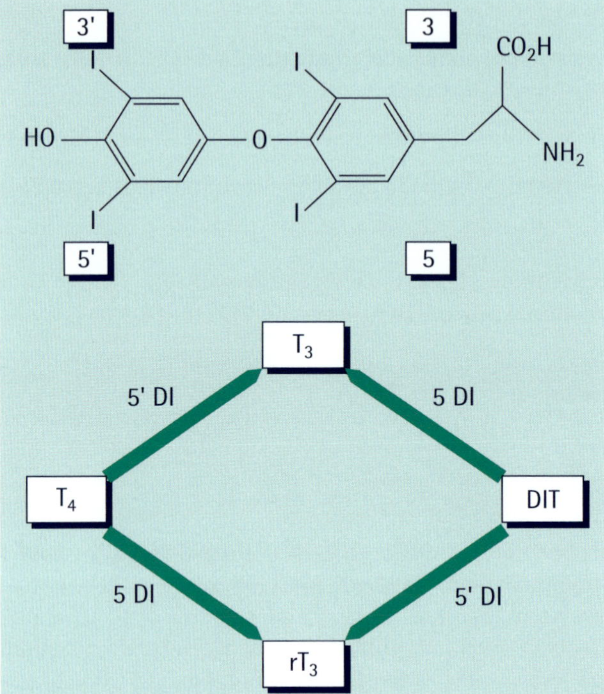

Fig. 4.1 Thyroxine metabolism. Thyroxine, the major hormone product of the thyroid gland is iodinated at the 3,5, 3′ and 5′ positions. Deiodination at the 5′ position yields triiodothyronine (T_3), the major active hormone. Deiodination at the 5 position yields reverse T_3 (rT_3) which is metabolically inactive but is a marker for severe illness. Further deiodination of either T_3 or rT_3 yields diiodothyronine (DIT). DI = deiodinase.

retinoids. Congenital excess is responsible for the rare syndrome of familial euthyroid hyperthyroxinaemia. TTR is of considerable interest because of its association with neurodegenerative disease. The protein is highly expressed in the central nervous system, being produced by the choroid plexus. It forms a major component of the protein deposits in the microvascular lesions and neurofibrillary tangles of senile amyloid. Changes in serum albumin accompany acute severe illness and also occur in patients with hepatic and renal disorders.

The deiodinase (DI) enzymes are selenoproteins that catalyse the removal of iodine at the 5′ position of thyroxine to produce the active hormone triiodothyronine (T_3) (see Figure 4.1). Three separate genes for DI have been identified: DI1 (chromosome 1p33) is the major enzyme of liver and kidney, the major peripheral sites of T_3 production; DI2 (chromosome 14q24) is selectively expressed in the anterior pituitary and is key to the regulation of TSH expression in relation to circulating thyroxine; DI3 (chromosome 14q32) is the placental form and is involved in fetal thyroid hormone homoeostasis, although it is also expressed in other tissues during adult life.

In health, around 30% of circulating T_4 undergoes 5′-deiodination to produce T_3, 40% undergoes 5-deiodination to produce rT_3, and the remainder undergoes oxidative deamination and decarboxylation to produce triiodo- and tetraiodo-thyroacetic acid.

These products of deiodination undergo further deiodination and are eliminated in bile following conjugation to glucuronate or sulphate. The activity of DI enzymes and of TSH expression in the pituitary is influenced by circulating and locally produced cytokines (interleukin-6, tumour necrosis factor-α and interferon-β), levels of which are increased during acute or chronic illness.

Thyroid hormones enter the cell through organic anion transporters and L-amino acid transporters. Mutations in one transporter molecule, MCT8, has recently been associated with psychomotor retardation and increased circulating T_3—essentially a form of thyroid hormone resistance.[1] Thyroid hormone receptors are members of the nuclear receptor superfamily. They are hormone-activated transcription factors that modulate expression of a range of genes through binding to short repeated sequences of DNA known as T_3 response elements. The receptors are products of two genes, α and β, each of which is expressed as two different isoforms (α_1 and α_2, β_1 and β_2) and they function as heterodimers. β_2 does not bind thyroid hormone, β_2 has a restricted distribution (hypothalamus and anterior pituitary). The syndrome of thyroid hormone resistance is due to mutations in the β gene that decrease its ability to bind thyroid hormone. Mild hypothyroidism, including cognitive and behavioural problems in children, is associated with goitre and increased thyroid hormone levels, while TSH is normal or modestly increased.

Following acute myocardial infarction (AMI), there is a rapid downregulation of the thyroid hormone system.[2] This occurs in spite of the beneficial effects of thyroid hormone in improving cardiac function and lowering systemic resistance, but may be important in protecting the myocardium. Changes in thyroid hormone receptors at the tissue level mean that circulating thyroid hormone status may not exactly reflect the thyroid status of individual tissues. The level of T_3 (decreased) and rT_3 (increased) after AMI could be a valuable prognostic indicator.[2,3] The changes in thyroid function have also been reported to be of prognostic significance in other conditions including sepsis.[4]

Recent Developments

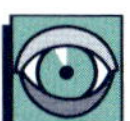

1 In patients with cardiac failure, low T_3 is an independent risk factor for death.[5] T_3 measurement could be of considerable clinical value in managing patients with cardiac failure as the test is cheap and widely available. It remains to be seen whether reversing this risk factor with thyroid replacement therapy would be of clinical value.

2 The thyroxine analogue 3,5-diiodothyropropionic acid (DITPA) has been shown to influence prognosis favourably in animal models of cardiac ischaemia and failure. In an animal model, DITPA facilitated angiogenesis (perhaps through increased expression of basic fibroblast growth factor) and decreased the size of the akinetic region produced by infarction.[6]

3 Peeters *et al.*[7] investigated thyroid hormone status in a large series of intensive care unit (ITU) patients. They confirmed that low TSH and T_3, along with increased rT_3 were markers for poor prognosis. Intensive insulin treatment, which may improve prognosis in ITU patients, had no effect on thyroid hormone levels. In patients who died, post-mortem tissue levels of DI1 correlated with T_3/rT_3 and negatively with rT_3. Liver and skeletal muscle levels of DI3 were positively correlated with circulating rT_3.

Conclusions

The patient's thyroid hormone changes may be a response to his acute illness. Mild hypothyroidism could have contributed to his symptoms prior to admission. Equally, he may have been tired because of his cardiac illness. The changes in thyroid hormone and TSH are part of his physiological adaptation to the acute illness, and may not reflect altered thyroid status at the tissue level. On present evidence, there is no justification for starting thyroid replacement in the acute phase of his illness and there is a risk of provoking cardiac dysrhythmias with thyroid hormone treatment. His abnormal thyroid test results should be noted (see Figure 4.2) and the thyroid tests repeated 6–8 weeks after he has recovered from the acute illness.

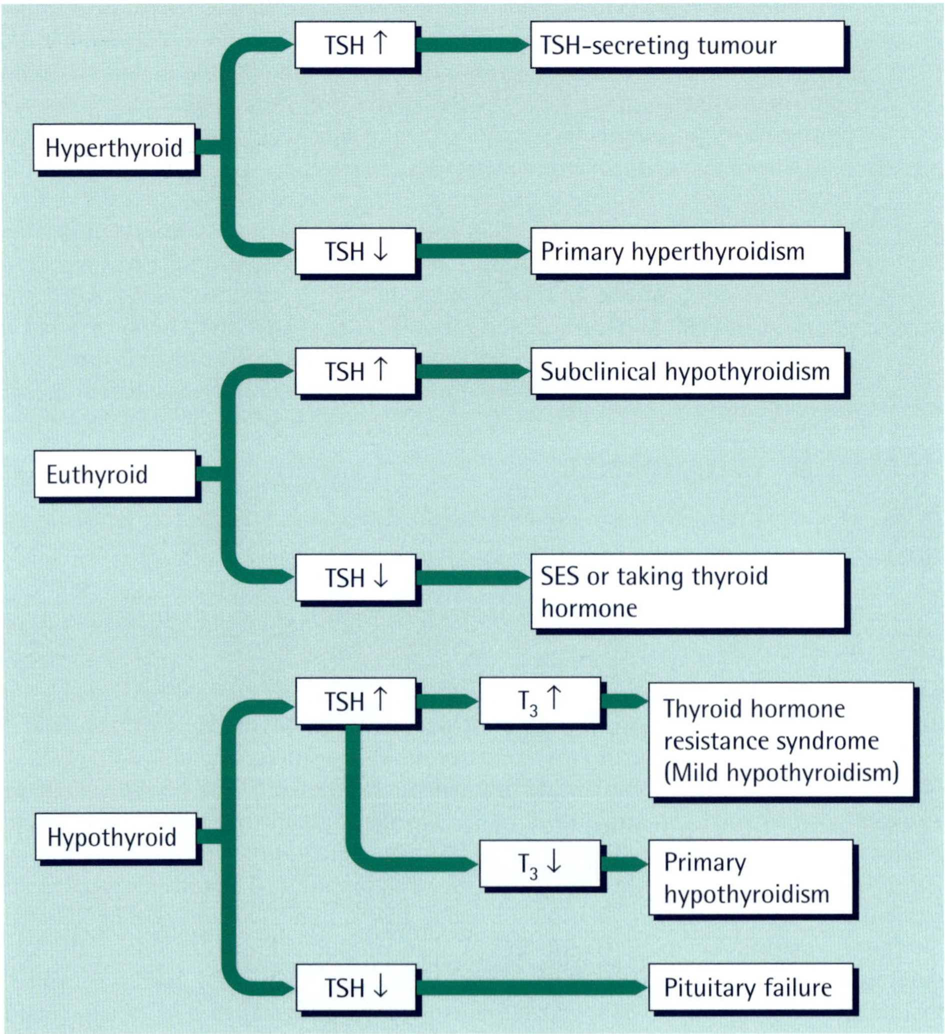

- Hyperthyroid
  - TSH ↑ → TSH-secreting tumour
  - TSH ↓ → Primary hyperthyroidism
- Euthyroid
  - TSH ↑ → Subclinical hypothyroidism
  - TSH ↓ → SES or taking thyroid hormone
- Hypothyroid
  - TSH ↑
    - T_3 ↑ → Thyroid hormone resistance syndrome (Mild hypothyroidism)
    - T_3 ↓ → Primary hypothyroidism
  - TSH ↓ → Pituitary failure

Fig. 4.2 Interpretation of thyroid tests (SES = sick euthyroid syndrome).

Further Reading

1 Jansen J, Friesema ECH, Milici C, Visser TJ. Thyroid hormone transporters in health and disease. *Thyroid* 2005; **15**: 757–68.

2 Friberg L, Werner S, Eggertsen G, Ahnve S. Rapid down-regulation of thyroid hormones in acute myocardial infarction: is it cardioprotective in patients with angina? *Arch Intern Med* 2002; **162**: 1388–94.

3 Pavlou HN, Kliridis PA, Panagiotopoulos AA, Goritsas CP, Vassilakos PJ. Euthyroid sick syndrome in acute ischemic syndromes. *Angiology* 2002; **53**: 699–707.

4 Yildizdas D, Onenli MN, Yapicioglu H, Topaloglu AK, Sertdemir Y, Yüksel B. Thyroid hormone levels and their relationship to survival in children with bacterial sepsis and septic shock. *J Pediatr Endocrinol Metab* 2004; **17**: 1435–42.

5 Pingitore A, Landi P, Taddei MC, Ripoli A, L'Abbate A, Iervasi G. Triodothyronine levels for risk stratification of patients with chronic heart failure. *Am J Med* 2005; **118**: 132–6.

6 Zheng W, Weiss RM, Wang X, *et al.* DITPA stimulates arteriolar growth and modifies myocardial postinfarction remodeling. *Am J Physiol Heart Circ Physiol* 2004; **286**: H1994–2000.

7 Peeters RP, Wouters PJ, van Toor H, Kaptein E, Visser TJ, Van den Berghe G. Serum 3,3′,5′-triiodothyronine (rT3) and 3,5,3′-triiodothyronine/rT3 are prognostic markers in critically ill patients and are associated with postmortem tissue deiodinase activities. *J Clin Endocrinol Metab* 2005; **90**: 4559–65.

PROBLEM

05 Amiodarone and the Thyroid

Case History

AP is a 65-year-old man who started amiodarone (200 mg per day) 6 months ago when he developed ventricular tachycardia following a myocardial infarction. He also takes a β-blocker, nitrate and aspirin. He has lost 3.2 kg in weight and his general practitioner is concerned that his free T_4 is elevated at 35 pmol/l (normal 12–25 pmol/l) and his thyrotropin (TSH) is suppressed. There is no previous history of thyroid disease and thyroid antibodies are not present.

How would you investigate his possible hyperthyroidism?

If you decide that he has hyperthyroidism, what is the best treatment option?

Should he stop taking amiodarone?

Background

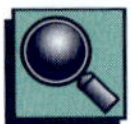

Amiodarone was developed in the 1960s as a coronary vasodilator and is the most widely prescribed antiarrhythmic drug after β-blockers and digoxin. It is a class III antiarrhythmic agent, acting principally by prolonging the repolarization phase of the action potential. It is useful in a range of supraventricular and ventricular arrhythmias, although it is only licensed for the latter in the USA. The greatest benefit from the drug is in monomorphic and polymorphic ventricular tachycardia, and in conditions associated with high risk of sudden death. Unlike many other antiarrhythmic agents, it does not depress cardiac function.

Amiodarone may be given intravenously (150–300 mg) or orally (maintenance dose 200–400 mg per day). It is highly fat soluble and protein bound, accounting for its long half-life of up to 100 days, and the fact that oral loading may take some days. Amiodarone is metabolized in the liver to desethylamiodarone which also has some antiarrhythmic activity. Amiodarone should not be used during breastfeeding. It also crosses the placenta, although there has been no evidence of teratogenicity. It is contraindicated in patients with nodal bradycardia or heart block, unless a pacemaker is *in situ*. As it inhibits members of the cytochrome P450 superfamily, it can potentiate other drugs including warfarin, digoxin, simvastatin, theophylline, sildenafil, ciclosporin, and class I antiarrhythmic drugs.

Side effects of amiodarone limit its use: changes in liver enzymes are common and it can cause florid hepatitis and cirrhosis; pulmonary fibrosis is one of the most serious side effects; it can cause peripheral neuropathy, including optic neuropathy. Corneal microdeposits arise because of the insolubility of the drug—these are usually asymptomatic but may cause light-scattering effects. The drug sensitizes users to ultraviolet-A light and use of a high sun protection factor (SPF) barrier is recommended. It may also cause a blue-grey discoloration of the skin. Amiodarone may cause sleep disturbances and nightmares. Recommendations for surveillance of patients taking amiodarone are summarized in Table 5.1.

Table 5.1 Surveillance of patients taking amiodarone

Time period	Recommendation
Before starting	Clinical examination
	Electrolytes
	Liver tests
	Thyroid tests and antibodies*
	ECG and chest X-ray
Every 6 months	Electrolytes
	Liver tests
	Thyroid tests
Annually	Slit lamp examination†

*Patients with thyroid antibodies should have thyroid tests every 3 months. †Some specialists would only request this if there were ocular symptoms.

Patients taking amiodarone should be warned that drinking grapefruit juice may potentiate the action of the drug. Furanocoumarins in grapefruit inhibit the CYP3A4 enzyme in the gastrointestinal tract and liver. This enzyme is important in the clearance of drugs including amiodarone, some statins (atorvastatin, simvastatin, lovastatin), ethinylestradiol, ciclosporin, some calcium-channel blockers (felodipine and nisoldipine), sertraline and benzodiazepines.

Amiodarone is 37% iodine by weight, 10% of which is released as free iodine. This is 7.5 mg of iodine per day for a patient taking a maintenance dose of 200 mg. Amiodarone increases plasma and urinary iodine by 40-fold. Recommended daily intake of iodine is 150 μg per day for individuals over 12 years of age and 200 μg per day for pregnant and lactating women. The main dietary sources of iodine are dairy foods (in iodine-replete areas), seafood and iodized salt (2 g provides daily iodine requirement).

The effects of amiodarone on thyroid function are complex and variable.[1] By inhibiting the enzyme 5′-deioidinase, amiodarone decreases conversion of T_4 to T_3. As a consequence, T_4 increases by around 40% and T_3 decreases by around 20%. There is an accompanying increase in reverse T_3. These changes take place within days of commencing the drug. Decreased thyroid hormone feedback on the thyroid leads to early increase in TSH which returns to normal within 3 months. These changes mean that around 50% of patients taking amiodarone have abnormal thyroid tests; thyroid function is difficult to assess if baseline tests were not done before starting the drug; and thyroid disorders can be difficult to diagnose. Amiodarone may have local effects, decreasing T_3 binding to its receptor and thus inducing partial local hypothyroidism.

Amiodarone-induced hypothyroidism is about four times more common in iodine-replete areas, and may affect up 15% of patients. It is often transient and will resolve quicker if the drug can be stopped. Amiodarone-induced hypothyroidism is more common in women (F:M = 1.5:1), and in those with pre-existing thyroid antibodies or increased TSH. Those with underlying autoimmune disease are more likely to have goitre and to develop permanent hypothyroidism. A woman with thyroid antibodies has a relative risk of 13 of developing amiodarone-induced hypothyroidism. The inhibitory effect of iodine (Wolff–Chaikoff effect) and direct thyroid damage with autoantigen exposure are important in pathogenesis. Symptoms are similar to hypothyroidism from other causes, although they may be masked by underlying cardiac disease and exacerbate symptoms of the latter. Thyroxine can be given concurrently with amiodarone if necessary.

The incidence of amiodarone-induced thyrotoxicosis (AIT) varies from 2% in iodine-sufficient areas to 12% in iodine-insufficient areas. Two types are recognized depending on whether there is underlying thyroid disease or whether it is due to destructive thyroiditis (see Table 5.2). Colour flow Doppler has been used by a number of investigators as a way of demonstrating the increased blood flow associated with underlying Graves' disease or toxic nodular disease. Symptoms of thyrotoxicosis may be partly masked because of the β-blocking effect of amiodarone. It seems unlikely that amiodarone predisposes to cancer but a case of thyroid cancer has been reported in association with AIT.[2] Continuing amiodarone treatment does not influence the outcome of antithyroid drug therapy, and if the drug is stopped many experts feel that it is safe to restart when the thyrotoxicosis has been treated. Some would suggest ablating the thyroid with radioactive iodine prior to restarting the drug where the risk from recurrent thyrotoxicosis is high.

Table 5.2 Two types of amiodarone-induced thyrotoxicosis

	Type 1	Type 2
Pre-existing thyroid disease	Graves' disease Multinodular goitre	No
Duration of amiodarone use	<2 years	Usually longer
Local tenderness	Absent	Sometimes
Goitre	Usually	Usually not
Iodide uptake	Low	Very low
Autoantibodies	If Graves' disease	No
Serum interleukin-6	Normal	Increased
Colour flow Doppler	Increased flow	Normal
Thyrotoxicosis	Non-transient	Transient
? Stop amiodarone	If possible	Not necessary
First line therapy	High-dose antithyroid drugs	Prednisolone
Subsequent hypothyroidism	Unusual	Frequent, but often transient

High-dose steroids are usually recommended for type 2 AIT, particularly if there is pain and tenderness around the gland. Most practitioners would not stop amiodarone. A proposed scheme for managing AIT is shown in Figure 5.1.

For type 1 AIT, high-dose carbimazole or methimazole is the treatment of first choice. Patients are relatively resistant, and may require higher than normal doses (e.g. carbimazole 20 mg four times daily). Most practitioners would stop amiodarone. Perchlorate is useful as a second line of treatment, discharging the excess iodine from the thyroid. Doses of 200–1000 mg per day are used for up to 2 months. Rarely, this can cause aplastic anaemia—monitoring of blood count twice per week is recommended. Radioactive iodine is of limited use because of the low uptake in the gland.

Recent Developments

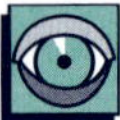

1. A meta-analysis of amiodarone use following cardiac surgery[3] showed that it decreased incidence of atrial fibrillation and ventricular rhythm disturbances, reduced risk of stroke and shortened hospital stay. It also remains extremely useful in patients with refractory or recurrent troublesome supraventricular arrhythmias.

2. Our current reliance on amiodarone may diminish as newer antiarrhythmic drugs become available: for example, bepridil[4] is a calcium antagonist with a distinctive cellular mode of action and some sodium-channel blocking activity. The drug is highly effective in converting atrial fibrillation to sinus rhythm. Other class III agents are under investigation including ibutilide,[5] and dronedarone[6] is a non-iodine containing analogue of amiodarone that lacks many of its side effects, including those that affect thyroid function.

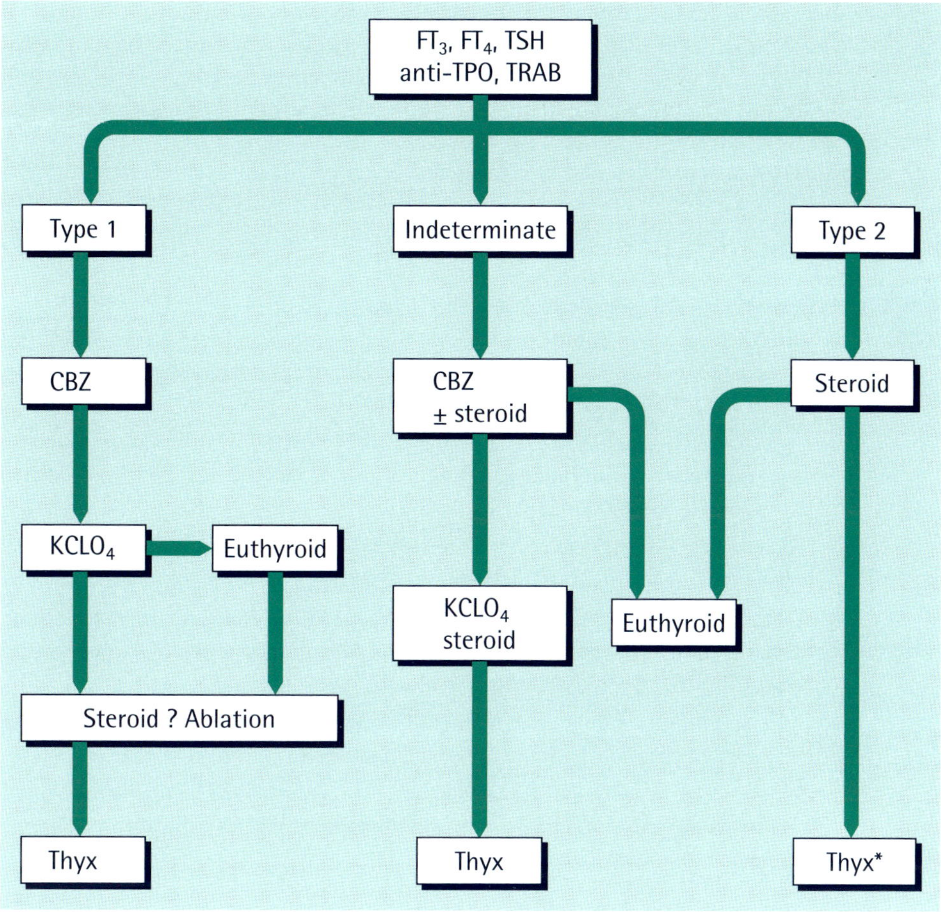

FT_3, FT_4, TSH
anti-TPO, TRAB

Type 1 | Indeterminate | Type 2

Type 1 → CBZ → $KCLO_4$ → Euthyroid
$KCLO_4$ → Steroid ? Ablation; Euthyroid → Steroid ? Ablation
Steroid ? Ablation → Thyx

Indeterminate → CBZ ± steroid → $KCLO_4$ steroid → Thyx
CBZ ± steroid → Euthyroid

Type 2 → Steroid → Thyx*
Steroid → Euthyroid

Fig. 5.1 Management of suspected amiodarone-induced thyrotoxicosis (AIT). Ablation is by means of radioactive iodine therapy. Iopanoic acid, a contrast medium containing iodine, would be used by some practitioners for refractory cases. *Rarely required. Many cases of type 2 AIT resolve with no treatment—careful monitoring is an option if the patient has mild or no symptoms and is cardiac stable. CBZ = carbimazole; $KCLO_4$ = perchlorate; Thyx = thyroidectomy; TRAB = TSH receptor antibodies.

3 Non-pharmacological management of arrhythmias has become sophisticated in recent years. This includes the use of radiofrequency ablation surgery for patients with atrial fibrillation.[7] This can be used effectively with pharmacotherapy if necessary. For patients with dangerous ventricular rhythm disturbances, implantable cardiac defibrillators are safe and highly effective.

Conclusions

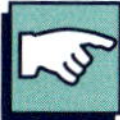

Thyroid tests are difficult to interpret in patients taking amiodarone. It is important that they are requested before starting the drug and at regular intervals during treatment. In addition to thyroid tests, the investigation of the above patient may include thyroid antibodies (antithyroid peroxidase) and TSH receptor antibodies), thyroid ultrasound, and colour flow Doppler (if available). It can be difficult to decide whether the patient is thyrotoxic if symptoms are not marked. This patient is most likely to have type 2 AIT. His amiodarone should not be stopped. He may not require any treatment in the short term but his thyroid function should be carefully monitored. If treatment is thought to be needed, high-dose corticosteroids should be considered (e.g. prednisolone 60 mg per day).

Further Reading

1 Basaria S, Cooper DS. Amiodarone and the thyroid. *Am J Med* 2005; **118**: 706–14.

2 Saad A, Falciglia M, Steward D, Nikiforov YE. Amiodarone-induced thyrotoxicosis and thyroid cancer. Clinical, immunohistochemical, and molecular genetic studies of a case and review of the literature. *Arch Pathol Lab Med* 2004; **128**: 807–10.

3 Aasbo JD, Lawrence AT, Krishnan K, Kim MH, Trohman RG. Amiodarone prophylaxis reduces major cardiovascular morbidity and length of stay after cardiac surgery: a meta-analysis. *Ann Intern Med* 2005; **143**: 327–36.

4 Nakazato Y, Yasuda M, Sasaki A, *et al.* Conversion and maintenance of sinus rhythm by bepridil in patients with persistent atrial fibrillation. *Circ J* 2005; **69**: 44–8.

5 Fragakis N, Papadopoulos N, Papanastasiou S, *et al.* Efficacy and safety of ibutilide for cardioversion of atrial flutter and fibrillation in patients receiving amiodarone or propafenone. *Pacing Clin Electrophysiol* 2005; **28**: 934–61.

6 Touboul P, Brugada J, Capucci A, Crijns HJG, Edvardsson N, Hohnloser SH. Dronedarone for prevention of atrial fibrillation: a dose-ranging study. *Eur Heart J* 2003; **24**: 1481–7.

7 Geidel S, Ostermeyer J, Lass M, *et al.* Three years experience with monopolar and bipolar radiofrequency ablation surgery in patients with permanent atrial fibrillation. *Eur J Cardiothorac Surg* 2005; **27**: 243–9.

PROBLEM

06 Subclinical Hypothyroidism

Case History

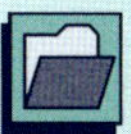

A 26-year-old woman presents complaining of feeling tired and heavy periods. She got married 18 months ago and has been trying to become pregnant. She is a smoker. Her general health is very good and she is not taking any medications. Her mother developed hypothyroidism in her 40s and she has a cousin with coeliac disease. Her serum thyrotropin level (TSH) is mildly raised at 7.2 mIU/l (normal range up to 4.5 mIU/l), but thyroid hormone levels are within the normal range.

Does she require any further investigations?

Do her thyroid tests have any bearing on fertility?

Should she be started on thyroxine replacement?

If she becomes pregnant, will her requirement for thyroxine change?

Background

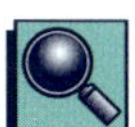

Hypothyroidism is common. Subclinical disease usually manifesting as high TSH and mild symptoms is extremely common, particularly in older people:[1] in the Whickham survey, carried out in the north-east of England, high serum TSH was reported in 7.5% of women and in 2.8% of men. Similarly, in the National Health and Nutrition Examination Survey (NHANES) II study, 4.6% of North American subjects had increased TSH. Studies in older people report mild or subclinical hypothyroidism in 10–15%.

Treatment of subclinical hypothyroidism has been controversial, although some studies in the 1980s and 1990s suggested improved neuropsychological performance.[1] For people with TSH less than 10 mIU/l, symptomatology is generally indistinguishable from normal individuals and the major argument for treatment has been to improve lipid profile and thus decrease the risk of cardiovascular disease. US consensus guidelines in the early years of the twenty-first century did not recommend routine treatment of those with TSH less than 10 mIU/l; did not advocate universal screening; and did not support a role for thyroid antibody measurement in the decision-making process. A recent review[2] by a panel of experts concluded the literature relating to subclinical hypothyroidism was deficient in a number of areas. In particular, evidence relating the condition to adverse cardiac endpoints was lacking from large population-based studies, and evidence to support use of thyroid antibody testing routinely was poor. However, it was acknowledged that progression rate to overt hypothyroidism was 2–5% per year, and that presence of thyroid antibodies and higher levels of TSH (>10 mIU/l) were markers for likely progression.

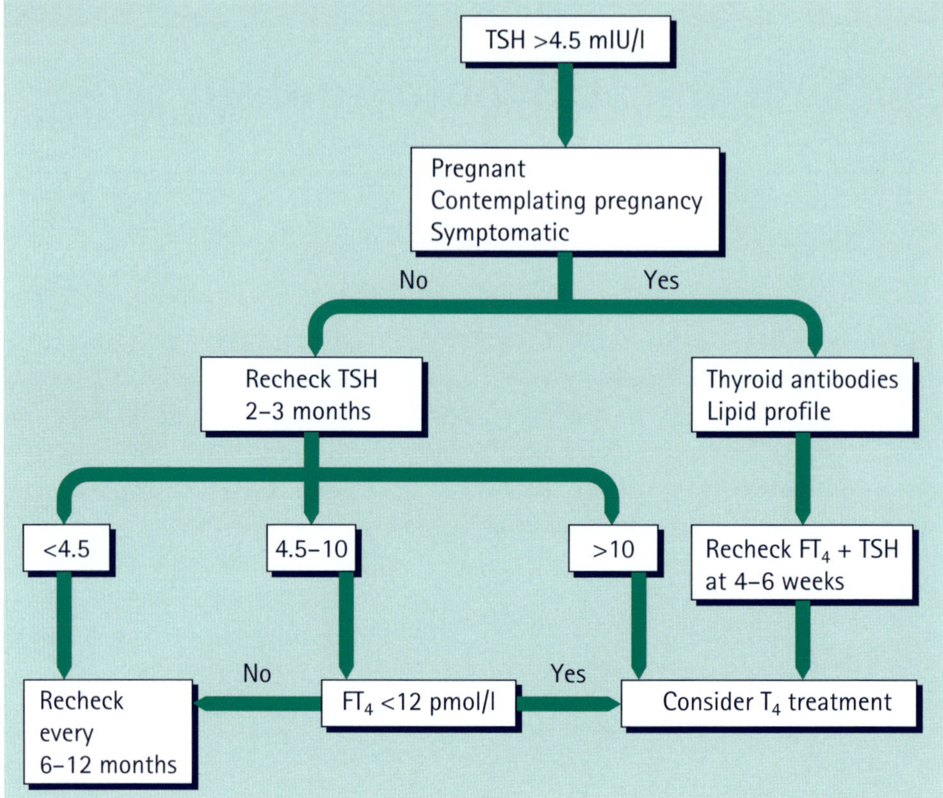

Fig. 6.1 Diagnosis and management of subclinical hypothyroidism.

For asymptomatic individuals with TSH >10 mIU/l, no treatment and repeat tests at 6–12 months were recommended. The group felt that evidence linking subclinical hypothyroidism to poor outcome of pregnancy was 'fair', and recommended treating women who were planning pregnancy and increasing the dose of thyroxine during pregnancy. A management algorithm based on the deliberations of this group of experts has been produced.[2] We present a modified version in Figure 6.1.

Menstrual irregularities, subfertility and anovulation are recognized in severe hypothyroidism.[1] However, there is a lack of systematic studies investigating the possible link between subclinical hypothyroidism and subfertility. Available data suggest that mild hypothyroidism is not associated with marked menstrual irregularities, gross disturbances in prolactin levels or marked corpus luteum dysfunction. An Austrian study[3] of women referred with subfertility and treated with finely tuned thyroxine replacement adjusted according to thyrotropin-releasing hormone (TRH) testing achieved a high level of pregnancy. It seems prudent to treat women who are contemplating pregnancy as their thyroxine requirements will increase if they do become pregnant and thyroxine treatment is both safe and inexpensive.

The link between gross thyroid deficiency in the mother and neurological development of the child was recognized in the late nineteenth century. Evidence relating to the

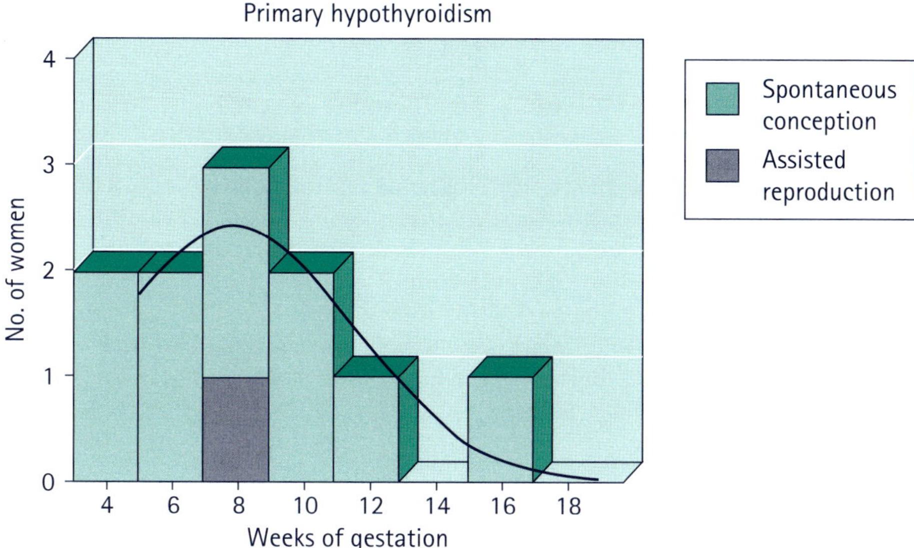

Fig. 6.2 Timing of increased thyroxine during pregnancy (from the study by Alexander *et al.*[5]). Figure shows the week of gestation at which increased thyroxine dose was needed in a small series of women followed from before conception through pregnancy.

effect of more subtle degrees of thyroid dysfunction has been relatively slow to accumulate. Haddow *et al.*[4] examined the children of 47 women who had TSH above the 99.7th centile. Their children were examined using a battery of tests to investigate language, reading ability, visuomotor skills, school performance and intelligence. These children were compared with 124 control children whose mothers had normal TSH during pregnancy. The children of mothers with high TSH performed significantly less well on the battery of tests; 19% of the mildly hypothyroid mothers had children with IQ less than 85, compared with only 5% of the controls.

Recent Developments

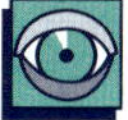

1 Alexander *et al.*[5] measured thyroid function, human chorionic gonadotropin and oestrogen sequentially before and during pregnancy. Thyroxine dose had to be increased in 17 out of 20 pregnancies, the mean increase being 47%. The increase was required as early as the fifth week and had to be maintained until delivery (Figure 6.2). The abnormalities associated with under-treatment of subclinical hypothyroidism in pregnancy are subtle, but significant—there are no gross changes in maternal or fetal outcome.

2 Polychlorinated biphenyls are pesticides that are universally present as environmental contaminants. Higher levels of these substances in pregnant women are associated with lower levels of thyroid hormones.[6] These effects are also present in animal models, and the compounds have been shown to influence the transcription of thyroid hormone responsive genes in the nervous system.

3 Available evidence suggests that untreated subclinical hypothyroidism is a risk factor for vascular disease with studies confirming increased low-density lipoprotein cholesterol

and increased carotid intima–media thickness. Studies have shown variable effects of thyroxine replacement on the dyslipidaemia, but this may depend on the adequacy of replacement. Patients with subclinical hypothyroidism have been documented also to have increased levels of insulin and C-reactive protein–both also risk factors for vascular disease.[7]

4 Autoimmune diseases, notably systemic lupus erythematosus, are associated with increased risk of miscarriage. In a recent meta-analysis, Prummel and Wiersinga[8] demonstrated an association between thyroid antibodies and risk of miscarriage. Combining data from eight case–control and ten longitudinal studies, they found an odds ratio of 2.73 among patients with autoimmune thyroid disease. It is not clear whether this is due to metabolic effects of altered thyroid hormone or to an altered immune state affecting the fetal allograft, or to demographic factors.

Conclusions

This patient should be investigated initially with free thyroid hormone and TSH measurements along with assessment of thyroid antibody status (antithyroid peroxidase and anti-thyroglobulin [anti-Tg]). She does not require thyroid imaging (isotope or ultrasound scanning). We would not initiate fertility investigations at this stage, but would seek to correct her hypothyroidism. It is not certain that subclinical hypothyroidism impairs fertility but correction of the hormone abnormality is definitely indicated prior to, and during, pregnancy. Her TSH should be checked on a second occasion before commencing thyroxine (if TSH is again elevated). In pregnancy, dose of thyroxine usually needs to be increased by the equivalent of two daily doses per week—generally 25–50 μg per day. The aim is to keep TSH between 0.5 mIU/l and 2.0 mIU/l with free thyroxine in the upper third of the normal reference range.

Further Reading

1 Roberts CG, Ladenson PW. Hypothyroidism. *Lancet* 2004; **363**: 793–803.

2 Surks MI, Ortiz E, Daniels GH, *et al.* Subclinical thyroid disease. Scientific review and guidelines for diagnosis and management. *JAMA* 2004; **291**: 228–38.

3 Raber W, Nowotny P, Vytiska-Binstorfer E, Vierhapper G. Thyroxine treatment modified in infertile women according to thyroxine-releasing hormone testing: 5 year follow-up of 283 women referred after exclusion of absolute causes of infertility. *Hum Reprod* 2003; **18**: 707–14.

4 Haddow JE, Palomaki GE, Allan WC, *et al.* Maternal thyroid deficiency during pregnancy and subsequent neuropsychological development of the child. *N Engl J Med* 1999; **341**: 549–55.

5 Alexander EK, Marqusee E, Lawrence J, Jarolim P, Fischer GA, Larsen PR. Timing and magnitude of increases in levothyroxine requirements during pregnancy in women with hypothyroidism. *N Engl J Med* 2004; **351**: 241–9.

6 Takser L, Mergler D, Baldwin M, de Grosbois S, Smargiassi A, Lafond J. Thyroid hormones in pregnancy in relation to environmental exposure to organochlorine compounds and mercury. *Environ Health Perspect* 2005; **113**: 1039–45.

7 Tuzcu A, Bahceci M, Gokalp D, Tuzun Y, Gunes K. Subclinical hypothyroidism may be associated with elevated high-sensitive C-reactive protein (low grade inflammation) *and* fasting hyperinsulinemia. *Endocr J* 2005; **52**: 89–94.

8 Prummel MF, Wiersinga WM. Thyroid autoimmunity and miscarriage. *Eur J Endocrinol* 2004; **150**: 751–5.

PROBLEM

07 Thyroid Function in Early Pregnancy

Case History

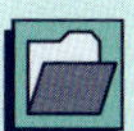

You are asked to see a 30-year-old woman who is 10 weeks pregnant. She has hyperemesis gravidarum and her free T_4 is increased at 32 pmol/l (normal 12–25 pmol/l) and her thyrotropin (thyroid-stimulating hormone [TSH]) is suppressed. She has no previous history of thyroid disease and this is her first pregnancy.

Is her thyroid function within normal limits, or does she have hyperthyroidism?

If hyperthyroid, what is the likely cause?

Does she require antithyroid drug therapy?

Background

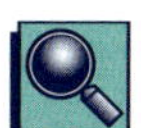

Major changes occur in thyroid tests during early pregnancy. Under the influence of oestrogen, thyroxine-binding globulin (TBG) increases, giving rise to increased total thyroid hormone concentrations. This is not of major physiological significance. However, free T_3 and free T_4 also increase and TSH decreases. TSH is undetectable in 10–15% of women in late first trimester. Increased hormone production may relate to increased metabolic rate, altered equilibrium with binding proteins, and the needs of the foetus for thyroid hormone until the fetal pituitary–thyroid axis has developed at around 20 weeks. The thyroid gland volume also increases in pregnancy perhaps because of altered iodine status with increased turnover and urinary loss.

TSH and human chorionic gonadotropin (hCG) share structural similarity: They have a common α chain and homologous β chains. The peak of hCG in the first trimester of pregnancy coincides with the trough of TSH and the highest levels of thyroid hormones. There is convincing evidence from *in vitro* and *in vivo* studies that the increase in thyroid

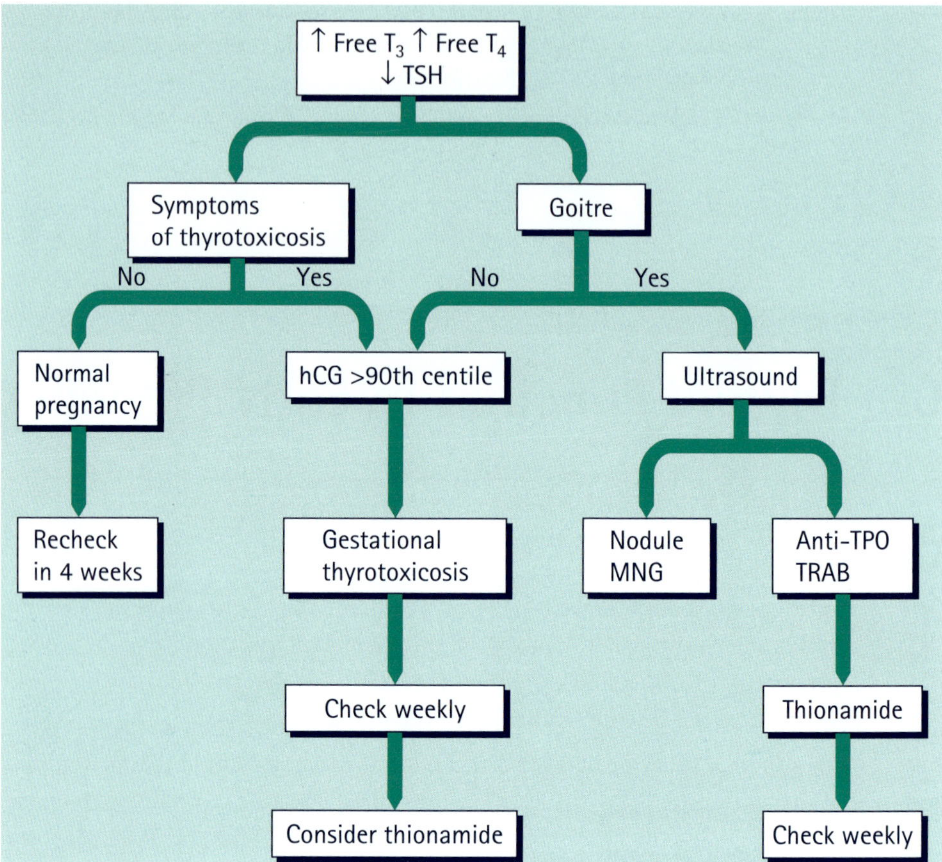

Fig. 7.1 Hyperthyroidism in early pregnancy. Gestational thyrotoxicosis should be considered if the human chorionic gonadotropin (hCG) level is above the 90th centile for the stage of pregnancy although cases with variant hCG but relatively low total hCG have been observed. MNG = multinodular goitre; TPO = thyroid peroxidase; TRAB = TSH receptor antibody.

function during early pregnancy is driven by hCG acting at the TSH receptor on thyroid cells. Women with trophoblastic disease have high circulating hCG (Figure 7.1) with variants that show enhanced TSH receptor stimulating activity.

Although nausea and vomiting are common in pregnancy, symptoms severe enough to warrant intervention occur in fewer than 20 cases per 1000. Hyperemesis gravidarum may present with weight loss, dehydration, acidosis (due to low food intake), alkalosis (due to vomiting) and hypokalaemia. Abnormalities in liver tests occur in up to 20% of cases. Reported risk factors include previous multiple parity, high saturated fat intake prior to pregnancy, and *Helicobacter pylori* infection. Severe complications are rare—these include oesophageal rupture, renal failure, retinal haemorrhage, central pontine myelinosis, and Wernicke's encephalopathy. Treatment includes attention to fluid and electrolyte balance and anti-emetics (e.g. chlorpromazine). For refractory cases, newer anti-emetics such as ondansetron should be considered, as should the use of corticosteroids. Enteral or parenteral feeding is required in severe cases. Hyperthyroidism occurs in about 60% of patients with hyperemesis. It is not usually severe enough to cause symptoms, and thus seldom requires treatment with antithyroid drugs. The hyperthyroidism generally resolves by around the 18th week of pregnancy.

Thyrotoxicosis occurs in 1 in every 2000 pregnancies, and is most commonly due to Graves' disease. Like other autoimmune diseases, Graves' disease is usually quiescent in pregnancy and can become more active in the post-partum period. The disease can become more active in the first trimester when most women are relatively hyperthyroid in any case. The major risk to the mother is of cardiac failure—hyperthyroidism induces dysfunction of cardiac muscle and there is expansion of plasma volume during pregnancy. The risks to the foetus are greater: the chance of fetal death or spontaneous abortion is increased; increased risk of developmental abnormalities has been reported; the fetus is more likely to be small for gestational dates and to require premature delivery.

It is essential that Graves' disease is effectively managed in women of reproductive age before they become pregnant. Radioactive iodine therapy is contraindicated during pregnancy. Surgery is seldom required but can be undertaken during the second trimester once the patient's symptoms have been carefully controlled with antithyroid drugs and β-blockers. The mainstay of treatment is antithyroid drugs. The dose of these should be kept to a minimum, particularly in early pregnancy. Infants of mothers with Graves' disease are at risk of neonatal hyperthyroidism due to the transplacental passage of TSH receptor antibodies (TBII). Plasma levels of these antibodies should be monitored during pregnancy in patients with Graves' disease. Those who remain antibody positive should have ongoing thionamide treatment to suppress TBII production.

A distinct entity, early gestational thyrotoxicosis is almost certainly due to excessive stimulation of the thyroid by hCG. The syndrome usually presents with hyperemesis along with the typical symptoms of hyperthyroidism. The condition has not been extensively studied. Most patients are of Asian origin, and the reason for this is not known. The condition is self-limiting but carbimazole treatment is often required until at least the middle of the second trimester. The association of hyperemesis and hyperthyroidism is common in situations where the hCG is particularly high including in twin pregnancies and in patients with trophoblastic tumours.

Recent Developments

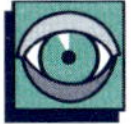

1 Carbimazole and, by implication, other antithyroid drugs are generally regarded as being relatively safe during pregnancy. However, a specific embryopathy with scalp defects, choanal atresia, and gastrointestinal abnormalities has been described.[1] This embryopathy may be related to prolonged severe thyrotoxicosis and to higher doses of the drug.

2 There is a strong argument that women should be routinely screened for thyroid disease during pregnancy.[2] Hypothyroidism is present in 2.5% of pregnancies. Both trophoblast function and fetal neurological development are highly dependent on thyroid hormone, and replacement should be started early in all pregnant hypothyroid women. Post-partum thyroid disturbance occurs in 5–9% of all pregnancies. Early pregnancy thyroid changes and thyroid antibodies are highly predictive.

3 Understanding the nutritional requirements of the pregnant woman is important in clinical and epidemiological terms. Lof *et al.*[3] measured basal metabolic rate (BMR)

in a series of pregnant women. Body weight and pre-pregnancy fat mass were major determinants of BMR, which also correlated highly with circulating thyroid hormone and insulin-like growth factor-1 levels.

4 A range of hormones has been implicated in causing hyperemesis but the underlying cause remains largely unknown.[4] Progesterone, oestrogen, prolactin, placental growth hormone, hCG, and leptin have all been implicated. Immunological and infectious triggers have also been considered. Leptin has recently been confirmed as a correlate of high body mass index in pregnancy and, in addition to a possible role in hyperemesis, it has also been considered as a potential early marker for pre-eclampsia.[5]

Conclusions

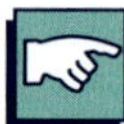

The above patient has increased thyroid hormone levels along with suppressed TSH. This is compatible with the changes in thyroid function seen in the first trimester of normal pregnancy. Some of the symptoms of hyperthyroidism are common in normal pregnancy (nausea, sweating). Careful enquiry should be made about symptoms. It would be useful to screen the patient for antithyroid peroxidase and TSH receptor antibodies. Although it is most likely that this patient is euthyroid, she could have early gestational thyrotoxicosis. Assuming she has no, or only mild, symptoms we would not treat her with antithyroid drugs but would check her thyroid function every 1–2 weeks until her tests are within normal limits and pregnancy is well established.

Further Reading

1 Foulds N, Walpole I, Elmslie F, Mansour S. Carbimazole embryopathy: an emerging phenotype. *Am J Med Genet* 2005; **132**: 130–5.

2 Lazarus JH, Premawardhana LDK. Screening for thyroid disease in pregnancy. *J Clin Pathol* 2005; **58**: 449–57.

3 Lof M, Olausson H, Bostrom K, Janerot Sjöberg B, Sohlstrom A, Forsum E. Changes in basal metabolic rate during pregnancy in relation to changes in body weight and composition, cardiac output, insulin-like growth factor I, and thyroid hormones and in relation to fetal growth. *Am J Clin Nutr* 2005; **81**: 678–85.

4 Verberg MFG, Gillott DJ, Al Fardan N, Grudzinskas JG. Hyperemesis gravidarum, a literature review. *Human Reprod Update* 2005; **11**: 678–85.

5 Baksu A, Ozkan A, Goker N, Baksu B, Uluocak A. Serum leptin levels in preeclamptic pregnant women: relationship to thyroid-stimulating hormone, body mass index, and proteinuria. *Am J Perinatol* 2005; **22**: 161–4.

PROBLEM

08 Post-partum Thyroid Disturbance

Case History

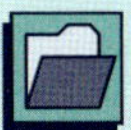

EF is a 33-year-old woman who delivered a healthy son 6 months ago. She presents with symptoms of depression. Her general health is good and her previous pregnancy was uncomplicated. Free T_4 is low at 9 pmol/l (normal 12–25 pmol/l) and her thyrotropin (thyroid-stimulating hormone [TSH]) is mildly increased at 7.2 mIU/l (normal 0.15–2.50 mIU/l).

Is she likely to have thyroid disease?

Would you offer her thyroid replacement?

What arrangements would you make for her follow-up?

Background

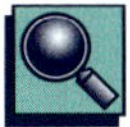

Disturbances of thyroid function in the post-partum period are extremely common, occurring in 5–9% of pregnancies.[1] The underlying pathology is thyroiditis similar to Hashimoto's disease with lymphocytic infiltration and follicle formation in the gland. Post-partum thyroid disturbance (PPTD) is an autoimmune disease caused by interplay between predisposition to autoimmunity and the effects of pregnancy on accelerating immune disturbances with a shift towards a T helper 2 pattern of cytokine expression. Almost all patients with PPTD are positive for antithyroid peroxidase (anti-TPO) during second trimester. However, anti-TPO is a poor predictor of the condition as only 50% of positive women will develop PPTD. Antithyroid antibodies are not a feature and, if present, suggest a diagnosis of Graves' disease. Around 50% of new cases of Graves' disease occur within 1 year (peak 3–6 months) after delivery. Increased prevalence of HLA-DR3, DR44, and DR5 has been reported in Graves' disease.

Presentation of PPTD is extremely variable and is often entirely asymptomatic. The common pattern is transient thyrotoxicosis followed by hypothyroidism (Figure 8.1). Thyrotoxicosis begins between 6 weeks and 6 months after delivery (median 13 weeks). Symptoms are seldom severe and specific treatment is usually not required. Some patients require β-blocker for a few weeks to decrease palpitations. TSH receptor antibodies are not present and the uptake of iodide or pertechnetate by the gland is low. Hypothyroidism begins at a median of 19 weeks, is frequently symptomatic, and often requires treatment with thyroxine. Permanent hypothyroidism develops in 25–30% of patients, increasing to 50% at 7 years. In others, hypothyroidism may not be permanent but can last up to 1 year. It is reasonable to tail off and stop thyroid hormone replacement after a few months if the patient is asymptomatic and does not have very high levels of

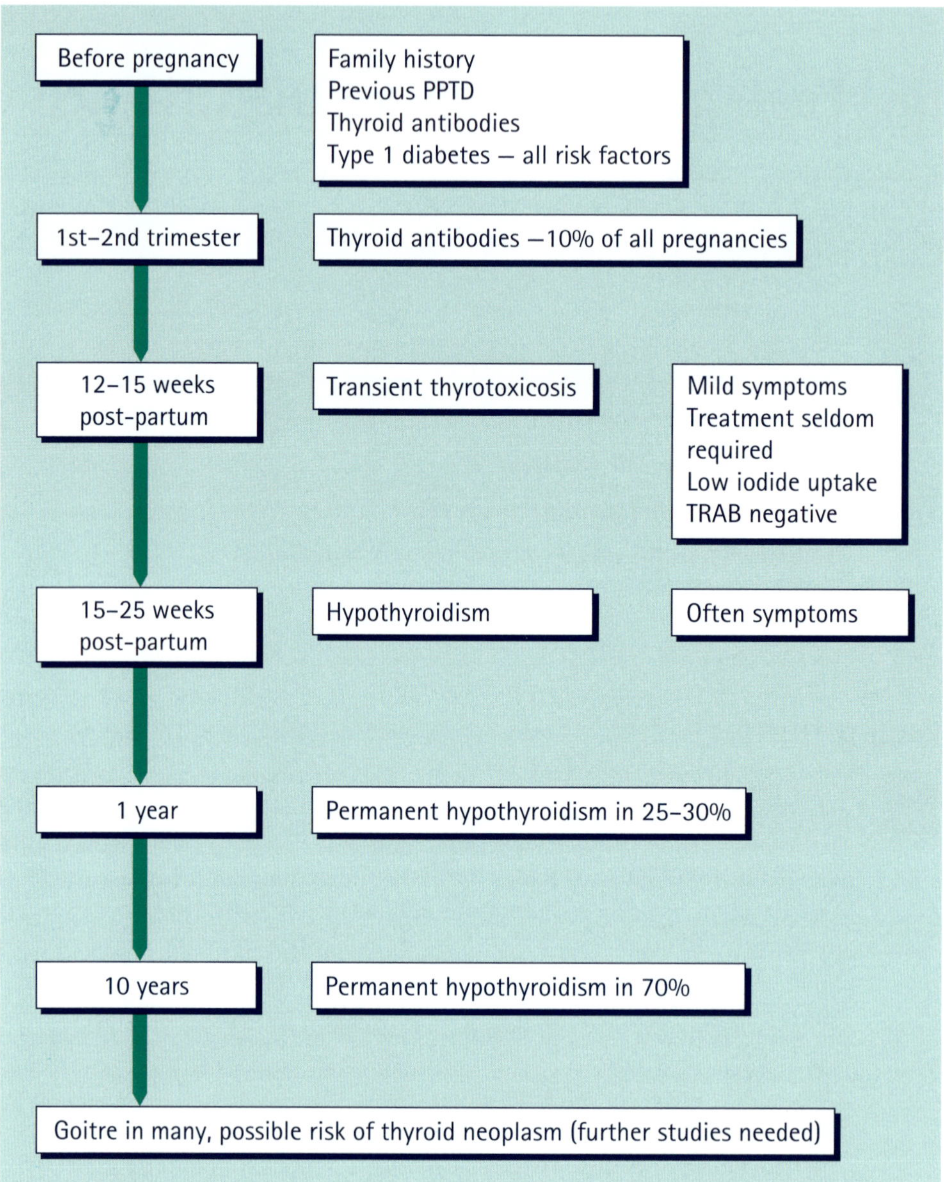

Fig. 8.1 Natural history of post-partum thyroid disturbance. TRAB = TSH receptor antibodies.

anti-TPO. Our practice is to continue with thyroxine if the patient is considering a further pregnancy.

Thyroid autoimmunity is, without doubt, the major predisposing factor for PPTD. Some of the changes in immune function associated with the condition pre-date pregnancy.[2] Other predisposing factors are a family history of thyroid disease or PPTD, type 1 diabetes, and a previous episode of PPTD. In fact, there is a 70% recurrence rate in patients who have an episode of PPTD. Smoking is an important predisposing factor for some thyroid disorders, especially Graves' disease and Graves' eye disease, but it does not appear to play role in PPTD.[3] Up to 1.5 billion people in the world are at risk of iodine deficiency. However, iodine status does not appear to influence risk of PPTD.

In most centres, women are not routinely screened for thyroid disease during and after pregnancy. Modern assay methods have reduced the cost of thyroid tests and made thyroid status easier to assess. There is a strong argument to consider universal screening for thyroid disorders during pregnancy:[4]

- Thyrotoxicosis occurs in 0.2% of pregnancies—this poses a considerable risk to both mother and fetus.
- Hypothyroidism is present in 2.5%—this increases the risk of fetal loss, and is associated with impaired neuropsychological development of the child.
- PPTD occurs in 5–9% of women following pregnancy—it is associated with considerable morbidity in the post-partum period and a highly significant incidence of permanent hypothyroidism.

Both thyroid antibody positivity and PPTD have been associated with depression in the post-partum period. A trial of thyroxine therapy in Wales[5] found no evidence that thyroxine therapy could prevent depression in thyroid antibody positive women.

Recent Developments

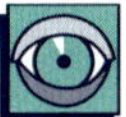

1 Microchimerism is defined as the presence of a small number of cells from one organism in the tissues of a host organism. It is considered a potentially important mechanism in the predisposition to autoimmune diseases that follows pregnancy.[6] The presence of fetal calls in maternal peripheral blood, skin, and thyroid has been demonstrated. Suppression of maternal immunity during pregnancy allows these cells to survive in potential autoimmune target organs. Following pregnancy, with the restoration of normal immune function and the shift back to a T helper 1 immune state, the fetal cells may trigger a graft-vs.-host reaction in tissues such as the thyroid.

2 Many forms of benign thyroid disease are more common in women and may be exacerbated by pregnancy. PPTD may be very common, although often undetected, in parts of the world where fertility rate and total birth rate are high. A recent population-based, case–control study from Kuwait has suggested that PPTD may increase the risk of thyroid cancer by up to ten-fold.[7]

3 Even patients with mild thyroid disturbance have a high incidence of permanent thyroid failure on follow-up: Azizi[8] followed up a large cohort of patients with PPTD who had either subclinical or overt hypothyroidism at presentation. The prevalence of thyroid failure after withdrawal of thyroxine treatment an average of nearly 2 years later was similar in both groups at around 60%.

Conclusions

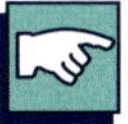

This patient is highly likely to have PPTD, and she almost certainly has an underlying predisposition to autoimmune thyroid disease. Enquiry should be made regarding symptoms of hypothyroidism, and she should be asked about mood disturbances. There is a high risk that she will develop permanent hypothyroidism. If she is asymptomatic, she could be followed up with thyroid tests at monthly intervals. Thyroid antibody (anti-TPO) levels would help to assess the likelihood that she will become permanently hypothyroid. If symptomatic, thyroxine therapy would be indicated. This should be continued for 6–12 months and then gradually withdrawn to assess her underlying thyroid function. If she were planning further pregnancy, we would continue thyroxine until 6 months or so after the delivery of her last child.

Further Reading

1. Nader S. Thyroid disease and other endocrine disorders in pregnancy. *Obstet Gynecol Clin North Am* 2004; **31**: 257–85.
2. Kokandi AA, Parkes AB, Premawardhana LDKE, John R, Lazarus JH. Association of postpartum thyroid dysfunction with antepartum hormonal and immunological changes. *J Clin Endocrinol Metab* 2003; **88**: 1126–32.
3. Vestergaard P. Smoking and thyroid disorders—a meta-analysis. *Eur J Endocrinol* 2002; **146**: 153–61.
4. Lazarus JH, Premawardhana LDKE. Screening for thyroid disease in pregnancy. *J Clin Pathol* 2004; **58**: 449–52.
5. Harris B, Oretti R, Lazarus J, *et al.* Randomised trial of thyroxine to prevent postnatal depression in thyroid-antibody-positive women. *Brit J Psychiatry* 2002; **180**: 327–30.
6. Ando T, Davies TF. Postpartum autoimmune thyroid disease: the potential role of fetal microchimerism. *J Clin Endocrinol Metab* 2003; **88**: 2965–71.
7. Memon A, Radovanovic Z, Suresh A. Epidemiological link between postpartum thyroiditis and thyroid cancer. *Eur J Endocrinol* 2004; **19**: 607–9.
8. Azizi F. The occurrence of permanent thyroid failure in patients with subclinical postpartum thyroiditis. *Eur J Endocrinol* 2005; **153**: 367–71.

PROBLEM

09 Thyrotoxic Crisis

Case History

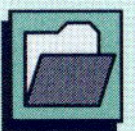

FP is a 46-year-old woman who has been taking carbimazole on and off for 10 years. She is poorly compliant with her treatment and follow-up. She presents with vomiting, is severely dehydrated and has a resting pulse rate of 120 beats per minute. On examination you find her to be extremely tremulous and emaciated, and she has an 80 g goitre with a loud overlying bruit.

What follow-up is normally recommended for a patient taking carbimazole?

How would you manage this patient during her acute illness?

How would you plan her longer-term management?

Background

Thyroid storm is diagnosed when patients present with the most severe manifestations of thyrotoxicosis. Although rare, the condition is important since it is fatal in up to 30% of hospitalized patients.[1] Hyperthyroidism severe enough to cause thyroid storm only commonly occurs in Graves' disease. Thyroid hormone values do not have to be particularly high, and may overlap substantially with those of patients with untreated thyrotoxicosis presenting to outpatient clinics. Other factors such as intercurrent infection, dehydration and the duration of untreated thyrotoxicosis are important factors. Thyroid storm most commonly occurs in older people. In patients with toxic adenomas, toxicosis may be predominantly due to T_3. Apart from the expected signs and symptoms of thyrotoxicosis, a number of other features may be present. Muscle symptoms include weakness from myopathy due to the thyroid hormone excess, muscle pain associated with increased levels of creatine kinase, and rhabdomyolysis in severe cases. Apathetic thyrotoxicosis usually occurs in older individuals who present with myopathy, hypotension, tachycardia, confusion and coma. Prolonged vomiting, poor oral intake and dehydration may account for the occasional association with Wernicke's encephalopathy due to thiamine deficiency. These patients present with nausea and vomiting, nystagmus and mental changes. Severe cases may have lactic acidosis, and multiple organ failure (cardiac, hepatic and renal). A differential diagnosis is shown in Box 9.1.

In the past, the commonest precipitating event was neck surgery in patients who had undiagnosed thyrotoxicosis or those who had been inadequately prepared for surgery. Now, common precipitating factors are undiagnosed thyrotoxicosis, poor patient compliance, surgery, trauma, childbirth and infection. Overdose of thyroxine is surprisingly

Box 9.1 Differential diagnosis of thyroid storm

- Delirium tremens
- Opioid withdrawal
- Amphetamine overdose
- Panic attack
- Mania
- Phaeochromocytoma

well tolerated with severe symptoms only when greater than 10 mg has been ingested. Symptoms start about 3 days after ingestion and reach their maximum at 10 days. Recent case reports of thyroid storm include cases precipitated by strangulation, aspirin toxicity, cytotoxic chemotherapy, and radioactive iodine treatment.

Treatment is summarized in Figure 9.1. The following measures should be considered:

- *Supportive treatment.* Intravenous fluids—normal saline or 5–10% dextrose as indicated; antibiotics for intercurrent infection; group B vitamins. Passive cooling using ice packs or cooling blankets. Avoid high doses of aspirin—it displaces thyroid hormones from binding sites. Digoxin, β-blockers, calcium-channel blockers or amiodarone to control cardiac rhythm and rate.
- *Antithyroid drugs.* Propylthiouracil is the drug of choice as it decreases conversion of T_4 to T_3. An initial dose of 150–200 mg orally or by nasogastric tube is adequate, repeated every 6 hours. Carbimazole 60–100 mg initially followed by 100–120 mg per day may be used.
- *Large doses of iodine* given acutely inhibit thyroid hormone synthesis within the thyroid (Wolff–Chaikoff effect). Iodine should be given 1 hour after antithyroid drugs; 30 drops of Lugol's iodine daily in divided doses can be given. Alternatively, potassium iodide 100–130 mg every 6 hours can be used. In emergency 500–1000 mg sodium iodide can be given every 8 hours.
- *β-blockers.* Propranolol is the preferred agent as it has an addition action decreasing deiodination of T_4 to T_3. They will help control tachycardia, tremor, sweating and agitation. Propranolol can be given at an initial dose of 40–120 mg, repeated at 6-hourly intervals. In an emergency, 1–3 mg can be given intravenously.
- *Dexamethasone.* Corticosteroids inhibit release of thyroid hormone and also inhibit peripheral conversion to triiodothyronine. Dexamethasone 2–4 mg every 6 hours should be given.
- *Lithium.* This inhibits outward transport of thyroid hormone in the thyrocyte. Lithium may be particularly useful in patients with severe thyrotoxicosis who are sensitive to iodine. An initial dose of up to 1000 mg should be followed by 300 mg every 8 hours. Toxic effects will be avoided if the plasma level of lithium is kept under 1.5 mmol/l.
- *Amiodarone.* The drug contains a large amount of iodine and, in addition, inhibits peripheral generation of T_3. It has occasionally been used to benefit in thyroid storm, even in the absence of cardiac rhythm disturbances.

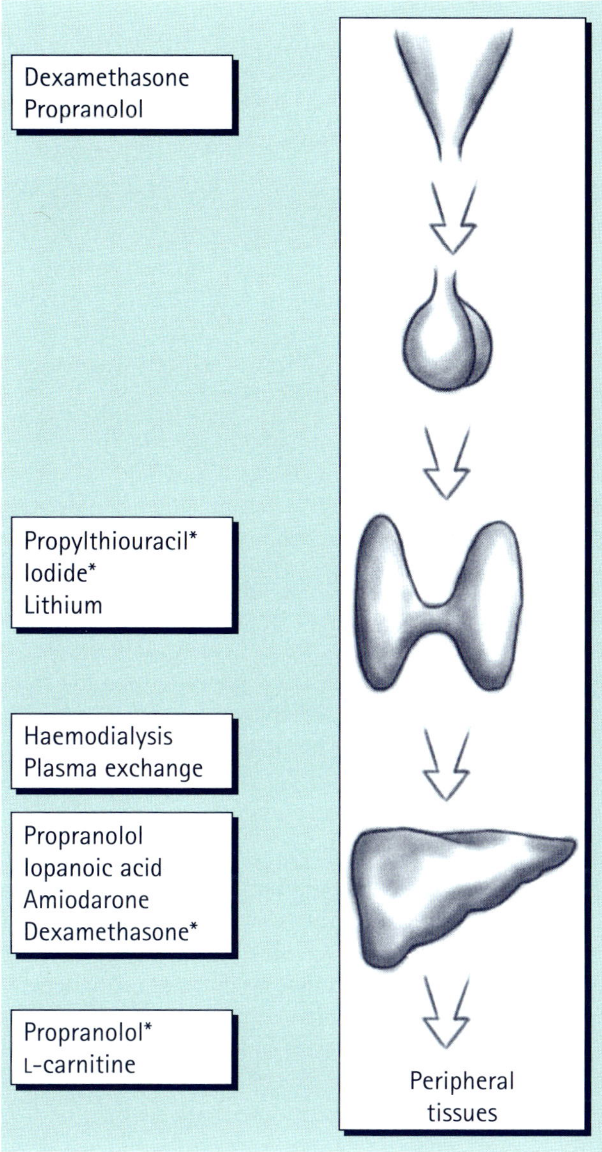

Fig. 9.1 Treatment of thyroid storm. *Main site of action of first-line drugs.

- *Radiographic contrast media*. Ipodate (Oragrafin) or iopanoic acid 1–2 g repeated daily help to decrease thyroid hormone generation in the thyroid and also to decrease peripheral generation of triiodothyronine.

Oral activated charcoal helps to remove thyroid hormone from the stomach in cases of overdose if given sufficiently early. Resins (colestipol, cholestyramine) that bind thyroid hormone may be useful in cases of overdose or as an adjunct in cases resistant to standard measures. Dantrolene, a drug used in malignant hyperpyrexia, has been used to effect in thyroid storm. The drug inhibits massive release of calcium from the endoplasmic reticulum of cells such as striated myocytes. Finally, thyroid hormone can be removed from the circulation by peritoneal dialysis, haemodialysis or by plasmapheresis. The latter is particularly useful since hormone that is protein bound is also removed.

Recent Developments

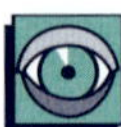

1. Lithium is probably underused as an antithyroid drug. Worsening of thyrotoxicosis can occur after radioactive iodine therapy due to radiation-induced damage and increased thyrotropin (thyroid-stimulating hormone [TSH])-receptor antibodies in patients with Graves' disease. A short course of lithium protects against worsening of hyperthyroidism following administration of radioactive iodine.[2]
2. Plasma exchange has been used occasionally in patients who do not respond rapidly to standard measures.[3,4] This treatment removes free and bound hormone, thus diminishing the overall pool. It will also reduce levels of TSH receptor antibodies in patients with Graves' disease, thus diminishing the stimulus to thyroid overactivity.
3. L-carnitine is an important molecule in cellular intermediary metabolism. It also inhibits nuclear uptake of triiodothyronine and thyroxine and has potential use in severe thyrotoxicosis.[5,6] All other measures used for this condition decrease the amount of thyroid hormone delivered to tissues. L-carnitine, by diminishing the action of thyroid hormone at cellular level, has a unique mechanism of action. Furthermore, it is a natural product and has a low risk of side effects. A suitable dose is 1–2 g every 12 hours.

Conclusions

Patients with newly diagnosed thyrotoxicosis should be seen every 4–6 weeks until their condition is stable. Once this is achieved, 3-monthly visits are suitable. If taking antithyroid drugs, they should be instructed to report any untoward side effects immediately. The mainstays of managing impending or actual thyroid crises are supportive measures including fluid and electrolyte balance, antithyroid drugs (preferably propylthiouracil), β-blockers (propranolol), steroids, and large does of iodine or iodine-containing compounds. ^{131}I should be considered after thyroid storm. The patient may well require thyroid hormone replacement afterwards but is not in any major danger in the short or medium term if compliance is less than ideal.

Further Reading

1. Sarlis NJ, Gourgiotis L. Thyroid emergencies. *Rev Endocr Metab Disord* 2003; **4**: 129–36.
2. Vannucchi G, Chiti A, Mannavola D, *et al*. Radioiodine treatment of non-toxic multinodular goitre: effects of combination with lithium. *Eur J Nucl Med Mol Imaging* 2005; **32**: 1081–8.
3. Kokuho T, Kuji T, Yasuda G, Umemura S. Thyroid storm-induced multiple organ failure relieved quickly by plasma exchange therapy. *Ther Apher Dial* 2004; **8**: 347–9.

4 Petry J, Van Schil PEY, Abrams P, Jorens PG. Plasmapheresis as effective treatment for thyrotoxic storm after sleeve pneumonectomy. *Ann Thorac Surg* 2004; **77**: 1839–41.

5 Benvenga S, Lapa D, Cannavo S, Trimarchi F. Successive thyroid storms treated with L-carnitine and low doses of methimazole. *Am J Med* 2003; **115**: 417–18.

6 Benvenga S, Amato A, Calvani M, Trimarchi F. Effects of carnitine on thyroid hormone action. *Ann N Y Acad Sci* 2004; **1003**: 158–67.

PROBLEM

10 Thyroid Eye Disease

Case History

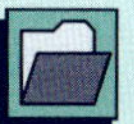

Mr AT, aged 53 years, seeks your advice. His wife has noticed that his right eye has become more prominent in recent months. He is generally well and has not noticed any visual disturbance. He smokes 20 cigarettes per day but does not take any medications. There are no symptoms of hyperthyroidism but his thyrotropin (thyroid-stimulating hormone [TSH]) level is suppressed and the free T_4 increased modestly at 27 pmol/l (normal 12–25 pmol/l).

Outline how you would carry out Mr AT's initial assessment?

What general advice would you give him?

Should he have antithyroid drugs or any other treatment?

Would you consider referring him for surgical management?

Background

Thyroid eye disease (TED) affects around 20% of Graves' patients. It is of variable severity and its onset may be before or after onset of thyroid dysfunction. It may occur in isolation, and in association with other autoimmune diseases, particularly Hashimoto's thyroiditis. It can be unilateral. The active phase generally lasts about a year, and most cases are burnt out within 18 months. Recurrence occurs in only 5% of cases. Its aetiology, clinical features and management have been reviewed recently.[1,2]

TED is regarded as an autoimmune disease on the grounds of histological features, association with the active phase of Graves' disease, and response to immunosuppressive therapy. The disease is probably initiated by immunological cross-reaction between antigens common to thyroid and orbital tissues. The immune response is both humoral and cellular. TSH receptor mRNA and protein is expressed in orbital fibroblasts and preadipocytes. These cell types in other locations also express TSH receptor, and it is not clear why the disease localizes only to the orbit (and skin in patients with Graves' dermopathy). TED is more likely to occur in patients with high levels of TSH receptor antibody. Other shared antigens include G2s, a 141 amino acid fragment of the transcription factor FOXP1, present in both thyroid and extraocular muscles. Anti-G2s is present in around 50% of patients with TED. Antibodies to Fp, formerly known as 64 kDa protein, are present in 30–60% of cases, and antibodies to collagen XIII have also been described recently. The pathogenesis of TED is summarized in Figure 10.1.

Clinical features are highly variable. The diagnosis is a clinical one. All patients should have thyroid function and autoantibody status checked. Measurement of degree of proptosis with an exophthalmometer is useful to document severity and progress. Patients should have visual acuity and visual fields documented. Magnetic resonance imaging (MRI) is preferred to computed tomography (CT) for imaging, both because of its higher resolution and also to protect the lens from the high doses of radiation associated with CT. Ultrasound and radiolabelled somatostatin analogue (Octreoscan) are useful in some cases, and the use of Doppler flow ultrasound to document the increased blood flow that accompanies orbital inflammation has been advocated by some. Males are relatively more predisposed, although the overall female:male ratio for TED is 4:1 compared with 10:1 for Graves' thyrotoxicosis. Males are at higher risk of optic neuropathy.

The NOSPECS classification is no longer considered precise enough for scientific studies but it remains useful as a mnemonic, and for teaching purposes:

- No eye signs.
- Only symptoms or signs: dry eyes, irritation, sensation of foreign body, excessive lacrimation, upper lid retraction, infrequent blinking, lid lag.
- Soft tissue involvement: periorbital oedema, conjunctival oedema, expansion of the lids, extrusion of orbital fat.
- Proptosis: exophthalmometry >22 mm, or >3 mm asymmetry. This is regarded as severe if greater than 28 mm.
- Extraocular muscle involvement: diplopia. Severity ranges from mild limitation at extremes of gaze to fixation of one or both globes. The disease affects inferior, medial, superior and lateral rectus muscle in that order with differing frequency.
- Corneal involvement: corneal stippling, ulceration, cloudiness, necrosis and perforation.
- Sight threatening: this is due to compressive optic neuropathy, and an indication for urgent referral to an ophthalmologist.

Treatment

A Local measures

- Artificial tears to moisten the cornea.
- Moisture shields fitted to the temporal side of spectacles to minimize tear evaporation.
- Punctal plugs to expand the volume of the lacrimal lake.
- Topical antibiotics if there is evidence of infection due to corneal exposure.

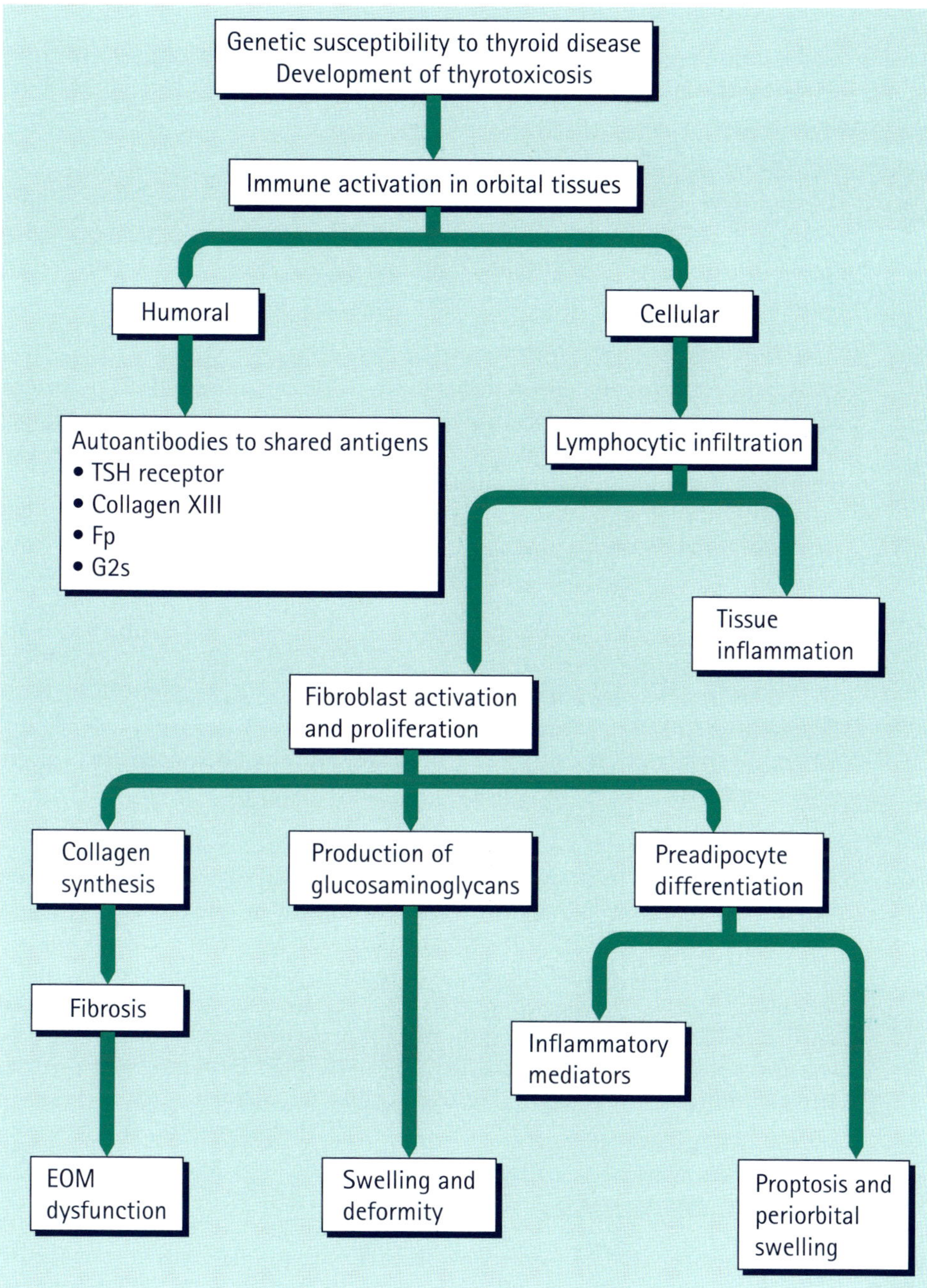

Fig. 10.1 Pathogenesis of thyroid eye disease. EOM = extraocular muscle.

B Stop smoking

TED is around seven times more likely to occur in smokers. Smoking may produce local hypoxia and can stimulate production of glycosaminoglycans. Smoking also diminishes the response to immunosuppressive treatment and radiotherapy. Stopping smoking decreases the risk of developing TED.

C Treat thyroid dysfunction

It is not clear whether the temporal relationship between thyroid dysfunction and the appearance of TED is purely due to immunological factors, or whether thyroid hormone status also plays a part.

D Immunosuppressive treatment

There has been no large randomized study with corticosteroids, but they are clearly effective in patients with marked periorbital inflammation and in optic neuropathy. They are of limited use in treating proptosis and extraocular muscle involvement. Intravenous methylprednisolone is probably more effective than oral prednisolone, and is the treatment of choice for patients with acute and severe disease. Ciclosporin, azathioprine and cyclophosphamide are also useful.

E Orbital radiotherapy

This has been controversial until recently but, with recent trial results, it is thought to be useful in patients with severe disease, particularly if used with corticosteroids A total dose of 20 Gy is generally used delivered in fractions over 2 weeks. There is increased risk of cataract – up to 12% on long-term follow-up – and the treatment is usually reserved for patients over 40 years. It may cause retinopathy and should only be used with caution in patients with diabetes. There is also a slightly increased risk of malignancy.

F Surgery

Tarsorrhaphy is the most commonly carried out surgical procedure and is mainly carried out for cosmetic reasons or to decrease risk of problems with corneal exposure. This, and eye muscle surgery to correct strabismus, are seldom carried out in the acute phase. The ultimate results are much more predictable when TED is no longer active. Botulinum toxin has been used for short-term treatment until definitive surgery is indicated. Orbital decompression is indicated for optic neuropathy, orbital subluxation and severe exophthalmos. This is now usually performed by removal of one of the four orbital walls rather than removal of retro-orbital fat. There is a risk of extraocular nerve palsy.

Recent Developments

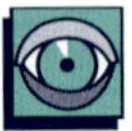

1. Boschi *et al.*[3] studied expression of TSH receptor antibody in extraocular muscle biopsies of patients with TED compared with non-thyroid patients undergoing surgery for strabismus. All of the biopsies from TED patients expressed TSH receptor and none of the control biopsies did so.

2. The critical role of increased adipose tissue in TED has been confirmed in a recently published study: orbital tissue from TED patients being treated by orbital decompression was studied using microarrays to investigate gene expression. There was increased

expression of adipocyte immediate early genes including the cysteine-rich angiogenic factor-61 (*CYR61*) and of the adipocyte marker stearoyl CoA desaturase.[4]

3 In a trial comparing intravenous methylprednisolone with oral prednisolone, Kahaly *et al.*[5] demonstrated that intravenous therapy was superior. Patients were followed up for 6 months. The response rate was 77% for IV therapy and 51% for oral therapy ($P > 0.01$). Patients treated with methylprednisolone had improved disease activity and severity, better quality of life, and less need for other interventions.

4 Somatostatin inhibits lymphocyte proliferation and activation, and accumulates in orbital tissues of patients with TED. In a 16-week trial[6] of the long-acting formulation of the somatostatin analogue octreotide (Octreotide-LAR), proptosis was significantly decreased. There were no changes in overall clinical activity score or measured extraocular muscle volume.

Conclusions

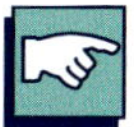

The patient should have thyroid function and thyroid antibodies (antithyroid peroxidase, anti-Tg, TSH receptor antibodies) measured. The imaging method of choice is MRI. This will help confirm the diagnosis, exclude other possible causes of his symptoms, and give an indication of the extent of disease. He should be advised to stop smoking, although the major documented effect of smoking on susceptibility to TED is in women. We would treat him with carbimazole to render him biochemically euthyroid, even though he does not have symptoms of thyrotoxicosis. Surgery is not indicated at this early stage in the absence of severe or sight-threatening features.

Further Reading

1 El-Kaissi S, Framan AG, Wall JR. Thyroid-associated ophthalmopathy: a practical guide to classification, natural history and management. *Intern Med J* 2004; **34**: 482–91.

2 Cawood T, Moriarty P, O'Shea D. Recent development in thyroid eye disease. *BMJ* 2004; **329**: 385–90.

3 Boschi A, Daumerie C, Spiritus M, *et al.* Quantification of cells expressing the thyrotropin receptor in extraocular muscles in thyroid associated orbitopathy. *Br J Ophthalmol* 2005; **89**: 724–9.

4 Lantz M, Vondrichova T, Parikh H, *et al.* Overexpression of immediate early genes in active Graves' ophthalmopathy. *J Clin Endocrinol Metab* 2005; **70**: 4784–91.

5 Kahaly GJ, Pitz S, Hommel G, Dittmar M. Randomized, single blind trial of intravenous versus oral steroid monotherapy in Graves' orbitopathy. *J Clin Endocrinol Metab* 2005; **90**: 5234–40.

6 Wémeau JL, Caron P, Beckers A, *et al.* Octreotide (long-acting release formulation) treatment in patients with Graves' orbitopathy: clinical results of a four-month, randomized, placebo-controlled, double-blind study. *J Clin Endocrinol Metab* 2005; **90**: 841–8.

SECTION TWO **02**

Adrenal

PROBLEM

11 Addison's Disease

Case History

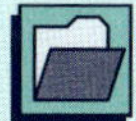

A 38-year-old Caucasian man complains of fatigue and light-headedness over the past 6 months. He has lost weight and is experiencing intermittent abdominal pain. On examination, his blood pressure is low at 100/80 mmHg, and he is generally pigmented. He has a cousin with insulin-dependent diabetes mellitus.

How should he be managed initially?

What is the differential diagnosis and likely cause of his adrenal failure?

How would you establish the diagnosis?

What management and follow-up would you initiate?

Background

Primary adrenal insufficiency arises because of destruction or inadequate function of the adrenal cortex. It affects between 110 and 140 people per million in developed countries, and females are more commonly affected. Over 90% of the cortex needs to be lost before symptoms of adrenal failure develop. Hypopituitarism causing secondary adrenal failure leads to

Table 11.1 Circulating concentrations and rates of production of adrenal steroids

Hormone	Production/day (g)	Production/day (mol)	Plasma concentration
Cortisol	15–30 mg	40–80 μmol	200–500 nmol/l
Aldosterone	70–180 μg	200–500 nmol	0–440 pmol/l (recumbent) 110–900 pmol/l (ambulant)
DHEAS	3.5–20 mg	10–60 μmol	3–12 μmol/l (male) 1–10 μmol/l (female)

DHEAS = dehydro-3-epiandrosterone sulphate.

similar symptoms but mineralocorticoid function is spared. Steroid hormones are synthesized in the three layers of the adrenal cortex—zona glomerulosa (mineralocorticoids), zona fasciculata and zona reticularis (glucocorticoids and androgens). Plasma levels and daily production rates are shown in Table 11.1. Glucocorticoid and mineralocorticoid are routinely replaced in patients with adrenal failure. The role of androgen replacement remains controversial but is beneficial in some cases.

In 80–90% of cases the cause is autoimmune destruction of the cortex. Tuberculosis is the second commonest aetiology and accounts for a greater proportion of cases in developing countries. In autoimmune adrenal failure, the endocrine cells of the adrenal cortex are destroyed predominantly by autoreactive T cells. There is also a humoral immune component, and circulating anti-adrenal antibodies are a useful marker for immune-mediated Addison's disease. Anti-adrenal antibodies, detected by immunofluorescence, are present in about 80% of patients at diagnosis, declining gradually to around 10% at 15 years after diagnosis. The antibodies are mainly directed at the enzyme steroid 21-hydroxylase. Using sensitive immunoassays for these antibodies, nearly all patients with autoimmune adrenal failure are positive at diagnosis, and 60% are still positive 15 years after diagnosis. Up to 5% of patients with associated autoimmune disease including thyroid disease and type 1 diabetes are also positive for the antibodies, although only a relatively small proportion may develop Addison's disease. The immunogenetics of Addison's disease and autoimmune polyendocrine deficiency syndromes (APS) is discussed in Chapter 12. Figure 11.1 is a diagnostic algorithm for differential diagnosis of adrenal failure. No specific diagnosis is made in up to 10% of patients with primary adrenal insufficiency. Several genetic syndromes causing adrenal failure have been better characterized in recent years:

- X-linked adrenoleukodystrophy is a peroxisomal disorder associated with a defect in an ATP-binding cassette protein leading to decreased metabolism, and increased accumulation of very long chain fatty acids. It is the commonest genetic cause of adrenal failure, accounting for up to 30% of cases in young males.
- X-linked adrenal hypoplasia congenita is due to a defect in the *DAX-1* transcription factor gene, and is frequently associated with other genetic abnormalities, including hypogonadotropic hypogonadism.

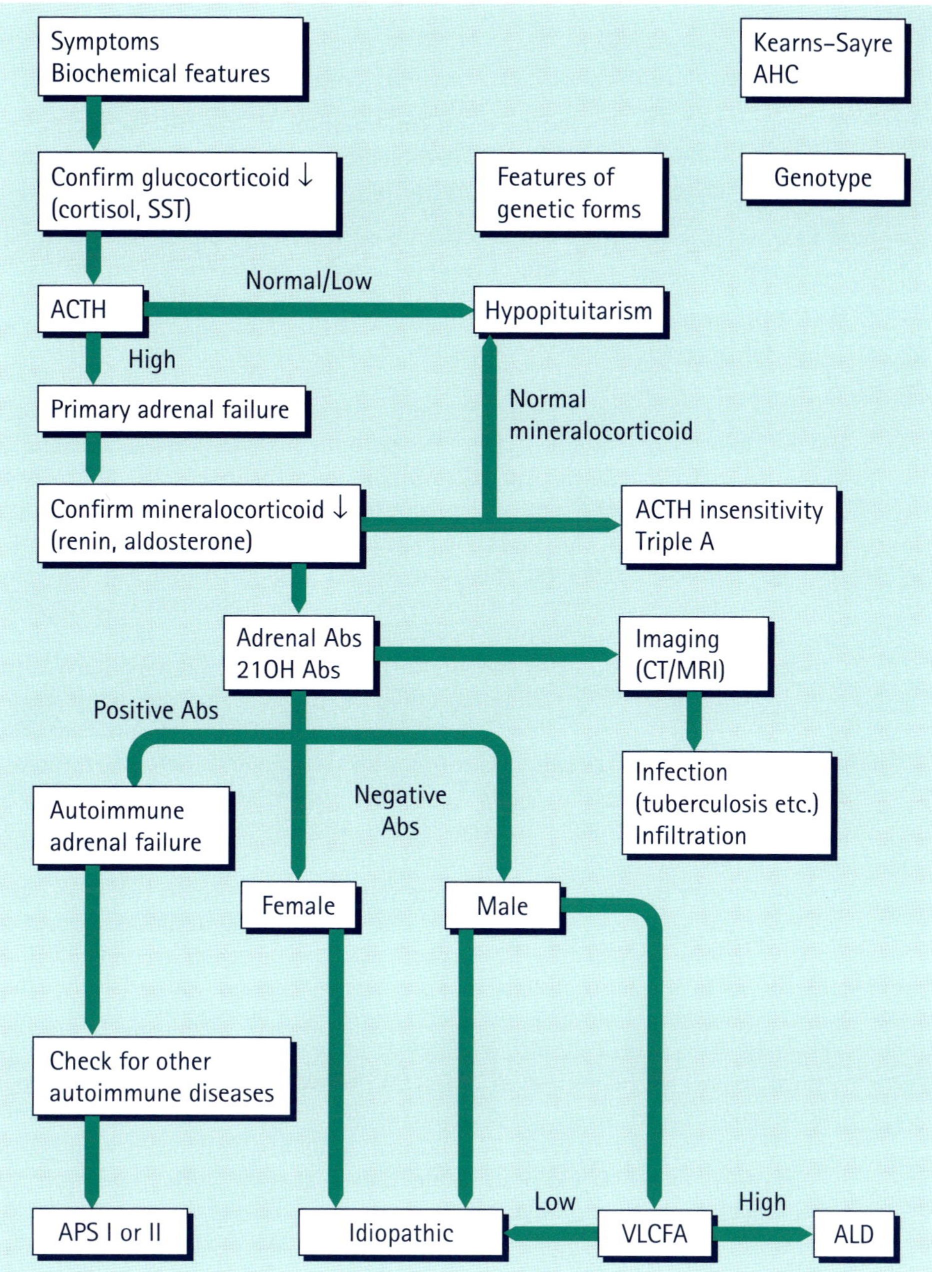

Fig. 11.1 Differential diagnosis of adrenal failure. Abs = antibodies; ACTH = adrenocorticotrophic hormone; AHC = adrenal hypoplasia congenita; ALD = adrenoleukodystrophy; APS = autoimmune polyendocrine deficiency syndromes (type I and II); CT = computed tomography; MRI = magnetic resonance imaging; VLCFA = very low chain fatty acids. Patients who are adrenal or 21-hydroxylase antibody negative on one occasion should have the measurement repeated on a second occasion before autoimmune disease can be excluded.

- Familial glucocorticoid deficiency is usually due to mutations in the gene for the adrenocorticotrophic hormone (ACTH) receptor leading to agenesis of the zona fasciculata and zona reticularis. It is inherited as autosomal recessive.
- Triple A (Allgrove's) syndrome is a combination of Adrenal insufficiency, Alacrima and Achalasia, along with various neurological deficits. Adrenal failure is due to ACTH insensitivity, and the mineralocorticoid axis is preserved.
- Kearns–Sayre syndrome due to deletion of mitochondrial DNA leads to pigmentary retinopathy, ocular myopathy, heart block, ataxia, and adrenal failure.
- IMAGe syndrome is a clinical clustering of Intrauterine growth retardation, Metaphyseal dysplasia, Adrenal hypoplasia, and Gonadal changes.

Symptoms of adrenal failure include chronic and progressive fatigue, postural hypotension, muscle weakness, loss of appetite and weight loss, nausea and vomiting, abdominal pain, diarrhoea, and skin pigmentation (primary adrenal failure). Onset is often insidious, and the diagnosis may not be made until the patient has impending or actual adrenal crisis. At this stage, the patient may be severely dehydrated and shocked, with hyponatraemia, hyperkalaemia, acidosis and hypoglycaemia. The immediate priorities are to restore plasma volume, correct electrolyte abnormalities, maintain blood glucose and to administer adequate doses of corticosteroid.

Adrenal crisis can occur in patients with undiagnosed adrenal failure or in patients with diagnosed disease who either omit their treatment or develop an intercurrent illness or stressful event. Normal saline is the mainstay of fluid resuscitation. Hypertonic saline should not be required as patients are both fluid and water depleted. In severely hypotensive and dehydrated patients, up to 1 l (10–20 ml/kg) may be given in the first hour, with the remainder over the next 24 hours. For an adult, typical fluid deficit would be 3–5 l. Blood pressure, urine output and jugular venous pressure should be monitored. A central venous line may be useful if the patient is very ill or at particular risk from over-replacement of fluid. Dextrose may be required to maintain blood glucose, which should be carefully monitored. Dextrose 10% is preferable to avoid water overload. Hydrocortisone is given 25–75 mg stat in children and 100–150 mg in adults followed by the same dose six hourly (intravenous) until circulation is restored and the patient is eating and drinking. At this stage, the patient should be commenced on oral hydrocortisone at three times the normal maintenance dose, as well as oral fludrocortisone (if they are judged to be mineralocorticoid deficient). Hyperkalaemia usually corrects itself with fluid and steroid replacement, but plasma levels and electrocardiogram should be carefully monitored.

If possible, blood should be withdrawn for a random cortisol measurement before replacement therapy is initiated. It is also helpful to carry out a short Synacthen test (SST) at baseline, if time and situation permit. Where hydrocortisone has been commenced, cortisol and SST can be measured after 24 hours of withdrawal if the period of replacement has been short. The standard SST uses 250 μg of synthetic ACTH given intramuscularly or intravenously. Blood is withdrawn for cortisol measurement at baseline and after 30 minutes. Cortisol should increase by 200 nmol/l or to greater than 520 nmol/l. Adrenal antibodies (particularly when an anti-21-hydroxylase immunoassay is used) are highly specific but, in an asymptomatic patient, may not always indicate that the patient will progress to adrenal failure. ACTH should be measured in all cases, and high levels are indicative of primary adrenal failure. When secondary adrenal failure seems possible, a long Synacthen test is indicated. Mineralocorticoid status is checked by measuring renin and aldosterone after overnight recumbency, and then following 30 minutes of being ambulant. Thyroid-stimulating hormone may be increased in patients with adrenal crisis, and initiation of thyroxine therapy in a hypothyroid patient may unmask latent adrenal failure.

Recent Developments

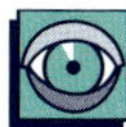

1. Prolonged duration of adrenal replacement therapy, mental problems, and sex steroid deficiency appear to be risk factors for adrenal crisis.[1] The relative risk with sex steroid deficiency was 3.7 (95% confidence interval 1.71 to 7.98), and the risk was decreased in those who had sex steroid replacement in Omori *et al.*'s study.[1]
2. Although autoimmune disease remains by far the commonest cause of adrenal failure in patients diagnosed in adult life, the range of diagnoses in younger patients (particularly males) is broader.[2] For those diagnosed in childhood autoimmune disease is the commonest cause in females, but genetic causes (adrenoleukodystrophy and congenital hypoplasia) are more common in males.
3. The molecular basis for adrenal gland differentiation, and thus of the rarer genetic forms of adrenal insufficiency, is now quite well understood.[3] The transcription factor WT-1 is responsible for development of the lineage that gives rise to adrenal, gonadal and renal cells. Congenital adrenal hypoplasia is usually caused by mutations in the *DAX-1* gene, although cases due to *SF-1* mutations are also described.
4. Tuberculosis can affect a variety of endocrine glands, but adrenal involvement is the commonest.[4] The mechanism of tuberculosis-induced adrenal destruction is complex, and includes a shift towards a T helper 2 immune response. Paradoxically, this change in immune response may be mediated by the high levels of cortisol and the decreased levels of DHEAS that accompany active mycobacterium infection.

Conclusions

A precise diagnosis should be established in all cases of suspected adrenal failure. Once investigations are complete, maintenance glucocorticoid and mineralocorticoid therapy should be initiated and reviewed at regular intervals. The patient should always carry identification—a bracelet or necklace with information regarding the diagnosis and treatment. They should also carry contact details for their attending physician. The patient should be aware that they should never stop their medication, that they should seek advice promptly if they are unable to take the medication or if they are vomiting persistently. Intercurrent illness or surgical procedures should be covered with increased doses of steroid. For minor illnesses or procedures, doubling the dose of hydrocortisone is sufficient. For major surgery, they should be covered with hydrocortisone 100 mg intravenously every six hours, preferably beginning the night before surgery. Patients travelling to areas with less well-developed medical services should know that 100 mg hydrocortisone can be given intramuscularly or intravenously in an emergency, and it may be useful for them to carry a vial of hydrocortisone with them. When patients are covered with higher doses of hydrocortisone, there is no need for them to increase mineralocorticoid replacement.

Further Reading

1 Omori K, Nomura K, Shimizu S, Omori N, Takano K. Risk factors for adrenal crisis in patients with adrenal insufficiency. *Endocrine J* 2003; **50**: 745–52.

2 Simm PJ, McDonnell CM, Zacharin MR. Primary adrenal insufficiency in childhood and adolescence: advances in diagnosis and management. *J Paediatr Child Health* 2004; **40**: 596–9.

3 Fujieda K, Tajima T. Molecular basis of adrenal insufficiency. *Pediatr Res* 2005; **57**: 62R–69R.

4 Kelestimur F. The endocrinology of adrenal tuberculosis: the effects of tuberculosis on the hypothalamo-pituitary-adrenal axis and adrenocortical function. *J Endocrinol Invest* 2004; **27**: 380–6.

PROBLEM

12 Autoimmune Polyglandular Syndromes

Case History

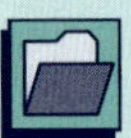

DS is a 23-year-old student with a strong family history of thyroid disease and diabetes. She developed type 1 diabetes at the age of 8 years, and Addison's disease at the age of 12. She is treated with insulin and steroid replacement (glucocorticoid and mineralocorticoid). She has married recently and consults you asking about risks of pregnancy and whether her children are likely to develop endocrine disease.

What kinds of polyendocrine deficiency syndrome are there?

How are they inherited?

How would you plan the follow-up and management of this patient?

Background

The existence of at least two distinct autoimmune polyglandular syndromes (APS) was first proposed in the 1980s. The distinct features of these syndromes are now well recognized, and a great deal is known about their clinical presentation and immunogenetics.[1,2]

The association of Addison's disease and autoimmune thyroid disease (Schmidt's syndrome) has been long recognized, as has the association between Addison's and type 1 diabetes (Carpenter's syndrome). The most frequently associated autoimmune endocrine disorders are type 1 diabetes and thyroid disease, accounting for nearly 50% of cases where multiple disorders are present.

- *APS I (autoimmune polyendocrinopathy-candidiasis-ectodermal dystrophy, APECED).* At least two of the following must be present: chronic mucocutaneous candidiasis; hypoparathyroidism; Addison's disease. Candidiasis usually appears before the age of 5, hypoparathyroidism before the age of 10, and Addison's before the age of 15. APECED may also be associated with autoimmune thyroiditis or Graves' disease, pernicious anaemia, hypogonadism, coeliac disease, and chronic active hepatitis. The ectodermal features that are variably associated include pitted nail dystrophy, alopecia, hypoplasia of the dental enamel, calcification of the tympanic membranes, and vitiligo.
- *APS II.* In this condition, the following are associated: Addison's disease; type 1 diabetes; autoimmune thyroid disease. Pernicious anaemia and vitiligo may occur. Gonadal failure and vitiligo are not found as commonly as in APS I.
- *APS III.* This is the association of autoimmune endocrine diseases as for APS II, but without Addison's disease.
- *APS IV.* This has been defined as the coexistence of Addison's disease and at least one other autoimmune disease, but not conforming to any of the above patterns.

In the recent large Italian series of patients with Addison's disease,[3] 83% overall were thought to be of autoimmune origin. APS I was present in 13% of the autoimmune cases, APS II in 41%, APS III in 5%, and isolated Addison's disease was present in 41%.

APS I is an autosomal recessive condition caused by a mutation of the autoimmune regulator (*AIRE*) gene at chromosome 21q21.3. Although it is autosomal recessive, patients have been described with mutations at only one allele. It remains possible that such cases have, as yet unidentified, mutations on the other allele. Some populations have particularly high prevalence of APS I—the prevalence is 1:25 000 in Finland due to the frequency of the R257X mutation, 1:14 500 in Sardinians due to the frequent occurrence of the R139X mutation, and 1:9000 in Iranian Jews because of the Y85C mutation. Higher frequencies of APS I have also been reported in Sweden and in northern Italy. APS I is slightly more predominant in females. The nature of the *AIRE* mutation does not appear to determine the pattern of disease. However, human leucocyte antigen (HLA) genotype does, to an extent, regulate the phenotype as in non-APS patients.

APS II is more common, occurring in up to 1:20 000 of population and tends to have its onset later in life. The female to male ratio is 3:1, and inheritance is autosomal dominant. It is a polygenic disorder, with contribution from the HLA locus, and from other disease susceptibility loci. The disorder has been linked strongly with the HLA-A1, B8, DR3, DQ2 haplotype. The DRB1*0404 genotype is associated with increased progression to Addison's disease among patients with diabetes, whereas the DRB1*0401 and DRB1*0402 subtypes appear to protect, even in individuals who are positive for 21-hydroxylase antibodies. The gene for cytotoxic T lymphocyte antigen-4 (*CTLA-4*) is an important susceptibility locus for autoimmune endocrine disease, including Addison's disease.

Table 12.1 Investigation in patients with autoimmune polyglandular syndromes

Endocrine/metabolic test	Autoantibody
T_3, T_4, TSH	TPO, thyroglobulin TSH receptor antibody
Fasting/random glucose, oGTT, HbA1c	GAD65, IA-2, insulin, islet cell
Cortisol, SST, aldosterone and renin	Steroid cell antibodies, 21-hydroxylase, SCC
Small intestinal biopsy	Transglutaminase, gliadin
Liver tests	Smooth muscle, Tryptophan hydroxylase
Elevated gonadotropins	Steroid cell antibodies, SCC
Macrocytic anaemia Vitamin B_{12}	Parietal cell antibodies, IF Anti H^+-K^+-ATPase
Genetic tests	
HLA typing	
AIRE genotyping	

HLA typing has little potential, at present, to influence clinical decision making and its routine use is not warranted. GAD = glutamic acid decarboxylase; IF = intrinsic factor; oGTT = oral glucose tolerance test; SCC = side chain cleavage; SST = short Synacthen test; TPO = thyroid peroxidase; TSH = thyrotropin.

Investigation of the patient depends on clinical presentation, age and other clinical features. Possible investigations are summarized in Table 12.1.

Recent Developments

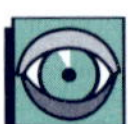

1 Soderbergh and colleagues[4] measured ten different antibody subtypes in a series of patients with APS I. Antibodies against side chain cleavage enzyme (SCC) provided the most specific marker for adrenal failure. Antibodies against tryptophan hydroxylase were markers for intestinal dysfunction and autoimmune hepatitis. The range of autoimmune markers now available is useful in research studies, but there is presently no justification for their routine use in clinical practice.

2 About 8% of the human genome consists of elements that were probably derived from retroviruses. The retrovirus-like long terminal repeat DQ-LTR13, located close to the *DQB1* gene has been linked with susceptibility to autoimmune diseases. A recent study[5] suggests that this association is simply due to linkage disequilibrium with DQB1 and DRB1 susceptibility genotypes.

3 Increased understanding of how the *AIRE* gene product functions is leading to a better understanding of the pathogenesis of autoimmune endocrinopathy syndromes and may lead to improved genotyping tests to quantify risks in patients.[6] Manipulating *AIRE* activity, perhaps genetically, is a possible strategy for future prevention of the development of multiple autoimmune disease.

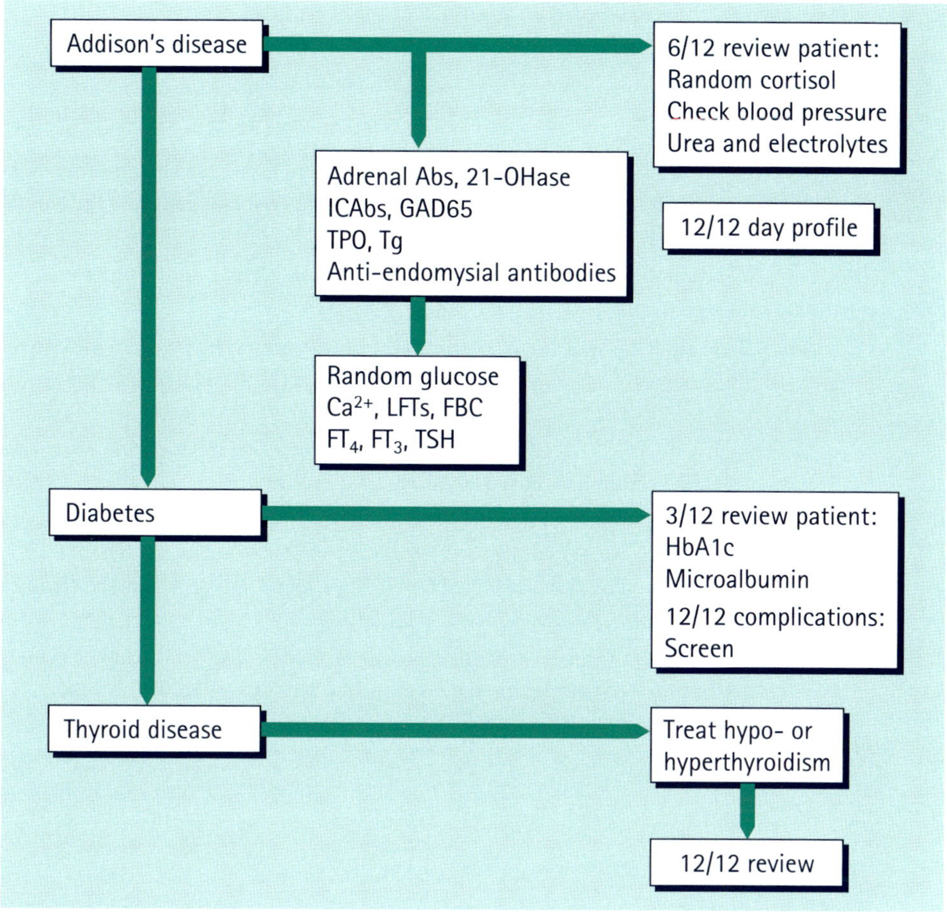

Addison's disease

6/12 review patient:
Random cortisol
Check blood pressure
Urea and electrolytes

Adrenal Abs, 21-OHase
ICAbs, GAD65
TPO, Tg
Anti-endomysial antibodies

12/12 day profile

Random glucose
Ca^{2+}, LFTs, FBC
FT_4, FT_3, TSH

Diabetes

3/12 review patient:
HbA1c
Microalbumin
12/12 complications:
Screen

Thyroid disease

Treat hypo- or
hyperthyroidism

12/12 review

Fig. 12.1 Monitoring and follow-up of a patient with autoimmune polyglandular syndromes. Annual screening for thyroid disease is important in all patients with either type 1 diabetes or Addison's disease. Coeliac disease is also a common accompaniment but often overlooked. 21-OHase = antibodies to 21-hydroxylase; FBC = full blood count; ICAbs = islet cell antibodies; LFTs = liver function tests; Tg = antibodies to thyroglobulin; TPO = thyroid peroxidase; TSH = thyrotropin (thyroid-stimulating hormone).

Conclusions

The recognition that autoimmune endocrine diseases are not associated in a random fashion, but that distinct genetic syndromes exist, and the sequence of developing conditions is somewhat predictable, greatly assist in planning follow-up and management. A suggested schema for this is shown in Figure 12.1. The above patient probably has APS II. Genotyping would be useful if she were thought to have APS I but there is currently no clinically useful genetic test to predict whether her child would be at risk of developing autoimmune disease. There is certainly an increased risk that the offspring of this patient will develop type 1 diabetes, autoimmune thyroid disease or adrenal failure. She should be monitored closely during pregnancy. There are probably no substantial risks beyond those associated with her diabetes, which should be tightly controlled prior to pregnancy. She will need increased steroid cover for labour.

Further Reading

1 Betterle C, Dal Pra C, Mantero F, Zanchetta R. Autoimmune adrenal insufficiency and autoimmune polyendocrine syndromes: autoantibodies, autoantigens, and their applicability in diagnosis and disease prediction. *Endocr Rev* 2002; **23**: 327–64.

2 Dittmar M, Kahaly GJ. Polyglandular autoimmune syndromes: immunogenetics and long-term follow-up. *J Clin Endocrinol Metab* 2003; **88**: 2983–92.

3 Buzi F, Badolato R, Mazza C, *et al.* Autoimmune polyendocrinopathy-candidiasis-ectodermal dystrophy syndrome: time to review diagnostic criteria? *J Clin Endocrinol Metab* 2003; **88**: 3146–8.

4 Soderbergh A, Myhre AG, Ekwall O, *et al.* Prevalence and clinical association of 10 defined autoantibodies in autoimmune polyendocrine syndrome type 1. *J Clin Endocrinol Metab* 2004; **89**: 557–62.

5 Gambelunghe G, Kockum I, Bini V, *et al*; Umbria Type 1 Diabetes Registry; Italian Addison Network. Retrovirus-like long-terminal repeat DQ-LTR-13 and genetic susceptibility to type 1 diabetes and Addison's disease. *Diabetes* 2005; **54**: 900–5.

6 Liston A, Gray DHD, Lesage S, *et al.* Gene dosage-limiting role of *Aire* in thymic expression, clonal deletion, and organ-specific autoimmunity. *J Exp Med* 2004; **200**: 1015–26.

PROBLEM

13 The Incidental Adrenal Nodule

Case History

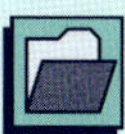

A 56-year-old woman with mild hypertension is investigated for episodes of abdominal pain. Her tests include an abdominal computed tomography (CT) scan on which a 2 cm nodule on the left adrenal gland is described. She is treated with lisinopril 10 mg per day and bendrofluazide 2.5 mg per day for her hypertension.

How should she be investigated further?

Are further imaging studies of the adrenal indicated?

Does she require surgery to remove the nodule from her left adrenal?

What follow-up should she have?

Background

Asymptomatic masses in the adrenal glands are now commonly detected on CT or magnetic resonance imaging (MRI) of the abdomen.[1,2] Most are innocent, but a significant proportion are either associated with hormonal disorders or malignancy. So-called 'incidentalomas' are found in up to 1% of abdominal scans, and are present in 5–10% of patients at post-mortem. They occur equally commonly in men and women. Incidental adrenal masses are commoner than abnormalities of adrenal function and now represent the commonest adrenal abnormality referred to endocrinologists for investigation. The prevalence rises from around 1% in young adults to 7% in the 70–80-year age group. The likelihood of malignancy also increases with age.

A differential diagnosis is presented in Table 13.1. The majority are benign and non-functioning. Together, functioning tumours (Cushing's, Conn's and virilizing tumours) account for only around 10% of cases. The adrenal is a very vascular organ, and therefore a common site for metastatic tumour (breast, bronchus, melanoma, lymphoma, etc.). Metastases are often bilateral and rarely can destroy enough adrenal tissue to cause adrenal failure, although patients often succumb to the underlying malignancy before they develop symptoms of steroid insufficiency. An adrenal incidentaloma in a patient with a previous history of malignant disease will prove to be malignant in up to 40% of cases. Adrenal carcinoma is a rare malignancy, with a prevalence of about 12 per million; 25% of adrenal tumours greater than 6 cm are malignant, compared with only 2% under 4 cm. Adrenal carcinomas may be functioning or non-functioning. Functioning tumours cause virilization or Cushing's syndrome (often with predominantly metabolic rather than

Table 13.1 Differential diagnosis of adrenal mass

Diagnosis	Per cent of cases
Non-functioning adenoma	60
Metastatic tumour	15
Functioning adenoma – cortisol producing	7
Functional adenoma – mineralocorticoid producing	3
Phaeochromocytoma	5
Adrenal carcinoma	5
Others (haemorrhage, cyst, myelolipoma)	5

somatic features) due to their rate of growth). Feminizing (oestrogen-producing) or aldosterone-producing malignant tumours are rare. Adrenal carcinoma has a poor prognosis with a mean survival of only 18 months with only 15% of patients still alive at 5 years. Myelolipoma is an unusual, benign lesion which contains fat, along with myeloid and erythroid components. It is generally found in the adrenal but may occur in the perinephric area outside the adrenal gland.

Incidental adrenal tumours may be detected by ultrasound, particularly if they affect the right adrenal. More commonly, however, they are picked up on CT or MRI—both these techniques have approximately equal sensitivity. Large tumours or irregularly shaped tumours are more likely to be malignant. High signal intensity on CT scanning (greater than 10–20 Hounsfield Units [HU]) is more likely with malignant lesions. Adenomas are typically lipid rich, and therefore of lower intensity. Delayed enhanced CT can also be of use since adenomas characteristically have a rapid washout of contrast because of their rich blood supply. Phaeochromocytomas show up as hyperintense lesions on T2-weighted MRI scanning. A diagnostic algorithm is presented in Figure 13.1. As with all tumours in endocrine glands, it is preferable to establish whether a state of hormone hypersecretion is present before proceeding to functional imaging. Clinical evidence of a high cortisol state should be sought, as should evidence of virilization or feminization. Hypertension, particularly if accompanied by hypokalaemia could be indicative of a state of mineralocorticoid excess or severe glucocorticoid excess. Two separate tests for high cortisol production should be carried out (see below). Measurement of urinary metanephrines is now the test of choice in screening for a phaechromocytoma (95% sensitive and 95% specific), whereas urinary catecholamines or vanillylmandelic acid (VMA) measurements are less sensitive.

Functional adrenal imaging should be considered when a state of hyperfunction has been demonstrated or is highly suspected. ^{131}I-, or more commonly used now, ^{123}I-metaiodobenzylguandine (MIBG) is 85% sensitive and 95% specific for phaeochromocytomas. ^{111}Indium-labelled octreotide is less sensitive but may detect tumours that are MIBG negative. For functioning cortical tumours (Cushing's, Conn's and virilizing tumours), ^{131}I-6-beta-iodomethylnorcholesterol (NP-59) scanning is the method that has found the widest usage. As with other ^{131}I-containing radiopharmaceuticals, prior blockade

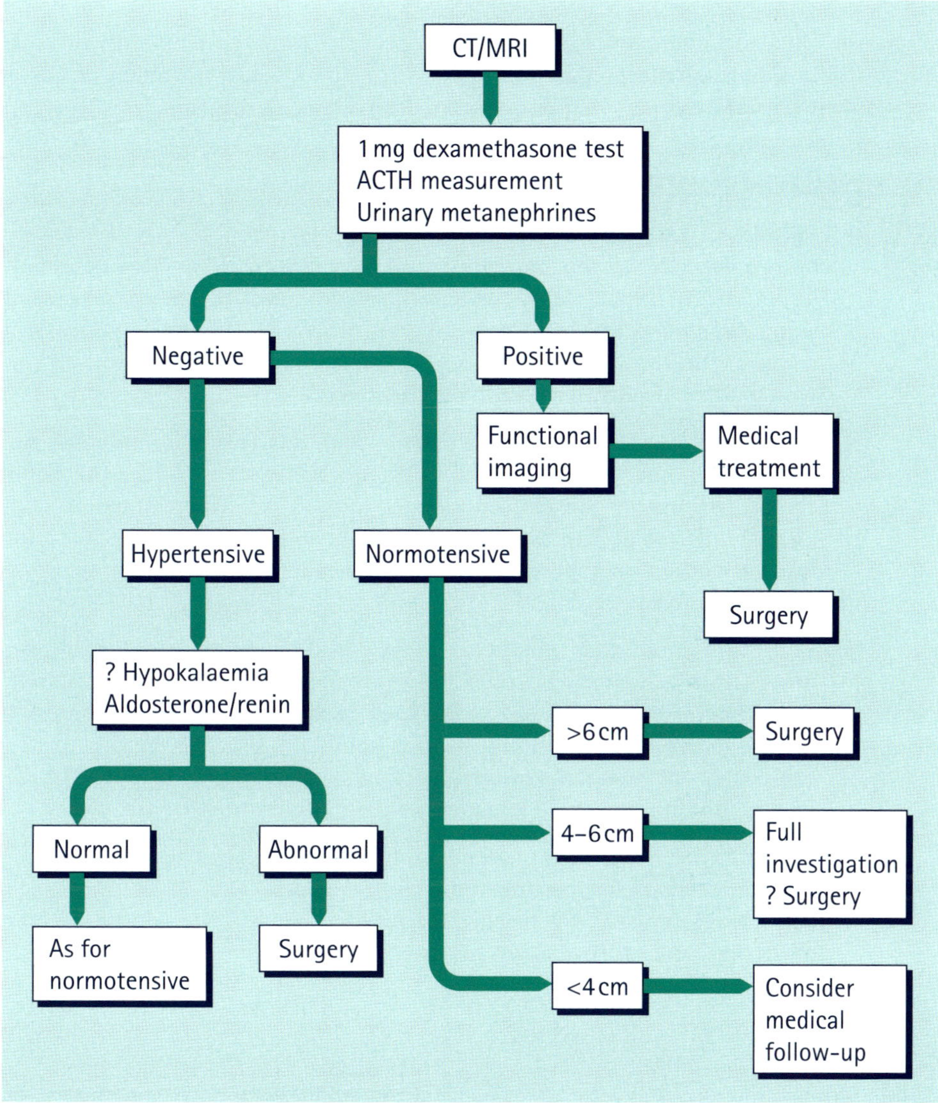

Fig. 13.1 Diagnosis and management of an adrenal mass. Two separate tests of hypothalamic–pituitary–adrenal function are indicated in all cases because of the relatively high prevalence of subclinical Cushing's in apparently non-functioning nodules. Functional imaging is carried out if a functioning tumour is suspected following biochemical investigation. ACTH = adrenocorticotrophic hormone.

of the thyroid with cold iodine is recommended. The sensitivity of NP-59 scanning is lower for lesions less than 3 cm. Single photon emission computed tomography (SPECT) with the above radiopharmaceuticals improves lesion definition. ^{11}C metomidate, an inhibitor of 11β-hydroxysteroid dehydrogenase, has been used to locate functioning cortical lesions.

In the past decade, development of laparoscopic surgery has revolutionized the management of adrenal nodules. Patients recover quicker, spend less time in hospital, and have less bleeding and wound infections and less pain than with laparotomy.

Laparoscopic surgery is generally not carried out for large lesions (greater than 8–10 cm) or where malignant disease is strongly suspected. Clearly, patients with phaeochromocytoma require careful preparation prior to surgery. Medical treatment of Cushing's syndrome prior to surgery may also shorten the overall recovery time.

Recent Developments

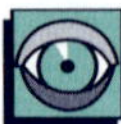

1 Subclinical autonomous glucocorticoid hypersecretion (SAGH) is a state of subtle, and sometimes variable, adrenocortical overactivity. It has been reported in up to 40% of adrenal incidentalomas and is associated with insulin resistance, hypertension, obesity and low bone mineral density. In a recent study,[3] increased midnight serum cortisol was a good marker for features of the metabolic syndrome in patients with incidentally discovered adrenal adenomas.

2 Reznik *et al.*[4] recently studied 21 patients with SAGH or autonomously functioning adrenal adenomas; 18/20 patients had cortisol increases in response to the vasopressin agonist terlipressin, and 17/20 responded to the 5-HT_4 receptor agonist cisapride. All 21 responded to at least one of eight stimuli, and 18 to multiple endocrine stimuli. Adrenal nodules may produce steroid hormones in response to a variety of neuroendocrine mediators.

3 In the future, molecular markers may help in differentiate functioning or malignant masses from benign and non-functioning masses.[1] Mutations of the tumour suppressor p53 or of the proliferation-associated protein ki67 can be present in malignant lesions. Increased insulin-like growth factor (IGF)-II or IGF-binding protein-2 gene expression may also be markers for lesions with high growth potential. Circulating chromogranin is increased in patients with phaeochromocytoma.

4 SPECT has been used to improve functional imaging of adrenal tumours. A recent study[5] has demonstrated that positron emission tomography with ^{18}F-fluorodeoxyglucose can detect malignant lesions with a high degree of accuracy. The resolution of this technique may prove to be a particular advantage.

Conclusions

When an incidental adrenal mass is discovered, further investigation to determine whether the mass is functioning and whether it might be malignant is indicated. Recent studies have demonstrated a high prevalence of subclinical hypercortisolism in lesions that might previously have been considered non-functioning. Multiple tests of adrenal function should be carried out and it may be that non-conventional stimuli such as vasopressin agonists or 5-HT_4 receptor agonists will be used in the near future. Surgery is definitely indicated for most lesions greater than 6 cm in diameter, as up to 25% will prove to be malignant. Most lesions less than 2 cm can be followed up medically, if they are not functioning and the patient is at low risk for malignancy. For lesions between 4 cm and 6 cm, the decision on surgery depends on the perceived risk that the mass is either functioning or malignant. The advent, and widespread use, of laparoscopic surgery has made surgical management less of a daunting option. For patients with small lesions who do not undergo surgery, follow-up should be undertaken at least every 6 months.

Further Reading

1 Nawar R, Aron D. Adrenal incidentaloma—a continuing management dilemma. *Endocr Relat Cancer* 2005; **12**: 585–98.

2 Dluhy RG, Maher MM, Wu C-L. Case 7—2005: a 59-year-old woman with an incidentally discovered adrenal nodule. *N Engl J Med* 2005; **352**: 1025–32.

3 Terzolo M, Bovio S, Pia A, *et al*. Midnight serum cortisol as a marker of increased cardiovascular risk in patients with a clinically inapparent adrenal adenoma. *Eur J Endocrinol* 2005; **153**: 307–15.

4 Reznik Y, Lefebvre H, Rohmer V, *et al*; REHOS study group. Aberrant adrenal sensitivity to multiple ligands in unilateral incidentaloma with subclinical autonomous cortisol hypersecretion: a prospective clinical study. *Clin Endocrinol* 2004; **61**: 311–19.

5 Tenenbaum F, Groussin L, Foehrenbach H, *et al*. 18F-fluorodeoxyglucose positron emission tomography as a diagnostic tool for malignancy of adrenocortical tumours? Preliminary results in 13 consecutive cases. *Eur J Endocrinol* 2004; **150**: 789–92.

PROBLEM

14 Cushing's Syndrome

Case History

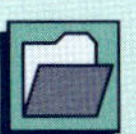

LB is a 40-year-old female schoolteacher. She has noticed weight gain, hirsutism and a tendency to bruise easily. These symptoms have been developing over the past 3 years. She has sought advice on a number of occasions and thinks, having researched her symptoms on the internet, that she may have Cushing's syndrome. A random serum cortisol is elevated at 700 nmol/l (normal 250–450 nmol/l).

How should she be investigated further?

At what stage should she be referred to hospital?

She would like to know what treatment she may require.

What is her prognosis?

Background

Investigation of a patient with suspected Cushing's syndrome frequently proves to be challenging. Furthermore, although sometimes difficult to diagnose, it is a condition that

Table 14.1 Differential diagnosis of Cushing's syndrome

		Per cent of cases
ACTH dependent	Pituitary adenoma	70
	Ectopic ACTH secretion	10
	Ectopic CRH secretion	<1
ACTH independent	Adrenal adenoma	10
	Adrenal carcinoma	8
	Macronodular hyperplasia	1
	Micronodular hyperplasia	<1

ACTH = adrenocorticotrophic hormone; CRH = corticotrophin-releasing hormone.

is often even more difficult to exclude. The first step is always to confirm that cortisol excess is present, and that cortisol production is not under normal control. This is easily done with the combination of urine free cortisol measurements, and an overnight dexamethasone suppression test (DST, with 1 mg dexamethasone). Further evaluation is indicated if the plasma cortisol fails to suppress below 50 nmol/l. In patients who are severely obese, depressed or have high alcohol intake plasma cortisol may fail to suppress adequately. The DST works on the principle that adrenocorticotrophic hormone (ACTH) production from a basophil adenoma will suppress with steroid but the threshold is higher than for normal pituitary tissue. Patients with ectopic ACTH or adrenal lesions show no change in ACTH levels. Cortisol suppression during a low-dose DST can occur, particularly if the Cushing's is cyclical.

Cushing's is relatively rare with an estimated incidence of 2–3 per million per year. It should be suspected in patients who present with bruising, round face, central obesity, hirsutism, proximal myopathy, striae, hypertension and glucose intolerance. The presentation is variable and it may take up to 5 years for patients to develop full-blown features of the syndrome. Patients with early-onset osteoporosis (age < 65 years) and with adrenal tumours should be screened. A differential diagnosis of Cushing's syndrome is presented in Table 14.1.

Once a state of cortisol excess is confirmed, and that it is ACTH dependent, the next investigations of choice are a prolonged DST and a corticotrophin-releasing hormone (CRH) test (Figure 14.1).[1] Performed together, these tests have virtually 100% sensitivity in detecting pituitary-driven Cushing's. Differences in test protocols, doses of dexamethasone, and the methods used to measure cortisol in different centres, along with the fact that no test performed alone even approaches 100% sensitivity and specificity, has given rise to uncertainty about which is the best test protocol. Care should be taken to distinguish between high-dose and prolonged DSTs. Some prefer to do the DST in a two-stage procedure where 1 mg dexamethasone is given to start with and then 8 mg is given on the following day or on a separate occasion. This protocol has the advantage of being shorter and lending itself to outpatient management. However, it has a sensitivity of only 68%, although it is virtually 100% specific, and there are inconsistencies between results of this test and the low-dose DST. Our preference is for a prolonged test where the patient is given 0.5 mg dexamethasone every 6 hours for 48 hours. This can be preceded by 48 hours of measuring diurnal cortisol and 24-hour urine free cortisol (UFC). Ectopic

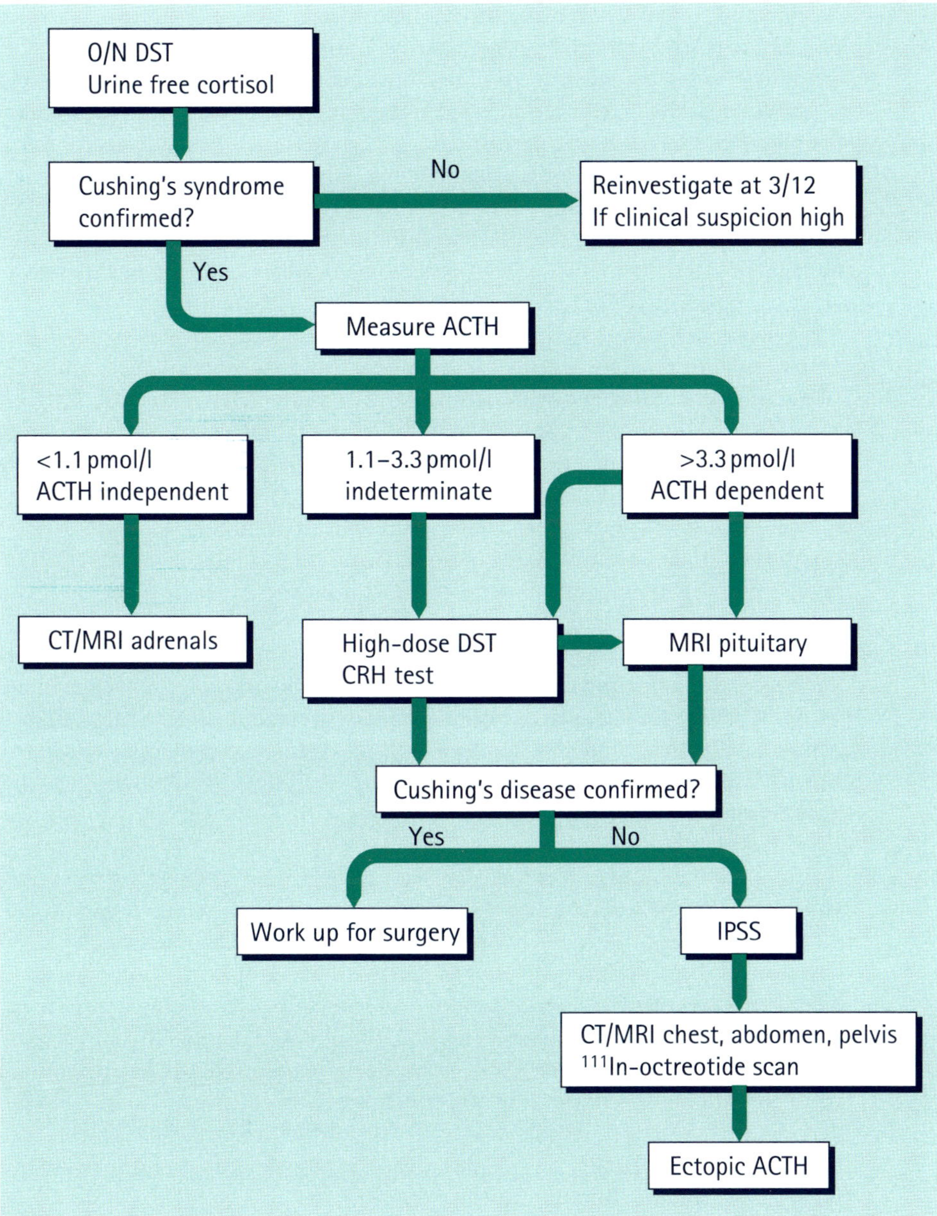

Fig. 14.1 Investigation of Cushing's syndrome. The first step is always to confirm the presence of cortisol excess, then to determine whether or not it is adrenocorticotrophic hormone (ACTH) dependent. In borderline cases, where there is a high index of suspicion, screening tests may have to be performed on multiple occasions. CRH = corticotrophin-releasing hormone; DST = dexamethasone suppression test; IPSS = inferior petrosal sinus sampling.

ACTH secretion most commonly comes from small cell lung tumour, pancreatic carcinoma, or from carcinoid tumours.

The CRH test formerly used ovine CRH but human CRH is now generally used (1 μg per kg or 100 μg is administered intravenously). The ACTH and cortisol is checked at baseline and for 60–75 minutes after. In Cushing's disease, ACTH increases by at least 35% and cortisol by at least 20%. Performed alone, the test has a sensitivity of between 70% and 90% for diagnosis of pituitary Cushing's. There is no response of either ACTH or cortisol in patients with ectopic ACTH secretion or Cushing's due to an adrenal lesion. The metyrapone test can be performed if there are difficulties with access to CRH, or in cases where there is diagnostic doubt. Metyrapone is an inhibitor of the enzyme 11β-hydroxylase. Administration of the drug leads to increased ACTH and cortisol precursors in patients with Cushing's disease. The desmopressin test is occasionally of use. The hormone, acting through its V_2 and V_3 receptors stimulates ACTH, and therefore cortisol, secretion in patients with Cushing's disease.

Magnetic resonance imaging (MRI) is the imaging method of choice for corticotroph adenomas. The lesions are hypodense and do not enhance, and MRI is only 70% sensitive. Lesions less than 6 mm may not be detected. A further difficulty is that up to 10% of the normal population have incidental pituitary adenomas, making it all the more important to be certain about the biochemical diagnosis before trying to interpret imaging studies and plan management. The technique of inferior petrosal sinus sampling (IPSS) is now widely available. It is highly accurate but technically demanding. It also carries risk of brain stem vascular damage, venous thrombosis pulmonary embolism and cranial nerve palsy. It is best used when there is proven ACTH-dependent Cushing's that may be due to ectopic ACTH secretion or where there is doubt whether a pituitary tumour is functioning. A ratio of central to peripheral ACTH in excess of 3.0 following CRH injection is diagnostic of basophil adenoma, and distinguishes Cushing's disease from other hypercortisolaemic states with a high degree of accuracy (sensitivity and specificity of 94%). Contrary to previous claims, it is unreliable in lateralizing tumour. Jugular venous sampling is safer and less technically demanding, but much less sensitive. Sampling from the cavernous sinus has also been advocated but carries high risk.

Transsphenoidal surgery is the treatment of choice for Cushing's disease, and leads to remission in 70–90% of cases. In cases with persistent or recurrent disease, repeat surgery leads to remission in 70%. Successful treatment is more likely with small tumours and if the lesion has been identified pre- or peri-operatively. Following successful removal there is a dramatic decrease in cortisol production and the patient requires careful weaning off steroid replacement as endogenous ACTH production recovers. This process can take up to 18 months, during which careful monitoring is required. Medical treatment may be useful in patients in preparation for surgery, or where surgery cannot be performed. Metyrapone has been the most commonly used drug. Ketoconazole is also widely used—this drug blocks the $P450_{SCC}$, 17,20 desmolase, 11β-hydroxylase, and the 17α-hydroxylase enzymes. Aminoglutethimide, mitotane, trilostane, and etomidate have all been used. Radiotherapy is useful in patients in whom surgery has failed or cannot be performed. The effect may be slow, necessitating interim medical therapy, and there is a high incidence of pituitary hormone deficiencies in the longer term.

Recent Developments

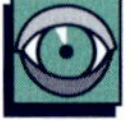

1 Silent corticotroph adenomas (SCA) are pituitary tumours that are not associated with clinical features of Cushing's disease, even though they are positive for ACTH on immunostaining.[2] Following surgery, up to a third of these tumours recur and up to a

fifth of patients with SCA go on to develop hypercortisolism. There is an argument for treating them with combined surgery and radiotherapy.

2 Although rare, nodular adrenal disease should be considered in the differential diagnosis of ACTH-independent Cushing's.[3] This disorder may be part of genetic syndromes including MEN type I, McCune–Albright syndrome, and the Carney complex. Cortisol secretion continues in the face of suppressed ACTH, and may be driven by other hormonal and neuroendocrine stimuli including vasopressin and gastric inhibitory polypeptide. The treatment of choice is surgical.

3 To date, long-term drug treatment of Cushing's has not been an option because of lack of complete effectiveness of drugs and the high incidence of side effects.[4] The drug RU-486 is a combined glucocorticoid, androgen and progesterone receptor blocker and has shown promise in preliminary studies. Other drugs of potential use in both decreasing ACTH secretion and inhibiting tumour growth are retinoic acid and peroxisome proliferator-activated receptor (PPAR)-γ agonists.

4 The recent review of 20 years' experience at the National Institutes of Health provides valuable information.[5] The authors confirmed the utility of IPSS for establishing the diagnosis. It is common to fail to localize the lesion initially, in which case the most likely diagnosis is pulmonary carcinoid. Survival rate is particularly poor in patients with small cell lung tumour, medullary thyroid carcinoma and gastrinoma.

5 Recovery following, even successful, treatment of Cushing's may take some time. Recently, quality of life has been assessed in series of patients with cured Cushing's.[6] Patients scored low on measures of fatigue, anxiety, depression, and other aspects of health and wellbeing. Development of hypopituitarism following treatment was a strong predictor of poor health. The duration of the illness prior to diagnosis, the need for surgery and the demands of follow-up may all be factors.

Conclusions

Investigation of suspected Cushing's syndrome should be carried out in stages. As Cushing's is relatively rare, we recommend that patients be referred at an early stage. The tests always need to be interpreted in the light of the clinical picture. There is, at present, no satisfactory medical treatment for the long-term treatment of Cushing's syndrome. The commonest diagnosis (70%) is Cushing's disease and the treatment of choice for this is surgery via a transsphenoidal route. Immediate re-operation is indicated for those who fail to respond immediately. With modern treatment and careful monitoring of the need for replacement hormones, the prognosis is very good, although many patients take up to 2 years to return to a normal, or near-normal, state of health.

Further Reading

1 Lindsay JR, Nieman LK. Differential diagnosis and imaging in Cushing's syndrome. *Endocrinol Metab Clin North Am* 2005; **34**: 403–21.

2 Baldeweg SE, Pollock JR, Powell M, Ahlquist J. A spectrum of behaviour in silent corticotroph pituitary adenomas. *Br J Neurosurg* 2005; **19**: 38–42.

3 Lacroix A, Bourdeau I. Bilateral adrenal Cushing's syndrome: macronodular adrenal hyperplasia and primary pigmented nodular adrenocortical disease. *Endocrinol Metab Clin North Am* 2005; **34**: 441–58.

4 Heaney AP. Novel medical approaches for the treatment of Cushing's disease. *J Endocrinol Invest* 2004; **27**: 591–5.

5 Ilias I, Torpy DJ, Pacak K, Mullen N, Wesley RA, Nieman LK. Cushing's syndrome due to ectopic corticotrophin secretion: 20 years' experience at the National Institutes of Health. *J Clin Endocrinol Metab* 2005; **90**: 4955–62.

6 Van Aken MO, Pereira AM, Biermasz NR, *et al.* Quality of life in patients after long-term biochemical cure of Cushing's disease. *J Clin Endocrinol Metab* 2005; **90**: 3279–86.

PROBLEM

15 Congenital Adrenal Hyperplasia

Case History

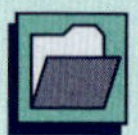

A 29-year-old woman seeks advice because of her embarrassing facial hirsutism. Her general health is good and she does not take any medications. Her sister has previously been diagnosed with congenital adrenal hyperplasia. She wonders whether she may also have this condition and if it is likely to affect her chances of becoming pregnant and whether it may affect her children.

How should the diagnosis be confirmed or excluded?

If she has the condition, what is the best approach to treatment?

Will it affect her chances of becoming pregnant?

What are the chances of a child being affected?

Background

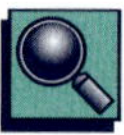

Congenital adrenal hyperplasia (CAH) is group of autosomal recessively inherited conditions where genes coding for one of the enzymes in the pathway leading to cortisol synthesis are defective. 21-hydroxylase deficiency is by far the commonest form, accounting for 95% of cases of CAH.[1] Defective production of cortisol and aldosterone with overproduction of adrenal androgens due to shunting of precursor steroids into the adrenal

Table 15.1 Biochemical changes in different forms of congenital adrenal hyperplasia

		Mineralocorticoid	Glucocorticoid	Sex steroid
21-OH	SW	↓↓	↓↓	↑↑
	Vir	↓	↓	↑↑
	Non-C	N	N/↓	↑
11β-OH		↑*	↓↓	↑↑↑
3β-HSD		↓↓	↓↓	↓†
17-OH		↑*	↓↓	↓↓
$P450_{SCC}$		↓↓↓	↓↓↓	↓↓↓

Non-C = non-classical; N = normal; SW = salt wasting; Vir = simple virilizing; *increased 11-deoxycorticosterone; †increased dehydroepiandrosterone.

androgen pathway account for the clinical features of the syndrome and for the hyperplasia of the adrenal cortex. In classic 21-hydroxylase deficiency, there is severe glucocorticoid and mineralocorticoid deficiency leading to hypotension, shock and salt wasting soon after birth. Females may be born with ambiguous genitalia because of the effects of excessive androgens. Advances in surgical reconstruction techniques have allowed near-normal genitalia to be refashioned in female patients early in life. Non-classic 21-hydroxylase deficiency is a milder form mainly diagnosed in women later in childhood or in young adulthood. They present with hirsutism, acne and menstrual irregularity. Males have normal genitalia at birth but grow excessively quickly, enter puberty early, and – if untreated – have short adult stature because of early and excessive exposure to androgens. The biochemical changes in different forms of CAH are summarized in Table 15.1.

21-hydroxylase deficiency

This has an incidence of 1:15 000 with a carrier rate of 1:60. There is considerable racial variation, e.g. the incidence in African-Americans is only one-third the incidence in white Americans. Neonatal screening is feasible but not carried out in most countries. This is mainly directed at detecting CAH in male children. Current methods do not detect the more subtle (non-classic forms). The gene for 21-hydroxylase is located on chromosome 6p21, within the human leucocyte antigen (HLA) complex. The active gene (*CYP21B*) and a highly homologous pseudogene (*CYP21A*) undergo recombination to produce a gene that does not effectively code for the enzyme. Most cases of CAH have different mutations on each of the two alleles.

Increased 17-hydroxyprogesterone (17-OHP) is the most widely available means of identifying and monitoring CAH. In untreated, or under-treated, cases ACTH will be increased. Chronic high levels of ACTH are responsible for the increased incidence of adrenocortical adenomas in patients with CAH. Secretion of corticotrophin-releasing hormone (CRH) is also increased. Increased central CRH may be responsible for the association of CAH with depression and anxiety, obesity and insulin resistance.

Glucocorticoid is necessary for the development and maintenance of the adrenal medulla, and defective catecholamine secretion has been documented in patients with classic CAH. Patients with non-classic CAH do not generally require replacement with glucocorticoid or mineralocorticoid.

Intrauterine diagnosis can be made with amniocentesis or chorionic villus sampling. Pre-natal treatment of the mother with dexamethasone can be used to suppress the fetal hypothalamic–pituitary–adrenal axis in affected females. In the neonatal period, salt and water balance (up to 80% are salt losers), along with glucocorticoid and mineralocorticoid replacement are essential. Feminizing surgery is also carried out in the neonatal period for affected females. Note that the internal genitalia are normal in these cases. During childhood, growth and development need to be managed carefully. Hydrocortisone is the preferred glucocorticoid, and the aim should be to suppress ACTH and 17-OHP into the physiological range but not to render them undetectable. The balance between achieving suppression of androgen excess and not exposing the patient to supraphysiological doses of glucocorticoid can be challenging.

11β-hydroxysteroid dehydrogenase deficiency

This is the second commonest form of CAH, accounting for about 3% of cases and with an incidence of around 1:100 000 births. The defect is in the *CYP11B1* gene located at 8q21. Increased deoxycorticosterone, a potent mineralocorticoid, leads to hypertension in this form of CAH. A mild late-onset form akin to non-classic 21-hydroxylase deficiency is recognized.

3β-hydroxysteroid dehydrogenase deficiency

This accounts for about 1% of all CAH and is due to defects in the *HSD3B1* gene at 1p13.1. There is decreased production of all three classes of steroids. Females require oestrogen replacement. Males require androgen replacement and genital abnormalities range from hypospadias to male pseudohermaphroditism. A non-classical form diagnosed in late teens or early adulthood is well recognized.

17β-hydroxylase deficiency

This is a rare form of CAH due to a defect in the *CYP17* gene at 10q24.3. Elevated deoxycorticosterone (DOC) leads to hypertension and hypokalaemia. Deficient adrenal and gonadal sex steroid production causes sexual infantilism in females and ambiguous genitalia in males. Polymorphisms of the *CYP17* gene have been linked with risk of breast, prostate and colon cancer.

$P450_{SCC}$ deficiency

This causes severe CAH with defective production of all steroids. The defect is in the *CYP11A* gene at 15q23–24, and the disorder is usually incompatible with life.

Non-classic 21-hydroxylase deficiency

The major presentation is in young women with hirsutism, acne and menstrual disturbances. It accounts for less than 5% of patients presenting with symptoms of androgen excess. Many patients (40%) with non-classic CAH have polycystic ovaries and

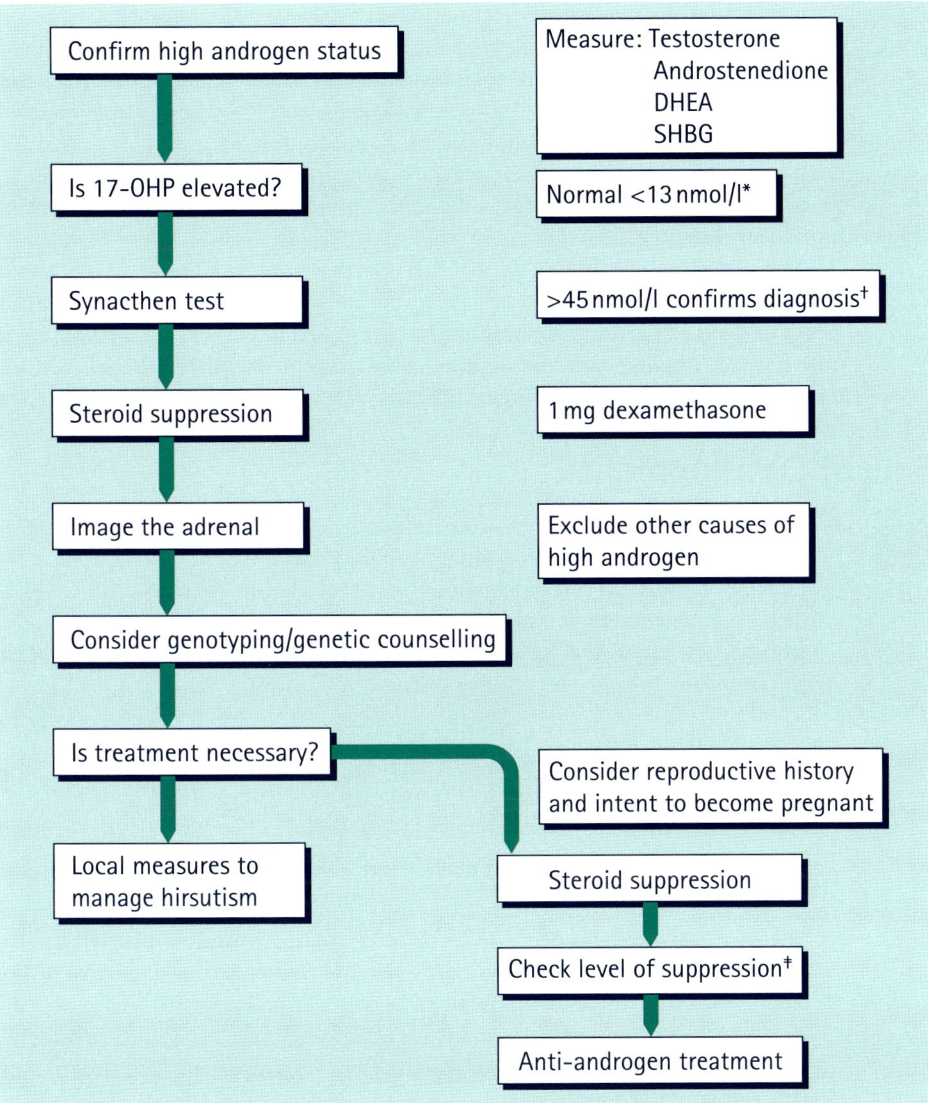

Fig. 15.1 Diagnosis and management of non-classical congenital adrenal hyperplasia (CAH). *Many patients with non-classical CAH have normal or near-normal 17-OHP at baseline. We routinely measure all three androgens as they are elevated to varying degrees in different patients. †We carry out short Synacthen test one morning, then ask the patient to take 1 mg dexamethasone late that evening, and repeat the short Synacthen test next morning. This routine both confirms that the high androgen levels are steroid suppressible and gives two confirmatory tests, one of which is carried out when adrenocorticotrophic hormone (ACTH) is not elevated. ‡While supraphysiological doses of steroid are needed to decrease ACTH sufficiently to decrease androgen production, patients do not need to be exposed to pharmacological doses of steroid. DHEA = dehydro-3-epiandrosterone; SHBG = sex hormone-binding globulin.

diminished fertility. Patients with non-classic CAH do not necessarily require treatment. A suggested algorithm for diagnosis and management is presented in Figure 15.1. The initial treatment is usually with corticosteroids given in a regimen that suppresses ACTH overnight (e.g. prednisolone 3–4 mg, or dexamethasone 1 mg) with a smaller dose of steroid during the day. 17-OHP levels should be monitored. If pregnancy is contemplated, and continuing steroid treatment is necessary, prednisolone is preferred as it does not cross the placenta. Anti-androgen treatment is also often required for patients with embarrassing acne or hirsutism.

Metformin may be useful, as in other women with symptoms of polycystic ovaries, although there are no systematic data in patients with CAH. Combined treatment with anti-androgen and aromatase inhibitor has been used in patients with classic CAH to minimize the dose of glucocorticoid required. Surgical removal of the adrenals with subsequent replacement therapy is an option for patients with severe problems of androgen excess.

Recent Developments

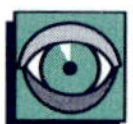

1 Weiss *et al.*[2] studied the hormonal response to exercise in patients with classic CAH. Adrenaline, but not noradrenaline, secretion was lower than in controls. The normal exercise-induced rise in blood glucose was blunted in patients with CAH, as was the increase in heart rate. It is clear that the decreased catecholamine state might interfere with normal physiological processes, and could be involved in disorders such as hypoglycaemia and blood pressure regulation.

2 High throughput genomic techniques can now be employed in neonatal screening programmes for 21-hydroxylase deficiency.[3] In conventional screening programmes, 17-OHP measurement is used. However, up to 1% of children have to be re-screened because of cross-reactivity between 17-OHP and other steroids that are increased in the neonatal period. Introduction of a second genetic screen for neonates who have high 17-OHP would reduce the rate of false positives.

3 The most severe form of CAH leads to decreased production of all three classes of steroid. Most cases are now thought to be due to deficiency of a transcriptional regulator, steroidogenic acute regulatory protein.[4] This protein, the gene for which is located at 8p11.2, participates in the acute response of steroid-producing cells to trophic factors. Mutations are particularly common in Palestinian, Korean and Japanese populations.

4 Patients with adrenal disorders may be insulin resistant and at risk of cardiovascular disease. Elevated plasma homocysteine, a marker for cardiac risk, has been described in women with polycystic ovarian syndrome but not in patients with non-classical CAH.[5] The latter patients also had no evidence of insulin resistance.

Conclusions

Congenital adrenal hyperplasia is the commonest recessively inherited disease. The diagnosis should be established by confirming that there is a state of hyperandrogenism and by measurement of baseline 17-OHP, which may be elevated in cases of CAH. A short Synacthen test will show an exaggerated rise in 17-OHP, as well as an increase in androgens. Many patients with non-classical CAH do not require treatment. If treatment is required, steroid suppression, just enough to normalize androgen levels, is the first line. Fertility is slightly diminished, and 40% of women have features of polycystic ovarian syndrome. The chance of the above patient's child being affected depends on the carrier status of her partner. She should have access to genetic counselling and genotyping if the diagnosis is confirmed biochemically. Note that, even is she is only a carrier; she could still have mild abnormalities in androgens, 17-OHP, and response to Synacthen. If both parents are carriers, there is a one in four chance of the child being affected. This increases to 50% if she has CAH (both alleles of the *CYP21* gene abnormal) and her partner is a carrier. If she has the disease and her partner is not a carrier, none of the children will have the disease but all will be carriers. The different types of 21-hydroxylase deficiency tend to breed true. The major concern in this case, therefore, is that a female child might develop features of non-classical CAH in early adulthood.

Further Reading

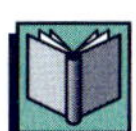

1 Merke DP, Bornstein SR. Congenital adrenal hyperplasia. *Lancet* 2005; **365**: 2125–36.

2 Weiss M, Mehlinger SL, Drinkard B, *et al.* Patients with classic congenital adrenal hyperplasia have decreased epinephrine reserve and defective glucose elevation in response to high-intensity exercise. *J Clin Endocrinol Metab* 2004; **89**: 591–7.

3 Kosel A, Burggraf S, Fingerhut R, Dorr HC, Roscher AA, Olgemoller B. Rapid second-tier molecular genetic analysis for congenital adrenal hyperplasia attributable to steroid 21-hydroxylase deficiency. *Clin Chem* 2005; **51**: 298–304.

4 Bhangoo A, Gu WX, Pavlakis S, *et al.* Phenotypic features associated with mutations in steroidogenic acute regulatory protein. *J Clin Endocrinol Metab* 2005; **90**: 6303–9.

5 Bayraktar F, Dereli D, Ozgen AG, Yilmaz C. Plasma homocysteine levels in polycystic ovary syndrome and congenital adrenal hyperplasia. *Endocr J* 2004; **51**: 601–8.

Pituitary

PROBLEM

16 Acromegaly

Case History

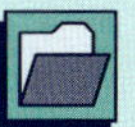

Mrs LD is a 36-year-old checkout operator. She complains of frequent headaches. Her family have commented on a coarsening of her facial features in recent years and her husband comments that she sleeps poorly and snores loudly at night. She had to have her wedding ring removed a few months ago as it was becoming very tight.

How should she be investigated further?

What are the treatment options if she has acromegaly?

What are the possible long-term complications?

Discuss her long-term follow-up.

Background

The annual incidence of acromegaly is 3–4 per million, and 99% of cases are caused by a pituitary somatotroph adenoma.[1] The vast majority arise sporadically but familial incidence is described, and it may occur in multiple endocrine neoplasia type 1, McCune–Albright syndrome, and in the Carney complex. Age of onset is usually 30–50 years, and it is equally common in men and women. Diagnosis is often delayed because of the variability of the symptoms, the insidious onset, and the frequent delay in definitive investigations.

Since the syndrome may be present for years before the diagnosis is made, even subtle changes in growth hormone secretion may lead to major clinical effects. Effective treatment rapidly reverses some of the symptoms including headache and sweating. In the longer term reversal of the soft tissue overgrowth contributes to reversing some of the changes in physical appearance and to improving cardiac and respiratory function. Increased morbidity and decreased life expectancy relate to hypertension and impaired glucose tolerance/diabetes—each occurring in about a third of cases and contributing to the increased risk of cardiovascular disease. There is controversy about whether risk of malignant disease is increased. About 30% of patients have colonic polyps and may be at risk of colon cancer.

Investigation and management of acromegaly are summarized in Figure 16.1. A random serum insulin-like growth factor (IGF)-1 level is a useful screening tool, particularly if the reference range is corrected for age. Random measurements of growth hormone (GH) are of limited use in diagnosing acromegaly. Measurement of IGF-1 should be followed by an oral glucose tolerance test in all cases. Glucose and GH are measured at baseline and every 30 minutes for 120 minutes following an oral 75 g glucose load. In normal people, and in those with cured acromegaly, GH will suppress to below 1 ng/ml. The test may yield indeterminate results in patients with chronic hyperglycaemia. An aberrant GH response to thyrotropin-releasing hormone (TRH) is present in up to 50% of patients. It is useful to carry out this test as it can help to detect residual or recurrent tumour following surgery. Prolactin measurements should also be carried out during the TRH test. A minority of acromegaly patients have tumours that secrete both prolactin and GH. These tumours may be more responsive to medical therapy, including dopamine agonists. Since 80% of somatotroph adenomas are macro tumours (>1 cm) and many are invasive, it is important to check other pituitary functions in all patients, particularly prior to surgery. Thyroid hormones and TSH should be measured. The diagnosis of secondary hypothyroidism is not always clear-cut in patients with complex pituitary diseases. It is, therefore, useful to carry out a TRH test, as described above, with measurement of TSH, prolactin and GH. Plasma electrolytes and osmolality should be checked. Gonadotropin levels may be in the normal range, even in patients with secondary hypogonadism. Normal menstrual function in women is reassuring. For men and non-menstruating women, levels of sex steroids should be checked. Post-menopausal women with hypopituitarism may not have the normal high levels of gonadotropins, although this is of no clinical significance. A short Synacthen test should be carried out in all patients and steroid replacement instituted prior to surgery where necessary.

There is no place for skull X-rays routinely although these will show frontal bossing and, in some cases, there will be erosion of the floor of the pituitary fossa. Magnetic resonance imaging (MRI) is the imaging modality of choice, although computed tomography (CT) will also demonstrate most of the tumours that cause acromegaly. All patients should have their visual fields formally assessed with perimetry. GH-secreting tumours express somatostatin receptor subtypes 2 and 5,[2] and ^{111}Indium-labelled octreotide can be used to image some tumours. This is not needed routinely but may be useful in cases where there is diagnostic doubt. The expression of somatostatin in somatotroph adenomas is important because it predicts response to somatostatin analogues.

Definitive surgical treatment is indicated in most cases and, with the exception of tumours that are very large or invasive, the trans-sphenoidal route is to be preferred. The outcome depends on the experience of the surgeon, the selection of surgical approach

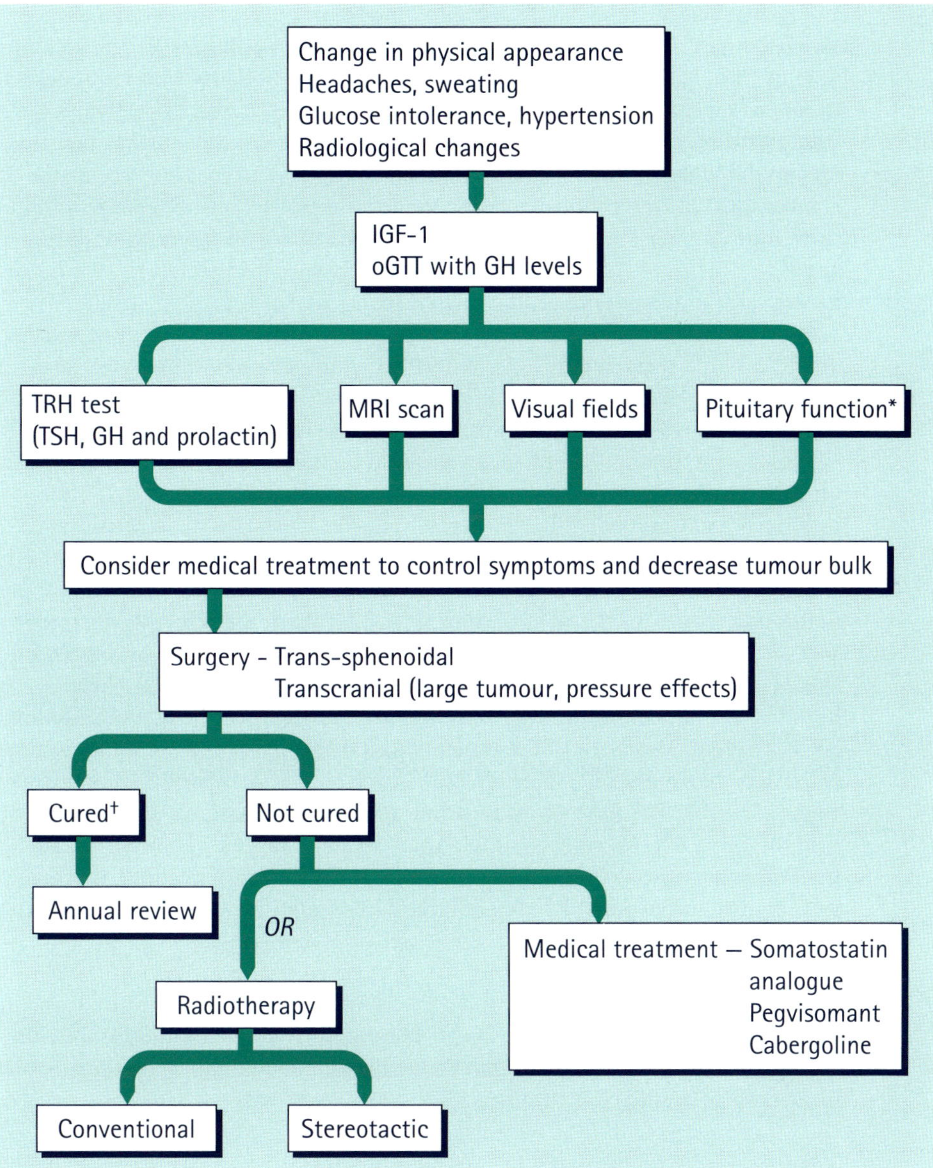

Fig. 16.1 Investigation and treatment of acromegaly. *All anterior pituitary functions should be checked—thyroid, gonadal and adrenal axes as well as posterior pituitary function (plasma osmolality and electrolytes). †Definition of a cure is that insulin-like growth factor (IGF)-1 is returned to normal for age and that growth hormone (GH) suppresses to below 1 ng/ml following an oral glucose load. oGTT = oral glucose tolerance test; TRH = thyrotropin-releasing hormone; TSH = thyrotropin (thyroid stimulating hormone).

and the baseline characteristics of the patient. Patients with very high levels of GH (>45 ng/ml) and those with large and invasive tumours are less likely to achieve cure. Suppression of GH to 1 ng/ml or below constitutes a cure. Treatment is generally regarded as satisfactory if the GH level suppresses to <5 ng/ml. In a recent large German series,[3] cure was achieved in 57.3% of patients undergoing trans-sphenoidal surgery. The risk associated with surgery in these patients was very low, and the recurrence rate over 10 years of follow-up was only 0.4%. The cure rate for patients who required transcranial surgery or repeat surgery was much lower at 5.2% and 21.3%, respectively.

Radiotherapy is an option for patients who either are not suitable for surgery or are not cured by surgery. Since most tumours are macroadenomas and invade the dura, bone or cavernous sinus, it is not surprising that cure is not achieved by surgery in many cases. Conventional radiotherapy is typically delivered in 20–30 fractions and may take up to 20 years to achieve its maximum effect. Suppressed GH secretion is achieved in over three-quarters of patients at 15 years, and up to 85% develop progressive hypopituitarism.[4] Focused, stereotactic methods achieve a much more rapid cure and can be delivered in a single treatment. These methods include gamma knife, linear accelerator and proton beam radiotherapy. They are not suitable for tumours that come within 5 mm of the optic chiasma, since they may cause visual loss in such cases.

Medical treatment should be considered in patients in whom surgery cannot be undertaken, those who are not cured by surgery, elderly patients and those with small tumours, and following radiotherapy until biochemical remission is achieved. Somatostatin analogues have become the mainstay of medical treatment. Two long-acting preparations given by intramuscular injection every 14–28 days are particularly useful—octreotide LAR and lanreotide. IGF-1 levels are significantly decreased in at least 70% of patients. The effect on tumour shrinkage can be disappointing, with less than 50% of patients having decreased tumour volume, and the mean shrinkage being less than 20%. However, few tumours increase in size during treatment. A recent meta-analysis[2] has confirmed the efficacy of these agents, and that long-acting octreotide is slightly more efficacious than lanreotide. Side effects include diarrhoea, abdominal cramps and biliary stones or sludge. For patients who cannot tolerate somatostatin analogues, or do benefit from their use, the GH receptor antagonist pegvisomant may be used. This drug binds to the GH receptor, preventing its dimerization and blocking signalling. It is given subcutaneously in an initial dose of 80 mg, followed by 10 mg/day, increased by 5 mg up to a maximum daily dose of 30 mg. Normal levels of IGF-1 are achieved in 90%. Dopamine agonists have been used in acromegaly for many years. In fact, only 30–50% of patients achieve satisfactory IGF-1 levels, and there is tumour shrinkage in a small proportion. Of these agents, the best evidence is with cabergoline, which should be used at a dose of 1–4 mg per week. Dopamine agonist therapy is most suitable for those with small or mixed (prolactin and GH) tumours.

Recent Developments

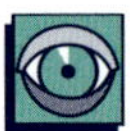

1. There is often a disparity between GH and IGF-1 levels,[5] making it difficult to define cure in some patients. Patients with such a disparity are more likely to have biochemical relapse following surgery, and require careful follow-up.

2. Quality of life is severely impaired in patients with acromegaly, particularly if they have had expensive and complex therapy beforehand.[6] AcroQol is a patient-friendly questionnaire with 22 health-related questions. This appears to provide a disease-specific means of assessing health status in patients with acromegaly.

3 A cyclo-hexapeptide (SOM230) has high affinity for the 1, 2 and 3 somatostatin receptor subtypes and has shown early promise in the treatment of acromegaly and in gastrointestinal neuroendocrine tumours.[7] Not only might such developments lead to more specifically targeted drug treatments, but they may also pave the way for improving local delivery of radiation treatment or chemotherapy by targeting cytotoxic agents to the site of tumours.

4 A recent multicentre Italian case–control study[8] demonstrated that 27.7% of patients with acromegaly had colonic neoplasia compared with 15.5% in controls presenting with non-specific abdominal complaints. The level of IGF-1 and the duration of acromegaly did not appear to be predictive of development of neoplasia.

Conclusions

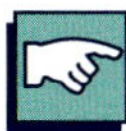

Measurement of circulating IGF-1 is a useful screening test so long as results are assessed against age-corrected normal ranges. The most definitive biochemical test is measurement of GH during a glucose tolerance test. Surgery to remove the pituitary tumour is indicated in most patients with acromegaly. Medical therapy is helpful in the time leading up to surgery and in those not cured by surgery. Radiotherapy should be considered in the latter. Long-term risks associated with the condition include hypopituitarism, diabetes, hypertension, increased risk of vascular disease and neoplasms of the colon. Patients may also have disability because of arthritis and dental deformity. There is also increased prevalence of respiratory disorders including sleep apnoea and obstructive pulmonary disease. Because of the latter, pneumococcal vaccine and annual influenza immunization should be considered. Annual checks of glucose tolerance test or GH day profile are advisory and other pituitary functions should be checked at the same time.

Further Reading

1 Park C, Yang I, Woo J, *et al.* Somatostatin (SRIF) receptor subtype 2 and 5 gene expression in growth hormone-secreting pituitary adenomas: the relationship with endogenous SRIF activity and response to octreotide. *Endocr J* 2004; **51**: 227–36.

2 Freda PU, Katznelson L, van der Lely AJ, Reyes CM, Zhao S, Rabinowitz D. Long-acting somatostatin analogue therapy of acromegaly; a meta-analysis. *J Clin Endocrinol Metab* 2005; **90**: 4465–73.

3 Nomikos P, Buchfelder M, Fahibush R. The outcome of surgery in 668 patients with acromegaly using current criteria of biochemical control. *Eur J Endocrinol* 2005; **152**: 379–87.

4 Minniti G, Jaffrain-Rea ML, Osti M, *et al.* The long-term efficacy of conventional radiotherapy in patients with GH-secreting pituitary adenomas. *Clin Endocrinol* 2005; **62**: 210–16.

5 Espinosa de los Monteros AL, Sosa E, Cheng S, *et al.* Biochemical evaluation of disease activity after pituitary surgery in acromegaly: a critical analysis of patients who spontaneously change disease status. *Clin Endocrinol* 2006; **64**: 245–9.

6 Rowles SV, Prieto L, Badia X, Shalet SM, Webb SM, Trainer PJ. Quality of life (QOL) in patients with acromegaly is severely impaired: use of a novel measure of QOL: acromegaly quality of life questionnaire. *J Clin Endocrinol Metab* 2005; **90**: 3337–41.

7 Oberg K. Future aspects of somatostatin-receptor mediated therapy. *Neuroendocrinology* 2004; **80**(suppl 1): 57–61.

8 Terzolo M, Reimondo G, Gasperi M, *et al.* Colonoscopic screening and follow-up in patients with acromegaly: a multicenter study in Italy. *J Clin Endocrinol Metab* 2005; **90**: 84–90.

PROBLEM

17 Prolactinoma

Case History

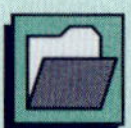

A 17-year-old girl attends with her mother. She had a normal menarche at the age of 13 but her periods stopped about 8 months ago. She has noted a milky discharge from her breasts, particularly when she is in the bath. Otherwise, she is fit and healthy and takes no medications. Her prolactin level is 6000 mU/l (normal up to 360 mU/l).

Discuss the further investigation of her high prolactin.

What is likely to be the favoured treatment?

How long should she be treated for?

How should she be followed up?

Background

Prolactinoma accounts for 40% of pituitary tumours.[1] A variety of physiological and pathological stimuli increase prolactin (see Table 17.1). Increases with physiological stimuli (except pregnancy) and drugs are usually modest (serum prolactin <800 mU/l). As a general rule, levels above 1000 mU/l require investigation. Values greater than 3000 mU/l nearly always indicate the presence of a prolactinoma. Intermediate levels can be due to stalk compression or to microprolactinoma. There is a reasonable correlation between tumour size and prolactin level. The exception can be with large tumours, which

Table 17.1 Differential diagnosis of hyperprolactinaemia	
Physiological	Pregnancy (up to ten times normal) Stress, eating, exercise Breast stimulation Lesions of the chest wall
Drugs	Metoclopramide, domperidone Phenothiazines, risperidone Monoamine oxidase inhibitors Tricyclics, serotonin selective reuptake inhibitors Verapamil, methyldopa Oestrogen Cimetidine Opioids, cocaine Protease inhibitors
Endocrine	Hypothyroidism Polycystic ovarian syndrome Prolactinoma – micro (<10 mm) macro (≥10 mm)
Pituitary stalk	Large pituitary tumours Cranial irradiation Craniopharyngiomas Stalk transection (trauma)
Other	Chronic renal failure (decreased clearance) Idiopathic

compress the pituitary stalk. Also, an assay artefact, the hook effect, can return falsely low levels unless samples are serially diluted. During the past 20 years, improved biochemical and radiological diagnosis, along with understanding of the condition have greatly improved management of patients with prolactinoma. Several key facts should be borne in mind:

- The vast majority (90%) are micro-tumours, and only a small proportion of these (1%) grow following diagnosis.
- Medical therapy with dopamine agonists is the treatment of choice, and both decreases prolactin and shrinks the tumour in most cases.
- Serum prolactin is a good marker for tumour size and, following initial investigation, can be used to adjust the dose of dopamine agonist therapy.

Women with prolactinoma present with oligomenorrhoea or amenorrhoea, and 80% have galactorrhoea. Men present with impotence or decreased libido. Fertility is decreased in men and women. Bone mineral density is decreased because of the hypogonadism. This may not recover completely following successful treatment. Men often present with larger tumours due to later diagnosis and probably because of underdiagnosis of small lesions.

Dynamic endocrine tests have a limited role to play in the diagnosis of prolactinoma. We usually carry out a thyrotropin-releasing hormone (TRH) test. Administration of intravenous TRH usually increases prolactin at 30 minutes. Patients with prolactinoma show high basal levels and no response to TRH. A similar test with dopamine antagonists (e.g. domperidone or metoclopramide 5–10 mg intravenously) is carried out in some centres. Both tests may show blunted response in patients with suprasellar lesions. Gadolinium-enhanced magnetic resonance imaging (MRI) is the imaging modality of choice, although most lesions will also be detectable with contrast-enhanced computed tomography.

Dopamine is the dominant physiological regulator of prolactin release, and its effect is inhibitory. Dopamine agonist drugs are the first line of treatment for most patients with prolactinoma. Bromocriptine normalizes prolactin in 80% of cases, and restores normal menses and fertility in 90%. Side effects include nausea, postural hypotension, depression and other psychoses. Treatment should be started gradually, and increased, according to response over several weeks. An initial dose of 0.625 mg/day is suitable. Micro-tumours typically require 5–7.5 mg/day. In patients with micro-tumours, when bromocriptine is discontinued after 24 months, 25% will have lasting remission. Because of its short half-life, bromocriptine is the drug of choice in a woman wishing to become pregnant. She should be instructed to continue with mechanical contraception until she has had two normal periods when starting the drug, and it should be stopped as soon as she has missed a period and pregnancy is confirmed.

The long-acting D_2 receptor agonist cabergoline is now the most widely used drug.[2] It is a non-ergot drug, has a lower incidence of side effects than bromocriptine, and need only be given twice weekly. It should be commenced at a dose of 0.25 mg once a week. Doses of 1 mg twice a week, or less, are usually sufficient to treat microprolactinomas. The drug may be tolerated by those who cannot tolerate bromocriptine, and it may be effective in patients who prove to be resistant to bromocriptine. Colao *et al.*[3] studied patients after withdrawal of long-term cabergoline. The drug was stopped if prolactin level was normal and there was no tumour, or there had been greater than 50% shrinkage of tumour. Recurrence rate was 24% in non-tumour hyperprolactinaemia, 31% in patients with microprolactinoma and 36% in patients with macroprolactinoma. Recurrence rate is small particularly when the MR scan is negative at the time of withdrawal.

Medical treatment is the first line, even in large tumours. Surgical debulking is indicated in women who are considering pregnancy because of the risk of tumour enlargement under the influence of oestrogen in pregnancy. Otherwise surgery and radiotherapy are reserved for those who either cannot tolerate or do not respond to medical treatment. Estimates of risk of progression from microadenoma to macroadenoma vary, but this may occur in up to 7% of cases, according to some authors. Thus, patients who are not deemed to require treatment should still be evaluated clinically, biochemically and radiologically at intervals. Patients with large tumours are at risk of hypopituitarism and visual field abnormalities, and should have checks performed at least every 6 months. An algorithm for management of patients with prolactinoma is presented in Figure 17.1.

Recent Developments

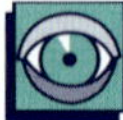

1 Hyperprolactinaemia is frequently caused by medications, particularly antipsychotic drugs.[4] These drugs exert their therapeutic action by blocking D_2 and D_4 receptors in the mesolimbic area of the brain. Extrapyramidal side effects are caused by blockade of D_2 receptors in the striatal area. Hyperprolactinaemia is due to blockade of D_2 receptors in the tuberoinfundibular system and on pituitary lactotrophs. If the drug cannot be stopped, hypogonadism may be treated with oestrogen or testosterone

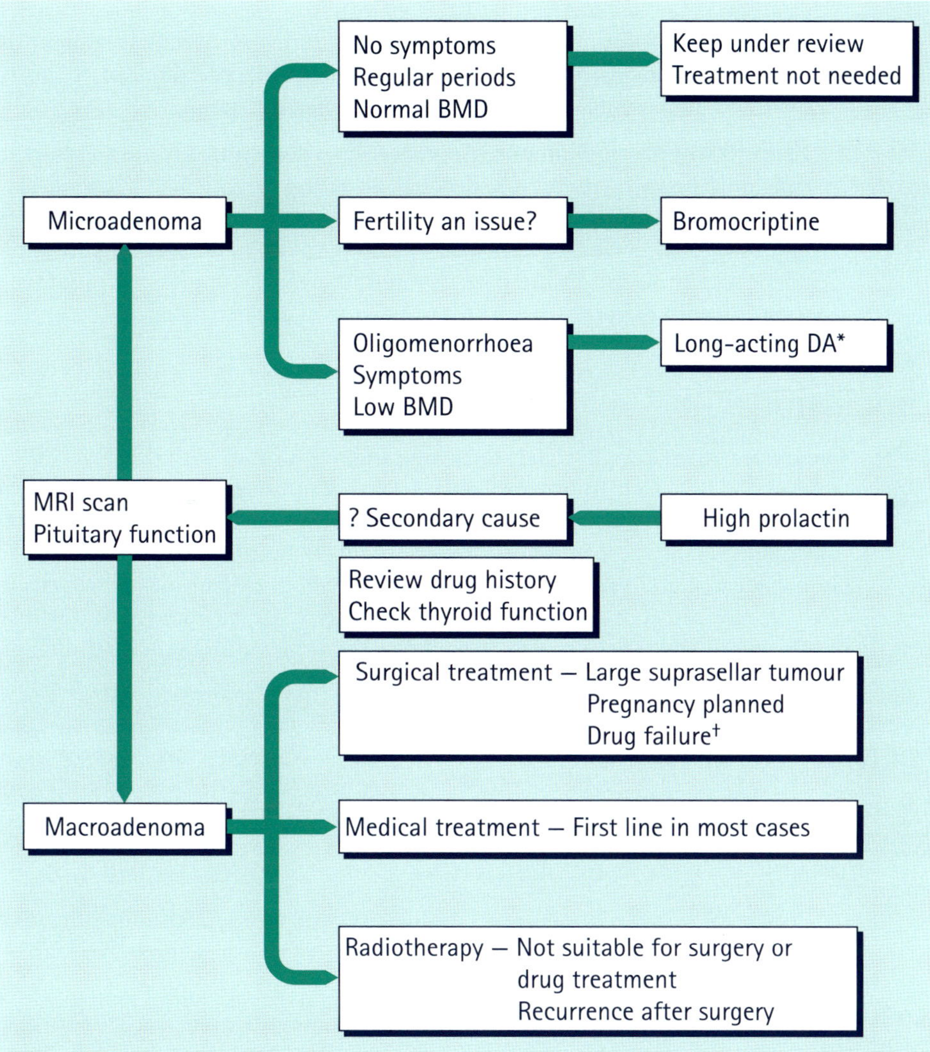

Fig. 17.1 Management of prolactinoma. *In patients who are intolerant or do not respond to dopamine agonist, oestrogen or testosterone replacement should be considered. †Surgery should be considered in patients who either cannot tolerate, or do not respond to, drug treatment. BMD = bone mineral density; DA = dopamine agonist.

replacement. Alternatively, dopamine agonist therapy may normalize prolactin levels in some cases, although there is a small risk of exacerbating the underlying psychosis.

2 Hormone tests should always be interpreted in the light of the clinical picture. Isoforms of prolactin can cause confusion, and the laboratory may need to take this into account, by taking steps to measure only the 23 kDa monomeric and biologically active form. Macroprolactin is monomeric or dimeric prolactin bound to IgG. It may lead to overestimation of prolactin. Also big prolactin (50 kDa or big big prolactin

(150 kDa) may account for up to 25% of immunoreactive hormone.[5,6] Lack of awareness of these isoforms of prolactin may lead to inappropriate treatment of patients who do not, in fact, have symptomatic hyperprolactinaemia, or to over-vigorous treatment of patients who have hyperprolactinaemic states.

3 Up to 10% of prolactinomas respond poorly to dopamine agonists. Prolactin receptor antagonists may be useful for this difficult group of patients.[7] These drugs may also have a role in the treatment of hormone-responsive malignancies: prolactin is a significant growth factor for breast and prostate tumours. There is significant local production of prolactin in these lesions and, therefore, suppressing pituitary prolactin secretion with dopamine agonist is unlikely to prove beneficial.

Conclusions

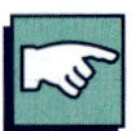

The above patient is highly likely to have a pituitary tumour with this degree of hyperprolactinaemia. It is likely to be a prolactin-secreting tumour, but at this level of prolactin it could be a non-functioning tumour causing high prolactin through stalk compression. Cabergoline is the most suitable unless she wants to become pregnant. Treatment should be re-evaluated at 2 years, and periodically thereafter. Dopamine agonist treatment can safely be stopped in many patients whose prolactin has normalized and whose tumour has shrunk. Patients with macro-tumours or those in whom there is residual tumour on MRI have a higher chance of recurrence.

Further Reading

1 Schlechte JA. Prolactinoma. *N Engl J Med* 2003; **349**: 2035–41.

2 Cook DM. Long-term management of prolactinomas—use of long-acting dopamine agonists. *Rev Endocr Metab Disorders* 2005; **6**: 15–21.

3 Colao A, Di Sarno A, Cappabianca P, Di Somma C, Pivonello R, Lombardi G. Withdrawal of long-term cabergoline therapy for tumoral and non-tumoral hyperprolactinaemia. *N Engl J Med* 2003; **349**: 2023–33.

4 Molitch ME. Medication-induced hyperprolactinaemia. *Mayo Clin Proc* 2005; **80**: 1050–7.

5 Suliman AM, Smith TP, Gibney J, McKenna TJ. Frequent misdiagnosis and mismanagement of hyperprolactinemic patients before the introduction of macroprolactin screening: application of a new strict laboratory definition of macroprolactinemia. *Clin Chem* 2003; **49**: 1504–9.

6 Mounier C, Trouilla J, Claustrat B, Duthel R, Estour B. Macroprolactinaemia associated with prolactin adenoma. *Hum Reprod* 2003; **18**: 853–7.

7 Goffin V, Bernichtein S, Tourraine P, Kelly PA. Development and potential clinical uses of human prolactin receptor antagonists. *Endocr Rev* 2005; **26**: 400–22.

PROBLEM

18 Non-Functioning Pituitary Adenoma

Case History

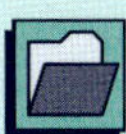

A 68-year-old man has noted a gradual decline in his vision with loss of his peripheral visual fields. He complains of feeling tired and of a diminished capacity for exercise over the past year or so. Examination confirms bitemporal hemianopia and a loss of body hair. Magnetic resonance imaging (MRI) shows the presence of a 4 cm pituitary mass extending superiorly and compressing the optic chiasma. Investigations confirm that he has hypopituitarism.

What treatment options are available?

What is the prognosis for his vision and his pituitary function?

How should he be followed up?

Background

Pituitary adenomas account for 10–15% of intracranial neoplasms. When they are non-secretory, or secrete minute amounts of hormone that do not produce clinically significant endocrine disturbances, they are referred to as non-functioning. They are symptomatic if large and if they produce pressure effects on nearby structures; occasionally they are asymptomatic and detected during routine imaging. Macroadenomas (>1 cm in diameter) are more likely to give rise to pressure symptoms.

The commonest presentations are with headaches, visual field defects and cranial nerve palsies. Headache is common in patients with large tumours. It is usually dull and increased with coughing. It may be at the vertex, fronto-occipital, retro-orbital, fronto-temporal or occipito-cervical areas. It perhaps results from stretching of the diaphragma sella by the tumour. The headache may present in a variety of clinical patterns, and is usually improved following hypophysectomy.[1] Dopamine agonist therapy may worsen headache. Rarely, the patient may present as an emergency with pituitary apoplexy. Symptoms of this include headache/meningism, vomiting, reduction in visual fields, diplopia and impaired consciousness. Pituitary apoplexy is most likely to occur with non-functioning pituitary adenomas. It may be missed with computed tomography (CT) in up to 50% of cases. Many cases can be managed conservatively but urgent decompression is indicated when pressure symptoms (Table 18.1) from the pituitary mass predominate.

Trans-sphenoidal surgery (Table 18.2) remains the treatment of first choice for large tumours. It provides a rapid relief of pressure effects including improvement in vision. Serious complications of surgery occur in less than 5% cases. The risk of complications is inversely proportional to the expertise of the surgeon. Post-operative complications

Table 18.1 Pressure effects of non-functioning pituitary tumors

Optic tract and chiasma (visual field defects)	Bitemporal hemianopia – commonest (8% patients develop complete loss of vision in one eye with a temporal defect in the other) Bitemporal scotomas – rapidly growing tumour with prefixed chiasma Monocular field defects – superior temporal; central scotoma All patients with visual field defects also have sellar enlargement
Cavernous sinus	Involvement of the cranial nerves due to lateral extension; visual field defects – usually absent III – commonest; pupillary function preserved like diabetic neuropathy IV, VI, V (pain and numbness in its distribution) Compression or obstruction of the carotid artery
Hypothalamus	Hyperphagia, abnormal temperature regulation, loss of consciousness, loss of hormonal input from the hypothalamus
Third ventricle	Obstructive hydrocephalus (less common than with craniopharyngiomas)
Temporal lobe	Complex partial seizures
Frontal lobes	Alteration in mental states Frontal lobe release signs
Posterior fossa	Brainstem dysfunction

Table 18.2 Surgical evaluation and follow-up

Pre-operative evaluation	Check for hormone deficiencies and replace Identify a marker such as α-subunit that can be used to monitor the response to surgery
Post-operative care	Immediate (within a few days): SIADH or diabetes insipidus may develop and urine volume and sodium should be closely monitored Short term (few weeks): Check for residual adenoma – MRI and/or α-subunit Check for hormonal status – free T_4, cortisol (metyrapone or somatostatin followed by insulin tolerance test), water deprivation is required Replace hormone deficiencies Long term: MRI and hormonal evaluation for adequacy of replacement or to identify subsequent hormone deficiencies

SIADH = syndrome of inappropriate antidiuretic hormone secretion.

include worsening vision, haemorrhage, cerebrospinal fluid rhinorrhoea and meningitis. Hormone deficiencies may occur as a consequence of surgery even if function was preserved pre-operatively. Diabetes insipidus may be transient or permanent. Post-operative radiotherapy may be given but carries a high risk of hypopituitarism.

Radiotherapy to the pituitary is a useful adjunct to treatment if MRI scans after 6–12 months show tumour re-growth. Routine radiotherapy is no longer recommended as improved imaging techniques in recent years allow recurrent tumour to be identified if regular follow-up scans are undertaken. The MRI scan may be difficult to interpret if done early (<3 months) after surgery because of artefacts. Conventional radiotherapy is increasingly being replaced with stereotactic radiation methods (e.g. the 'gamma knife') as the scatter of radiation to the surrounding structures is minimal and there is less chance of hypopituitarism.

Medical therapy has a limited role in the management of non-functioning pituitary adenomas. Less than 20% of tumours show significant shrinkage with dopamine agonists. Of the available agents, cabergoline is the one most likely to produce a beneficial effect. Somatostatin analogues are worth trying where surgery is contraindicated or delayed but these agents only decrease the size of a minority of tumours.

Recent Developments

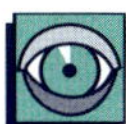

1. Radiosurgery has added to the range of treatment options for patients with pituitary adenomas.[2] Use of the linear accelerator or gamma knife allows radiotherapy to be delivered in a single fraction. Improved means of patient immobilization and imaging have contributed to the utility of these techniques. Long-term follow-up experience in patients with non-functioning tumours is, however, limited and surgery is still the treatment of choice.

2. A recent review[3] of a large series of pituitary apoplexy confirmed that conservative management is most appropriate for the majority, whereas patients with visual impairment are more likely to require early surgical intervention. The prognosis, including for visual field defects, is very good. Pituitary apoplexy is generally regarded as a rare complication. However, in a recent large Danish series, it was found to occur in 21% of patients with non-functioning pituitary tumours.[4]

3. Post-operative radiotherapy was previously considered to be required in many cases of non-functioning pituitary tumours following surgery. Clinical practice has changed, and only patients with clear evidence of residual tumour following operative treatment require radiotherapy in the early stages (Figure 18.1).[5] The obvious disadvantage of radiotherapy is the high incidence of progressive hypopituitarism in the years following treatment.

4. Non-functioning pituitary tumours are being detected with increasing frequency. They account for around 20% of pituitary tumours that present with clinical symptoms in adult patients less than 70 years old. However, the proportion of incidentally discovered tumours that are non-hormone secreting is about 40%, whereas approximately 80% of tumours diagnosed in elderly people are non-functioning.[6] Transsphenoidal surgery is both safe and effective in elderly patients.

5. Recovery of visual function following treatment is the major consideration for many patients. Rapid recovery (within days) occurs in some patients, including some who present with pituitary apoplexy. Most patients who make a complete, or virtually complete, recovery do so within 1–4 months.[7] A slower recovery phase is identifiable in some, but may be of limited clinical significance. Duration of disease is an important determinant of recovery. Hyperintensity of the optic nerves on T2-weighted MR images is associated with visual impairment, and may be a useful means of predicting visual symptoms and monitoring recovery.[8]

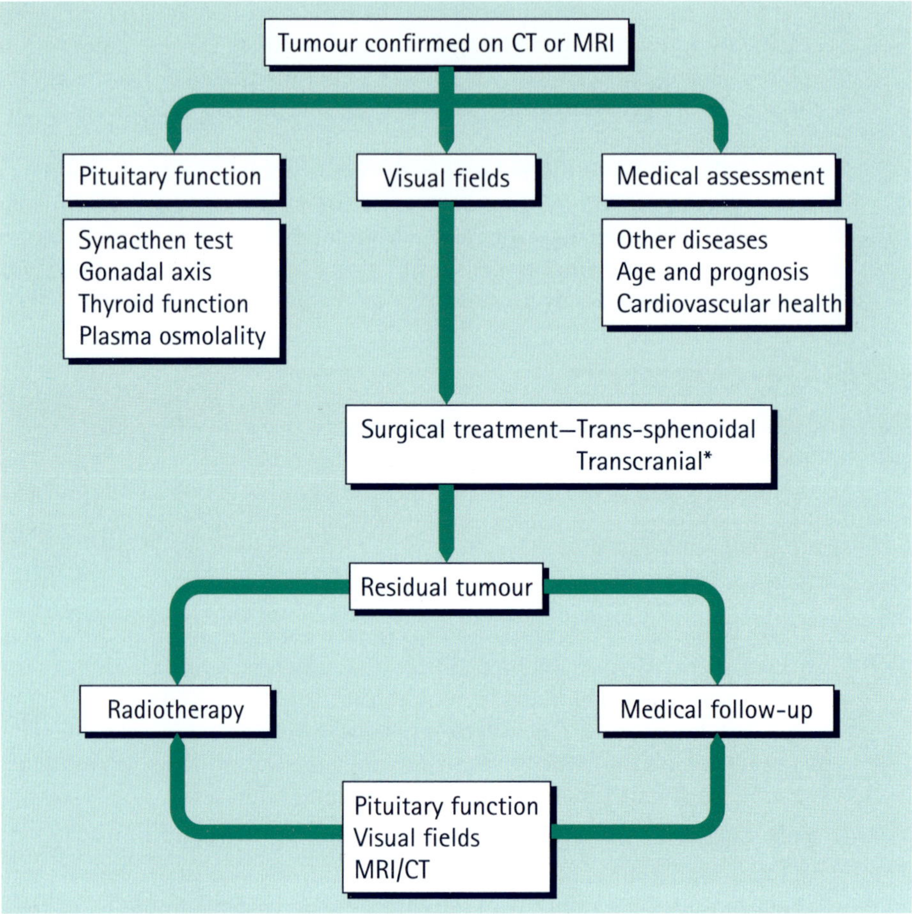

Tumour confirmed on CT or MRI

Pituitary function

Synacthen test
Gonadal axis
Thyroid function
Plasma osmolality

Visual fields

Medical assessment

Other diseases
Age and prognosis
Cardiovascular health

Surgical treatment—Trans-sphenoidal
Transcranial*

Residual tumour

Radiotherapy

Medical follow-up

Pituitary function
Visual fields
MRI/CT

Fig. 18.1 Investigation and treatment of non-functioning pituitary tumour. Treatment is more urgent in patients with visual symptoms. *Transcranial surgery is indicated in patients with tumours that are large or invasive and in some patients where there is visual impairment. Regular follow-up with imaging studies and visual fields is essential in all patients as there is no useful blood test to indicate the presence of residual or recurrent tumour.

Conclusions

Non-functioning pituitary tumours tend to present late and are more likely to present with hypopituitarism and visual failure than are functioning pituitary tumours. There is, at best, a limited response to medical therapy and surgery is indicated in most cases. For patients in whom surgery is not indicated, or not desired, and in those with incomplete response to surgery, radiation therapy should be considered. With modern treatment, prognosis for patients with hormonally silent pituitary adenomas is very good. Visual recovery depends on the duration of disease prior to surgery. After 4 months, those with poor recovery may not expect major improvements in vision. There is a high rate of recurrent/residual tumour and periodic imaging studies are required following initial surgery. In the absence of residual tumour, progressive pituitary failure is unusual after surgery but common after radiation therapy.

Further Reading

1 Levy MJ, Matharu MS, Meeran K, Powell M, Goadsby PJ. The clinical characteristics of headache in patients with pituitary tumours. *Brain* 2005; **128**: 1921–30.

2 Brada M, Alithkumar TV, Minniti G. Radiosurgery for pituitary adenomas. *Clin Endocrinol* 2004; **61**: 531–43.

3 Sibal L, Ball SG, Connolly V, *et al.* Pituitary apoplexy: a review of clinical presentation, management and outcome in 45 cases. *Pituitary* 2004; **7**: 157–63.

4 Nielsen EH, Lindholm J, Bjerre P, *et al.* Frequent occurrence of pituitary apoplexy in patients with non-functioning pituitary adenoma. *Clin Endocrinol* 2006; **64**: 319–22.

5 Almeda C, Lucas T, Pineda E, *et al.* Experience in management of 51 non-functioning pituitary adenomas: indications for post-operative radiotherapy. *J Endocrinol Invest* 2005; **28**: 18–22.

6 Minniti G, Esposito V, Piccirilli M, Fratticci A, Snatoro A, Jaffrain-Rea ML. Diagnosis and management of pituitary tumours in the elderly: a review based on personal experience and evidence of literature. *Eur J Endocrinol* 2005; **153**: 723–35.

7 Kerrison JB, Lynn MJ, Baer CA, Newman SA, Biousse V, Nemann NJ. Stages of improvement in visual fields after pituitary tumour resection. *Am J Ophtalmol* 2000; **130**: 813–20.

8 Tokamaru AM, Sakata I, Terada H, Kosuda S, Nawashiro H, Yoshii M. Optic nerve hyperintensity on T2-weighted images among patients with pituitary macroadenoma: correlation with visual impairment. *Am J Neuroradiol* 2006; **27**: 250–4.

PROBLEM

19 Hypopituitarism: Investigation and Treatment

Case History

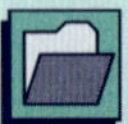

Mr TP is a 48-year-old accountant who suffered a severe head injury in a motor traffic accident two years ago. He has no residual neurological deficit but finds that his libido has not returned to normal and that he has difficulty in sustaining an erection. He is also generally tired and lacking in energy.

How should his pituitary function be investigated?

What are the most likely abnormalities?

Is spontaneous recovery of his pituitary function likely?

Discuss the approach to his long-term management.

Background

Hypopituitarism refers to the deficiency of one or more pituitary hormones. The common causes of hypopitutarism are listed in Table 19.1.

Table 19.1 Causes of hypopituitarism

Congenital	Pituitary hypoplasia Transcription factor defects Receptor defects Hormone mutation
Traumatic	Head injury, surgery, irradiation
Inflammatory	Primary hypophysitis, sarcoidosis' histiocytosis X, infections, Wegener's granulomatosis
Infiltrative	Haemochromatosis, leukaemia, lymphoma
Vascular	Post-partum haemorrhage, pituitary apoplexy, sickle cell disease, vasculitis
Neoplastic	Pituitary adenoma, neuroglial tumours, sphenoidal meningiomas, craniopharyngiomas, hypothalamic hamartomas, Rathke's cleft cyst, dermoid cyst

The clinical manifestations depend on the number and type of hormones impaired, the severity of hormone deficiency and the rapidity of onset. Features of pituitary failure are profound in infants with congenital pituitary failure who may also have other structural (possibly mid-line) defects. If pituitary failure is acute as in cases of pituitary apoplexy, the patient presents with hypotension, shock, hypoglycaemia, nausea, vomiting, severe asthenia and dilutional hyponatraemia. In many cases, hypopituitarism is insidious in onset and the manifestations depend on the hormones that are deficient.

Growth hormone (GH) is the first hormone to be affected in most cases of evolving hypopituitarism followed by gonadotropins (follicle stimulating hormone and luteinizing hormone and then thyrotropin (thyroid stimulating hormone [TSH] and adrenocorticotrophic hormone [ACTH]). Prolactin levels are usually elevated because of a loss of normal inhibitory tone of the dopaminergic neurones. Prolactin levels are low only when the pituitary is completely destroyed or aplastic (apoplexy, congenital). GH deficiency in children presents as failure to thrive. In adults features include obesity due to increased visceral fat, symptoms of tiredness and fatigability with increased insulin sensitivity in those with diabetes. Fine wrinkling around the mouth and eyes may be a prominent feature. Women with hypopituitarism are amenorrhoeic and infertile due to a lack of gonadotropins. Men often have decreased libido, diminished body hair and beard, gynaecomastia and increased body fat. Both men and women with gonadotropin deficiency may have a low bone mass. Deficiency of TSH presents as hypothyroidism with pale puffy skin, fatigue and cold intolerance without goitre. In hypopituitarism of insidious onset, ACTH deficiency manifests as fatigue, loss of appetite, weight loss, decreased skin and nipple pigmentation but without skin hyperpigmentation or hyperkalaemia. There is likely to be an abnormal response to stress with fever, hypotension and hyponatraemia. In cases where the posterior pituitary is involved, features are those of thirst (if preserved) polyuria and hypernatraemia. Hypopituitarism is insidious in onset and screening individuals at risk is important (Box 19.1).

Box 19.1 Conditions at high risk of hypopituitarism

- Patients with hypothalamic or pituitary mass lesions
- Infants with craniofacial abnormalities
- Previous irradiation to head and neck
- Systemic inflammatory disorders that may affect the pituitary and/or the hypothalamus
- Cerebral granulomatous diseases
- Following head trauma
- Previous skull-base surgery
- Incidental finding of an empty sella
- Post-partum haemorrhage with failure of lactation

Investigations should include baseline tests which are usually adequate to diagnose TSH and gonadotropin deficiency but further dynamic tests are necessary to assess ACTH and GH reserve (Table 19.2).

Glucocorticoid replacement should always precede thyroxine replacement in cases where both hormones are deficient. Thyroxine accelerates the degradation of cortisol and

Table 19.2 Investigations for pituitary reserve

Hormone	Baseline tests	Dynamic test
Growth hormone (GH)	GH, insulin-like growth factor-1, lipid profile	Insulin tolerance test Growth hormone releasing hormone + arginine Glucagon test
Thyrotropin (TSH)	TSH, free T_4	None necessary
Gonadotropin (FSH, LH)	FSH, LH, testosterone/oestradiol	None necessary
Adrenocorticotrophic hormone (ACTH)	Cortisol and ACTH	Short ACTH stimulation (Synacthen) test Metyrapone test

FSH = follicle-stimulating hormone; LH = luteinizing hormone.

can therefore precipitate adrenal crisis in patients with a low pituitary reserve. GH replacement is often not required. It is indicated in some cases where the individual remains symptomatic with tiredness, fatigue, lack of concentration with a general deterioration in quality of life despite adequate replacement of other hormone deficiencies. In some case of hypopituitarism, the concomitant hyperprolactinaemia causes relative hypogonadism and therefore treatment with dopamine agonists usually corrects the problem. In all other cases, testosterone (men) and oestrogen (women) replacement is necessary. In men, testosterone replacement reduces visceral fat and improves muscle strength. In both men and women, sex hormone replacement improves bone mass. Testosterone replacement should be monitored by serial prostate specific antigen (PSA) measurements.

Treatment involves correcting the underlying hormone defect:

- ACTH deficiency—prednisolone 5–7.5 mg once daily; hydrocortisone 10 mg (waking) and 5 mg (evening). An extra dose of 5 mg may be required at lunchtime.
- Gonadotropin deficiency—ethinyloestradiol with or without progesterone in women and testosterone in men
- Thyrotropin deficiency—L-thyroxine 100–200 μg/day
- Diabetes insipidus—nasal desmopressin—0.05–0.1 ml twice daily. The diagnosis and management of pituitary failure is summarized in Figure 19.1.

Recent Developments

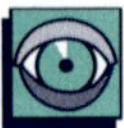

1 Congenital or genetic causes of pituitary failure are increasingly being recognized and characterized.[1] Failure of hormone secretion often arises because of mutations in the genes for key transcription factors.

2 Recent evidence[2] suggests that the state of apathy reported by many hypopituitary patients is a specific disorder and favourable response to stimulants such as methylphenidate has been reported. These drugs are normally reserved for patients with attention deficit/hyperactivity syndrome.

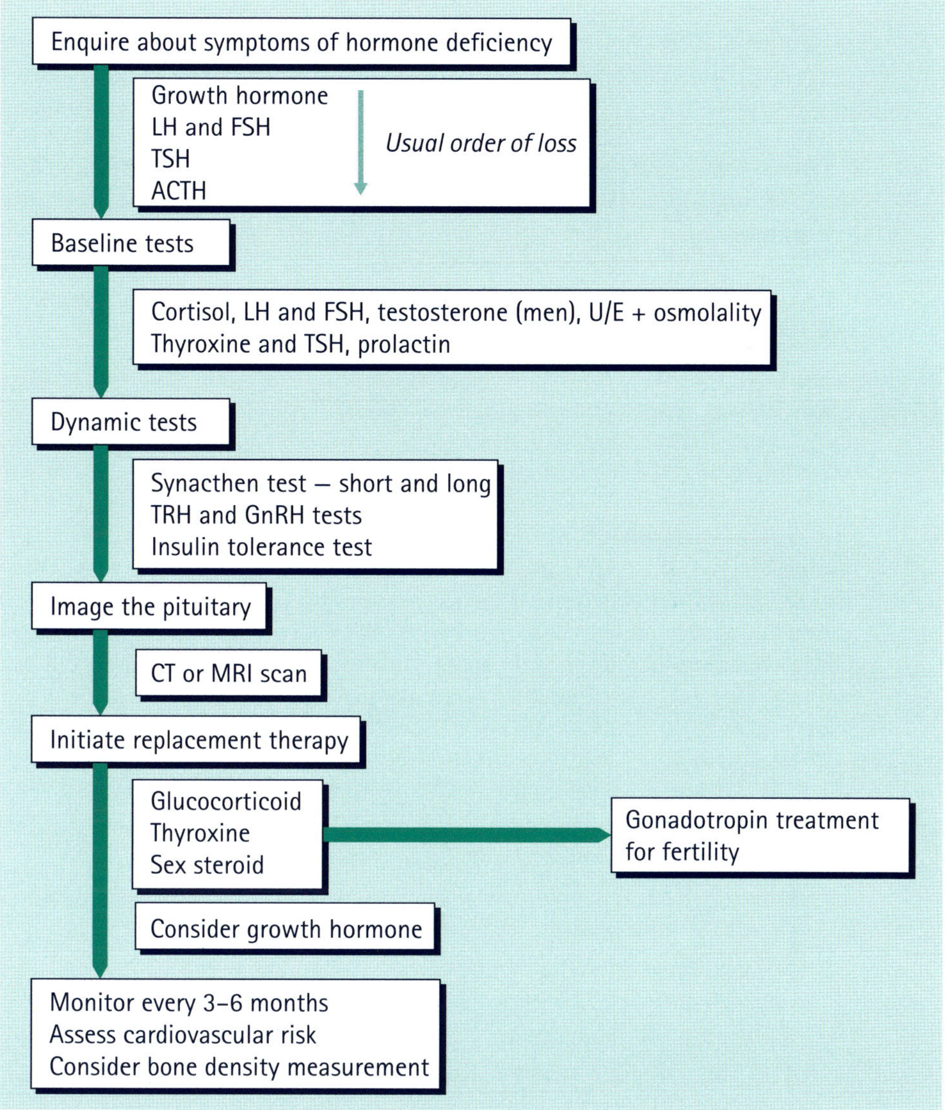

Fig. 19.1 Diagnosis and management of hypopituitarism. ACTH = adrenocorticotrophic hormone; FSH = follicle-stimulating hormone; GnRH = gonadotropin-releasing hormone; LH = luteinizing hormone; TRH = thyrotropin-releasing hormone; TSH = thyroid-stimulating hormone (thyrotropin); U/E = urea and electrolytes.

3 Traumatic brain injury (TBI) is a common clinical presentation affecting 1:1000 of the population each year. Pituitary dysfunction is common, affecting up to 30% and, although it usually is present in the post-acute phase, it may present in the chronic/recovery phase.[3] This complication of head injury is often overlooked. Diabetes insipidus is fairly common in people with TBI and is easy to recognize. Anterior pituitary hormone deficiencies are harder to recognize and often missed if specific tests are not carried out, and the effect of GH deficiency in particular is often not appreciated.

4 The use of GH in adults with relative deficiency associated with ageing remains controversial. However, it is no longer controversial to use GH in adults with proved deficiency.[4] GH replacement improves bone density, increases lean body mass, decreases fat mass, improves cardiac performance and exercise tolerance, and enhances mood and wellbeing. In the recent study by Arwert *et al.*[5] spinal bone mineral density (BMD) increased over 10 years of treatment and there was a favourable effect on lipid profile. However, hip BMD did not increase and there were no lasting benefits on body composition.

Conclusions

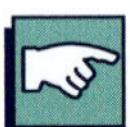

It is usually possible to make a diagnosis of the cause of pituitary failure. The above patient may well have hypopituitarism as a result of TBI. Typically GH secretion is lost, followed by (in order of decreasing frequency) gonadotropins, TSH, and ACTH. CT or MRI scan of the pituitary may well be normal but should be carried out to exclude pituitary tumour. It is unlikely that there will be spontaneous recovery in cases where there are hormone deficiencies for longer than 4–6 months after head injury. The patient's pituitary function should be carefully documented and necessary replacement should be instituted. Other deficiencies should be corrected before considering GH replacement. This is because of the cost and inconvenience associated with the treatment, and also because of lack of evidence regarding its long-term benefits. He should be seen at 3–6-monthly intervals to assess residual pituitary function and the adequacy of replacement therapy.

Further Reading

1 Dattani MT. Growth hormone deficiency and combined pituitary hormone deficiency: does the genotype matter? *Clin Endocrinol* 2005; **63**: 121–30.

2 Weitzer MA, Kanfer S, Booth-Jones M. Apathy and pituitary disease: it has nothing to do with depression. *J Neuropsychiatry Clin Neurosci* 2005; **17**: 159–66.

3 Schneider M, Schneider HJ, Stall GK. Anterior pituitary hormone abnormalities following traumatic brain injury. *J Neurotrauma* 2005; **22**: 937–46.

4 Popovic V, Aimaretti G, Casaneuva FF, Ghigo E. Hypopituitarism following traumatic brain injury (TBI): call for attention. *J Endocrinol Invest* 2005; **28**: 61–4.

5 Gharib H, Cook DM, Saenger PH, *et al*; American Association of Clinical Endocrinologists Growth Hormone Task Force. American Association of Clinical Endocrinologists medical guidelines for clinical practice for growth hormone use in adults and children—2003 update. *Endocr Pract* 2003; **9**: 65–76.

6 Arwert LI, Roos JC, Lips P, Twisk JWR, Manoliu RA, Drent ML. Effects of 10 years of growth hormone (GH) replacement therapy in adult GH deficient men. *Clin Endocrinol* 2005; **63**: 310–16.

SECTION FOUR 04

Reproductive

PROBLEM

20 Primary Amenorrhoea

Case History

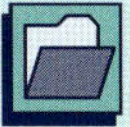

A 17-year-old girl attends seeking advice. She is very worried that her periods have not started yet. She is of normal height (1.6 m [5′ 6″]). Her breast development is limited and this is also a cause for concern. Apart from mild childhood asthma, there is no medical history of note. She is very active and competes at a high level in athletics. She does not take any medications.

Are investigations warranted at this stage and, if so, what?

What general advice would you give her?

Outline a plan for her follow-up.

Background

Primary amenorrhoea is the absence of menarche by the age of 16 years in presence of normal secondary sex characteristics. Investigations should be started by this age if the girl has not had any periods. Earlier age (12–13 years) for commencement of investigations is advised in cases where there is a history of cyclic pelvic pain or no secondary sex

Table 20.1 Common causes of primary amenorrhoea

Causes	Relative frequency (%)	Conditions
Chromosomal abnormalities and ovarian failure	50	Gonadal dysgenesis, commonly due to Turner's syndrome
Hypothalamic hypogonadism	20	Functional hypothalamic amenorrhoea
Mullerian dysgenesis	15	Mayer–Rokitansky–Kuster–Hauser (MRKH) syndrome
Transverse vaginal septum or imperforate hymen	5	
Hypothalamic and pituitary disease	5	Congenital gonadotropin-releasing hormone deficiency Hyperprolactinaemia Craniopharyngioma Haemochromatosis Sarcoidosis
Other causes	5	Androgen insensitivity syndrome 5α-reductase deficiency Congenital adrenal hyperplasia Polycystic ovarian syndrome

characteristics have appeared. All causes of secondary amenorrhoea can present as primary amenorrhoea. The common pathological causes that lead to primary amennorhoea are shown in Table 20.1.

Evaluation of the patient with primary amenorrohea should include a detailed history focusing on certain important aspects:

- pubertal development; growth velocity development of secondary sex characteristics
- family history of delayed puberty
- neonatal and childhood illness if any
- symptoms of virilization if any
- history of recent stress, extreme diet or exercise
- drugs
- symptoms of hypothalamic–pituitary disease—headache, visual defects, galactorrhoea.

Physical examination should include measurement of height and comparing it with rest of family members, breast development and examination of the external genitalia in addition to a thorough general examination. Baseline endocrine tests, follicle-stimulating hormone (FSH), luteinizing hormone (LH), thyroid-stimulating hormone, free T_4, oestradiol and testosterone should give clues for further testing. Pelvic ultrasound to detect the presence or absence of an intact uterus remains mandatory.

Functional disturbances are much more common than the above disease states. An approach to the assessment of the patient with primary amenorrhoea is shown in Figure 20.1. The

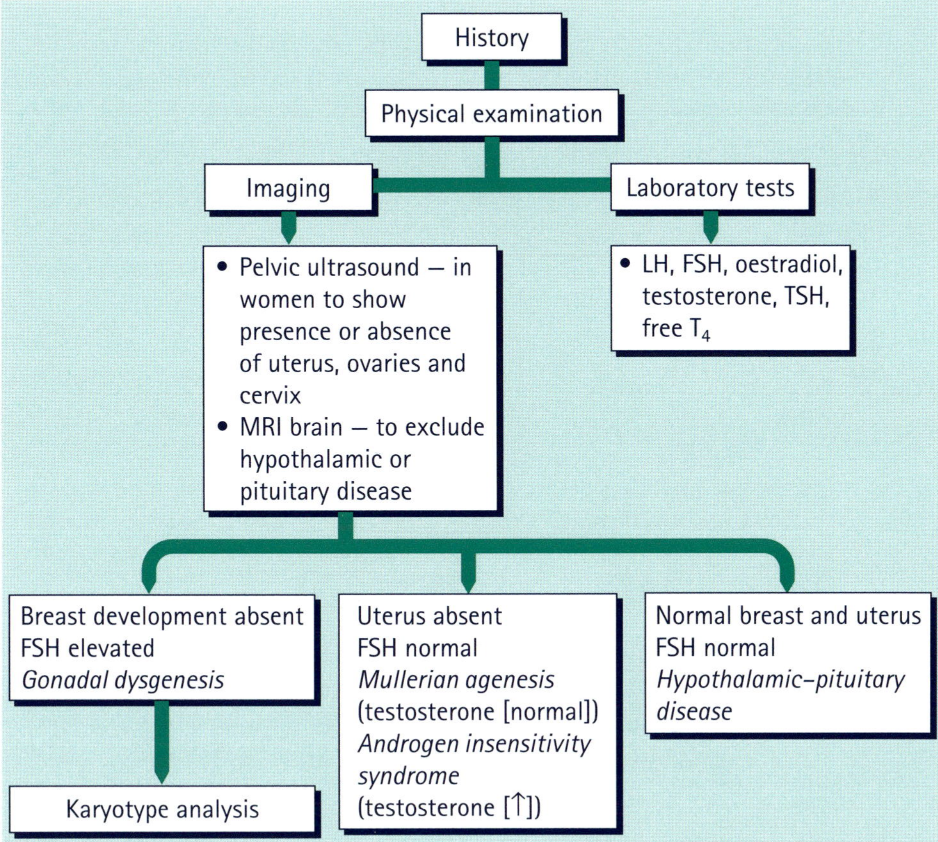

Fig. 20.1 Overview of assessment for amenorrhoea. Investigation should be undertaken in all cases after a careful clinical assessment. A precise diagnosis will allow the patient to be informed regarding the prognosis for development and fertility. FSH = follicle-stimulating hormone; LH = luteinizing hormone; TSH = thyroid-stimulating hormone.

clinical assessment should always include enquiry about diet and exercise. Body mass is probably the major trigger to puberty and the development of a normal menstrual cycle. In a recent study comparing female ballet dancers with age-matched controls,[1] the age at menarche was later in the ballet dancers and there was a higher prevalence of menstrual disorders, with 20% of the ballet dancers having amenorrhoea and 10% having oligomenorrhoea. The term 'female athlete triad' has been given to the combination of eating disorder, amenorrhoea and osteoporosis associated with a high level of participation in sporting activities.[2] The prevalence of primary amenorrhoea is less than 1% in the general female population compared with 20% in athletes performing at a high level. Women with the female athlete triad have a high prevalence of self-induced vomiting and purgative abuse. More subtle degrees of reproductive dysfunction are present in up to three-quarters of elite female athletes. These include anovulation and luteal phase disorders.

The possibility of an eating disorder should be borne in mind in all women with primary amenorrhoea. As with the female athlete triad, there is a disturbance of LH pulse frequency and amplititude. Anorexia nervosa occurs in 0.3–1% of the female population.[3]

There is often an association with compulsive exercise and patients frequently describe a fear of getting fat and have a disturbed body image. The disorder occurs in two patterns—food restriction and binging/purging. There is an increased frequency of other psychiatric diagnoses including depression, anxiety, obsessive–compulsive disorder and alcohol/substance misuse. The disorder commonly starts in adolescence and up to 70% make a full recovery. Of those who continue with anorexia into adulthood or develop the condition in adult life, less than 50% make a full recovery. There is considerable increased morbidity and an increased risk of premature death with the disorder. The focus of early treatment is usually on re-feeding, starting at 1200–1500 kcal/day. Patients are best managed by a multidisciplinary team, including a psychiatrist with special expertise in managing eating disorders. Drug treatments, including antidepressants and antipsychotic medications may have a role in some patients, particularly in preventing relapse.

Recent Developments

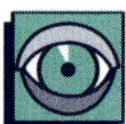

1. There is a question whether menstrual disturbance should be used as a diagnostic criterion for eating disorder.[4] Amenorrhoea or oligomenorrhoea are not only present in nearly all patients with anorexia nervosa, but also in a quarter of patients with eating disorder not specified and 15% of patients with bulimia nervosa.
2. Type 1 diabetes is associated with a high prevalence of menstrual and fertility disorders.[5] In a small percentage of cases this is due to associated autoimmune conditions such as hypophysitis and ovarian failure, but for most it is due to functional disturbances which are commoner in patients with poor glycaemic control. The coexistence of insulin deficiency and insulin resistance may be relevant in some patients.
3. Leptin is an exclusive product of the adipocyte and has a critical role in energy balance. Leptin receptors are present on the hypothalamic neurones that control energy balance and reproductive function. In a recent study,[6] administration of recombinant human leptin twice daily for up to 3 months restored feeding behaviour and normalized abnormalities in the pituitary–gonadal axis in a small number of women with hypothalamic amenorrhoea. Thyroid function was also returned to normal but abnormalities in cortisol secretion persisted.

Conclusions

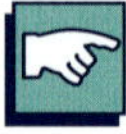

The above patient should undergo a thorough clinical assessment directed at detecting diseases of the hypothalamic–pituitary–gonadal axis. Attention should be paid to determining whether energy intake is meeting the requirements of her energy expenditure. When investigation is required it should be directed at establishing whether there is normal anatomy of the internal and external genitalia, normal function of the gonadal axis, no destructive or developmental lesions of the hypothalamus and pituitary, and a normal chromosomal complement. She should be advised to maintain or achieve a normal body weight and may need dietician input. Bone density measurement may be appropriate and may be followed by pharmacological measures to prevent further loss of bone mineral. Growth and development should be carefully followed until normal menstruation is established and has been present for at least a year.

Further Reading

1 Stokic E, Srdic B, Barak O. Body mass index, body fat mass and the occurrence of amenorrhea in ballet dancers. *Gynecol Endocrinol* 2005; **20**: 195–9.

2 Louks AB, Nattiv A. Essay: the female athlete triad. *Lancet* 2005; **366**: 549–60.

3 Yager J, Andersen AC. Anorexia nervosa. *N Engl J Med* 2005; **353**: 1481–8.

4 Abraham SF, Pettigrew B, Boyd C, Russell J, Taylor A. Usefulness of amenorrhoea in the diagnosis of eating disorder patients. *J Psychsomat Obstet Gynaecol* 2005; **26**: 211–15.

5 Arrais RF, Dib SA. The hypothalamus–pituitary–ovarian axis and type 1 diabetes; a mini review. *Hum Reprod* 2006; **21**: 327–37.

6 Welt CK, Chan JL, Bullen J, *et al*. Recombinant human leptin in women with hypothalamic amenorrhea. *N Engl J Med* 2004; **351**: 987–97.

PROBLEM

21 Secondary Amenorrhoea

Case History

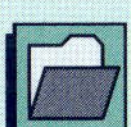

A 22-year-old married woman complains that her periods ceased 6 months ago. She had menarche at the age of 13 and her periods began to be irregular from the age of 18. She has never been pregnant in spite of having unprotected intercourse for 3 years. Her body mass index (BMI) is 31 kg/m^2. There is a strong family history of diabetes and hypertension. Her mother also had problems with irregular periods and had difficulty conceiving.

Discuss the differential diagnosis and investigation?

Is the family history relevant?

How would you manage this patient?

Background

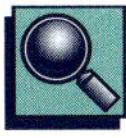

Secondary amenorrhoea is the absence of menses for more than three cycles or 6 months in women who previously had menses. Pregnancy remains the commonest cause of secondary amenorrhoea and should be excluded in all women who present with having lost their periods. Other causes are given in Table 21.1.

Table 21.1 Common causes of secondary amenorrhoea

Causes	Relative frequency (%)	Conditions
Ovarian disease	40	Polycystic ovarian syndrome Ovarian failure
Hypothalamic dysfunction	35	Functional hypothalamic amenorrhoea Anorexia nervosa Exercise and stress Congenital gonadotropin-releasing hormone deficiency Infiltrative disease—haemochromatosis, lymphoma, sarcoidosis
Pituitary disease	19	Hyperprolactinaemia Empty sella syndrome
Uterine disease	5	Asherman's syndrome
Other causes	1	Primary hypothyroidism

A pregnancy test (serum β-human chorionic gonadotropin) is the first step in all cases of secondary amenorrhoea. Physical examination should include measurement of height and weight (BMI), breast development and examination of the external genitalia in addition to a thorough general examination. The latter should include examination for acne, striae, vitiligo and acanthosis nigricans. Baseline endocrine tests, follicle-stimulating hormone (FSH), luteinizing hormone (LH), thyroid stimulating hormone, free T_4 and oestradiol are measured in all cases. Testosterone and dehydro-3-epiandrosterone sulphate should be measured if there are signs of virilization. Assessment of a patient with secondary amenorrhoea is summarized in Figure 21.1. Asherman's syndrome is an uncommon condition where extensive scarring within the uterine cavity leads to decreased menstrual function and reduced fertility. It may follow dilatation and curettage, uterine infection, or surgery to the uterus.

Polycystic ovarian syndrome (PCOS) is the commonest cause of menstrual irregularity and may be present in up to 3–5% of women.[1,2] It is associated with obesity but up to a fifth of women with the syndrome are of normal weight. The common clinical features of the syndrome are menstrual irregularity (oligomenorrhoea or amenorrhoea), hirsutism and other signs of androgen excess (acne and frontal balding) and decreased fertility. Patients usually have a normal menarche. The major biochemical abnormalities in PCOS are dysregulation of pulsatile release of LH and FSH leading to an increased LH/FSH ratio, insulin resistance, and increased androgen levels. Oestrogen levels are usually normal and high and the increased androgens arise both from enhanced ovarian secretion and increased peripheral conversion of oestrogen to androgen. The high levels of androgen and insulin contribute to decreased sex hormone-binding globulin (SHBG) levels which further increases the amount of free androgen available. Although signs of androgen excess are common, it is rare for patients to be virilized in PCOS. The combination of androgen excess and insulin resistance is also responsible for acanthosis nigricans—a pigmented thickening of the skin particularly on the neck and in other flexural areas.

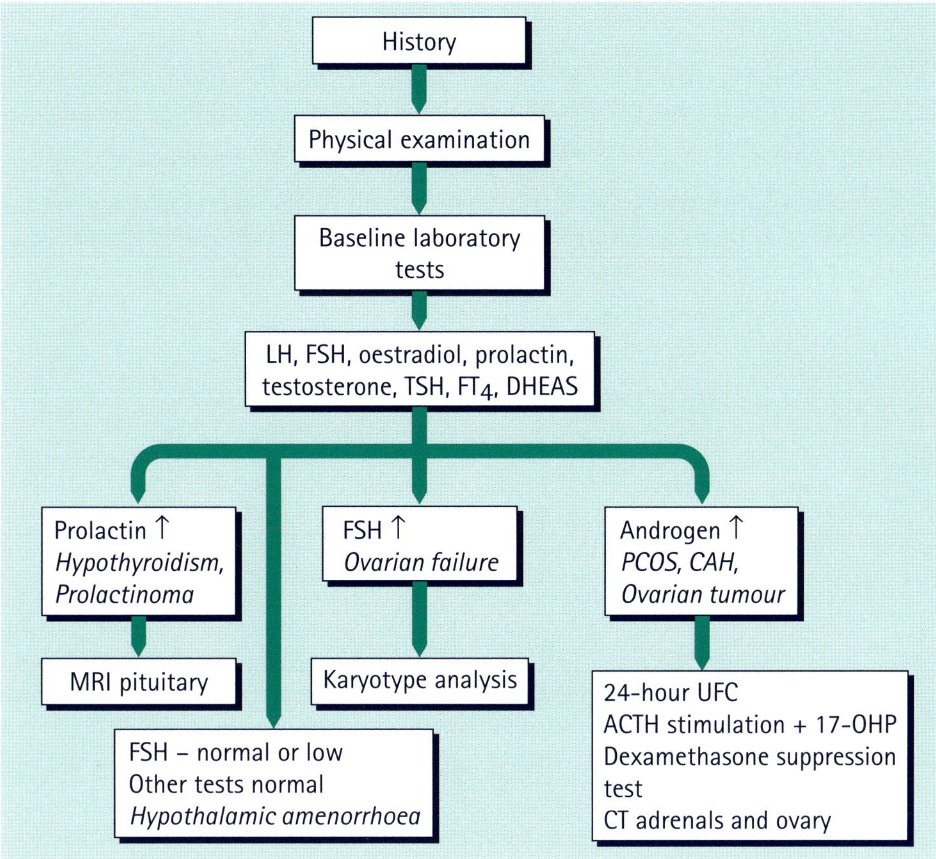

Fig. 21.1 Assessment of patient with secondary amenorrhoea. ACTH = adrenocorticotrophic hormone; CAH = congenital adrenal hypoplasia; DHEAS = dehydro-3-epiandrosterone sulphate; FSH = follicle-stimulating hormone; LH = luteinizing hormone; PCOS = polycystic ovarian syndrome; TSH = thyroid-stimulating hormone; UFC = urine free cortisol.

There are several important long-term complications which women with PCOS are at increased risk of. The prevalence of glucose intolerance and type 2 diabetes may be as high as 31% and 7%, respectively.[1] The risk of hypertension is also increased and this, along with glucose intolerance and dyslipidaemia, contribute to the reported threefold increase in risk of cardiovascular disease. There is increased risk of endometrial cancer due to prolonged, unopposed oestrogenic stimulation. Increased oestrogen exposure has also been implicated as a causative factor in breast cancer, the incidence of which may be slightly increased after the menopause in patients with PCOS. Further epidemiological evidence on the latter, and also to substantiate whether the incidence of ovarian cancer is increased, is required.

Treatment of women with PCOS is determined by what the predominant symptoms are. Lifestyle modification is a key element as weight loss and exercise will improve insulin sensitivity, and thus decrease many of the features of the syndrome. Oestrogen-containing contraceptive pills are used to regulate menstruation. However, in addition this oestrogen decreases ovarian androgen production and, by increasing SHBG level, decreases the amount of free androgen available. Combination oral contraceptive pill preparations should be used to ensure regular shedding of the endometrium. Women who opt not to take combination hormone treatment, or those in whom it is contraindicated, should be advised to use progesterone at least once every 6 months to prevent severe endometrial hyperplasia. Metformin has now been used for over a decade in women with PCOS. Improved insulin sensitivity may protect against development of diabetes and decrease androgen levels, although clinical benefit with regard to hirsutism is often limited. The drug has also been used to assist with induction of regular ovulation and thus restore fertility. The thiazolidinediones have similar clinical benefits and these are not limited to patients who are obese.

Recent Developments

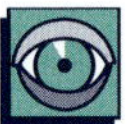

1. A recent trial compared the effect of metformin with lifestyle modification alone in obese women with PCOS.[2] Lifestyle modification improved body weight and menstrual function but there was no additional effect from metformin. The high usage of metformin in PCOS has, to an extent, been driven by patient demand.
2. In a recent trial,[3] both metformin and rosiglitazone were effective in improving insulin sensitivity, but rosiglitazone was more effective in decreasing androgen levels and improving menstrual function. Lemay *et al.*[4] have demonstrated that rosiglitazone may be very useful in combination with oestrogen/anti-androgen treatment in patients who have not benefited from simple lifestyle intervention.
3. Epilepsy occurs in 1–2% of the population, and female sufferers have decreased fertility. Valproate is a short-chain fatty acid that is used in the treatment of epilepsy and mood disturbances. Use of valproate is associated with development of features of PCOS, including hyperandrogenism and metabolic syndrome. The drug increases expression of genes in the theca responsible for androgen synthesis.[5]
4. Early fetal exposure to increased androgen may be one factor in determining future risk of developing PCOS.[6] Environmental and genetic factors interact. One extensively studied gene for susceptibility to insulin resistance and metabolic syndrome is the *PPAR-γ* gene. Certain alleles of this gene may protect women with PCOS and their first-degree relatives from development of type 2 diabetes.[7]
5. In a large cohort of PCOS patients,[8] type 2 diabetes was present in 6.6%. In the remainder, waist circumference of greater than 88 cm was present in 80%, low high-density lipoprotein cholesterol in 66%, high triglycerides in 32%, and blood pressure greater than 130/85 mmHg in 21%. Overall, 33.4% of patients without type 2 diabetes had three or more features of the metabolic syndrome.

Conclusions

PCOS is by far the commonest cause of secondary amenorrhoea. PCOS has been a hard condition to define, and the underlying causes have been poorly understood until recently. Polymorphisms in a number of genes have now been identified as altering susceptibility to PCOS and other high androgen states. The family history of the above patient is, therefore, likely to be relevant. Management of women with PCOS should always include consideration of lifestyle factors in the first instance. Insulin-sensitizing drugs are now widely used in practice, but they should be used in addition to diet and exercise. These drugs are most useful clinically in restoring menstrual function and ovulation. Modest weight loss with or without insulin-sensitizing drug may lead to success in a high proportion of patients.

Further Reading

1 Ehrmann DA. Polycystic ovary syndrome. *N Engl J Med* 2005; **352**: 1223–36.

2 Tang T, Glanville J, Hayden CJ, White D, Barth JH, Balen AH. Combined lifestyle modification and metformin in obese patients with polycystic ovary syndrome. A randomized, placebo-controlled, double-blind multicentre study. *Clin Endocrinol* 2006; **21**: 80–9.

3 Yilmaz M, Biri A, Karakoc A, *et al.* The effects of rosiglitazone and metformin on insulin resistance in obese and lean patients with polycystic ovary syndrome. *J Clin Endocrinol Metab* 2005; **28**: 1003–8.

4 Lemay A, Dodin S, Turcot L, Dechene F, Forest JC. Rosiglitazone and ethinyl estradiol/cyproterone acetate as single and combined treatment of overweight women with polycystic ovary syndrome and insulin resistance. *Hum Reprod* 2006; **21**: 121–8.

5 Wood JR, Nelson-Degrave VL, Jansen E, McAllister JM, Mosselman S, Strauss JF. Valproate-induced alterations in human theca cell gene expression: clues to the association between valproate use and metabolic side effects. *Physiol Genomics* 2005; **20**: 233–43.

6 Franks S, McCarthy MI, Hardy K. Development of polycystic ovary syndrome: involvement of genetic and environmental factors. *Int J Androl* 2006; **29**: 278–85.

7 Yilmaz M, Ergun MA, Karakoc A, *et al.* Pro12Ala polymorphism of the peroxisome proliferator-activated receptor-γ gene in first degree relatives of patients with polycystic ovary syndrome. *Gynecol Endocrinol* 2005; **21**: 206–10.

8 Ehrmann DA, Liljenquist DR, Kasza K, Azziz R, Legro R, Ghazzi MN. Prevalence and predictors of the metabolic syndrome in women with polycystic ovary syndrome. *J Clin Endocrinol Metab* 2006; **91**: 48–53.

PROBLEM

22 Polycystic Ovarian Syndrome – Subfertility

Case History

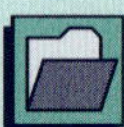

Mrs YT is a 34-year-old bank clerk who had polycystic ovarian syndrome (PCOS) diagnosed 8 years ago. She has been married for some time and is keen to have children but has never managed to conceive. She has read that metformin may be useful. She is not taking any medications. Her body mass index (BMI) is 32.8 kg/m^2. Her major worry is that she is approaching her mid-30s and if something is not done she may lose the chance to have children. She is also concerned about her long-term health.

Would you initiate infertility investigations at this stage?

Is metformin likely to help her conceive?

She accepts that her weight might be a major contributor. What strategies might be employed to help her lose weight and thus increase her chances of conceiving?

What are the risks to her future health?

Background

PCOS is the commonest diagnosed cause of menstrual irregularity and anovulatory infertility in women. It occurs in 3–5% of women, although there have been reports of incidence up to 10%. PCOS accounts for around 90% of women with oligomenorrhoea and 30% of women with amenorrhoea. The causes of anovulatory infertility are summarized as follows:

- Hypothalamic–pituitary failure (hypogonadotropic hypogonadism)—developmental abnormalities, pituitary tumours, trauma, irradiation.
- Hypothalamic–pituitary dysfunction—includes PCOS, luteal phase insufficiency, eating disorders, stress, and excessive exercise. Gonadotropins may be normal or low and, in PCOS, oestrogen levels are usually normal. This group accounts for the vast majority of anovulatory women.
- Ovarian failure—hypergonadotropic.
- Congenital or acquired disorders of the genital tract—do not respond to repeated oestrogen challenge (with or without progestagen).

- Hyperprolactinaemia—with or without pituitary space-occupying lesion. Levels of gonadotropin may be low or normal, with variable effects on menstruation depending on level of prolactin: may present with luteal phase insufficiency.

Even women who are only modestly overweight with PCOS may benefit from weight loss and exercise. A 5% weight loss may be sufficient to restore normal menses and ovulation. Weight loss also improves insulin resistance and lowers androgen levels. Many women with PCOS have tried a variety of means to induce weight loss and it can be very difficult to find an approach that is both acceptable to the patient and effective. A detailed assessment of the patient's food and exercise habits should be undertaken at the outset. It is useful for the patient to complete a food diary. In many centres, local and national guidelines do not recommend fertility treatment for patients with BMI greater than 30 kg/m^2. The optimal dietary approach for patients with PCOS is not known but may differ from dietary advice for the general population. The high insulin state sometimes drives hunger and stimulates desire for high carbohydrate foods. A hypocaloric state can be achieved either by decreasing food intake or by increasing energy expenditure. Drug treatment can be useful for some patients. Orlistat is a safe drug for women with PCOS, although it should be stopped if the patient becomes pregnant. Similarly, sibutramine should be discontinued as soon as pregnancy is confirmed and should not be used in women with uncontrolled hypertension.

The mainstay of treatment for ovulation induction in PCOS has been the non-steroidal oestrogen receptor antagonist clomiphene citrate (CC).[1] The drug is usually given at a dose of 25–50 mg for the first 5 days of the cycle, and it is usual to administer six cycles of treatment before other options are considered. CC can be given in doses of up to 250 mg/day, and regimens ranging from 3 to 10 days have been reported. CC is successful in inducing ovulation in up to 85% of women with PCOS. However, only half with successful ovulation induction become pregnant. It may be that the anti-oestrogen action of the drug contributes to the disparity between the rates of ovulation and pregnancy. CC is less effective in women with severe obesity or insulin resistance, and in those with markedly increased androgen levels. The effect of CC may be increased by adjunct treatment with an insulin-sensitizing drug (metformin). Human chorionic gonadotropin (hCG) may be used with CC to trigger ovulation induction. The risks of CC treatment include ovarian hyperstimulation syndrome and multiple pregnancies.

The use of metformin, either as first-line treatment or as adjunct therapy in women resistant to CC has increased markedly in the past decade.[2] When used as primary treatment, the effect appears to be comparable to that of CC. Metformin treatment has the potential to prevent, or retard the onset of, diabetes. Metformin can also be used with recombinant follicle-stimulating hormone (rFSH) to induce ovulation. There is debate whether metformin should be continued during pregnancy in women who successfully ovulate and conceive. Current practice is to stop the drug as soon as pregnancy is confirmed. Rosiglitazone has also been studied in women with PCOS, and has effects on androgens, menstrual function and ovulation, which are comparable to metformin. The latter is the preferred treatment in women who are trying to become pregnant as experience with rosiglitazone during pregnancy is limited. However, neither drug is licensed for use in PCOS.

Gonadotropin therapy to induce ovulation should be carried out in specialist centres because of the risk of ovarian hyperstimulation and multiple pregnancies. Women with PCOS are particularly sensitive to gonadotropins. Pure or recombinant FSH is now

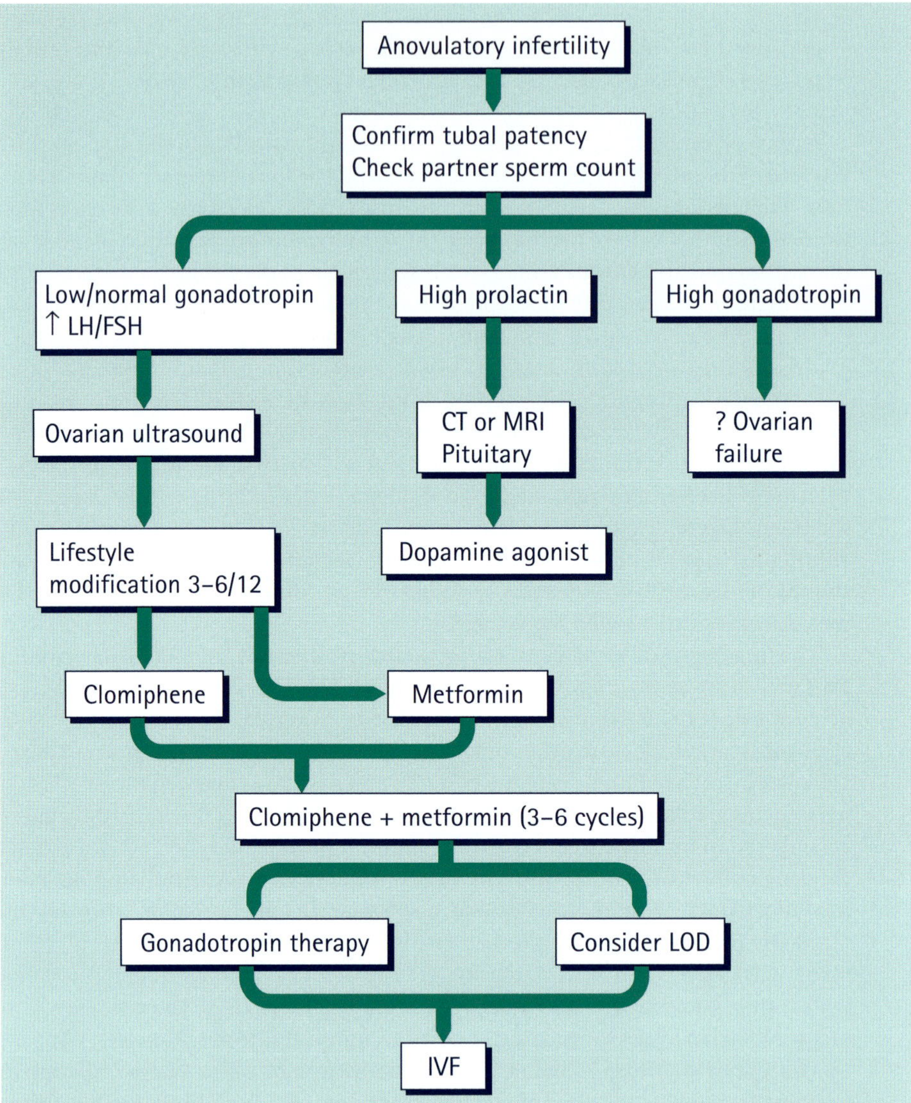

Fig. 22.1 Management of fertility in polycystic ovarian syndrome (PCOS). Weight management drugs (orlistat or sibutramine) may be considered in women who do not respond to lifestyle modification and do not immediately wish to become pregnant. Metformin may be the preferred primary drug treatment in women who have diabetes, are insulin resistant, or overweight. LOD = laparoscopic ovarian drilling.

preferred to human menopausal gonadotropin for inducing follicle development. A low-dose, step-up regimen is commonly employed. Follicle development is carefully monitored with ultrasound and with oestradiol levels. When a single follicle of 16–20 mm diameter has developed, ovulation can be induced with hCG. Older patients, those with increased body weight, and those who are severely insulin resistant are less likely to respond to gonadotropin therapy. Pulsatile gonadotropin-releasing hormone (GnRH) therapy is less widely used, and more complex but has a lesser risk of ovarian hyperstimulation, multiple pregnancies and miscarriage. GnRH agonists are widely used in *in vitro* fertilization and intracytoplasmic sperm injection (ICSI) protocols but not generally required for straightforward ovulation induction. The newer GnRH antagonists (cetrorelix and ganirelix) may also be useful to increase response to gonadotropins, particularly in patients who have high levels of luteinizing hormone.

Aromatase inhibitors (letrozole and anastrozole) can be used to decrease oestrogenic feedback at the pituitary level, and thus induce ovulation in women who are resistant to CC.[2] These drugs appear to be quite effective and safe. Their short half-life is an advantage as they are unlikely to affect the fetus. The management of fertility in patients with PCOS is summarized in Figure 22.1.

Surgical treatment is indicated in a minority of patients. Ovarian wedge technique is no longer in usage, and the most widely applied method is laparoscopic ovarian drilling (LOD) carried out with either an electrolysis needle or with laser—both give similar rates of success. In LOD, four to ten ports are made in each ovary. It is not entirely clear how the surgical techniques bring about clinical benefit. It may be through reduction in the hypersecreting ovarian parenchyma with lower androgen levels allowing for increased FSH secretion and thus maturation of ovarian follicles. It has also been hypothesized that injury to the ovary increased local insulin-like growth factor-1 secretion, and that this may sensitize the ovary to circulating FSH. Other techniques include ovarian diathermy and transvaginal ovarian drilling.

Recent Developments

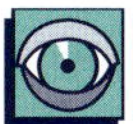

1 Metformin now has an established place in treatment of women with PCOS. Metabolic syndrome is present in up to 50% of patients.[2] The role of the thiazolidinedione drugs remains to be established and, for the present, they should probably be considered as second line drugs for women with insulin resistance.[3]

2 The effect of combined oral contraceptives on cardiovascular risk and long-term complications of PCOS remains uncertain.[4] In general, they do not appear to have any major effect in this regard, although insulin resistance may worsen in a proportion of women with certain preparations.

3 Gonadotropin therapy has been used since the 1930s. It is probably now only justifiable to use pure or recombinant preparations. The need for gonadotropins to be given as injections is a distinct disadvantage. Orally active non-peptide gonadotropin receptor agonists are in development.[5] These compounds may extend the use of gonadotropin therapy to induce ovulation in women with PCOS.

Conclusions

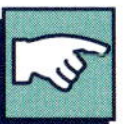

In women with suspected PCOS who wish to conceive, the diagnosis should be confirmed at an early stage both biochemically and with ovarian ultrasound. The sperm count of their partner should be checked and tubal patency assessed. Modest weight loss improves many of the features of PCOS including menstrual function and ovulation. The role of insulin resistance in PCOS is widely recognized and metformin is useful to improve glycaemic status and reproductive function. The major long-term risks of PCOS are type 2 diabetes, cardiovascular disease and endometrial cancer. Although women should be aware of these risks, and steps should be taken to prevent untoward outcomes, it is important not to cause undue alarm in healthy young women seeking fertility advice.

Further Reading

1 Cristello F, Cela V, Artini PG, Genazzi AR. Therapeutic strategies for ovulation induction in infertile women with polycystic ovary syndrome. *Gynecol Endocrinol* 2005; **21**: 340–52.

2 Kashyap S, Wells GA, Rosenwaks Z. Insulin-sensitizing agents as primary therapy for patients with polycystic ovarian syndrome. *Hum Reprod* 2004; **19**: 2474–83.

3 Checa MA, Requena A, Salvador C, *et al.* Reproductive Endocrinology Interest Group of the Spanish Society of Fertility. Insulin-sensitizing agents: use in pregnancy and as therapy in polycystic ovary syndrome. *Hum Reprod Update* 2005; **11**: 375–90.

4 Vrbikova J, Cibula D. Combined oral contraceptives in the treatment of polycystic ovary syndrome. *Hum Reprod Update* 2005; **11**: 277–91.

5 Lunenfeld B. Historical perspectives in gonadotrophin therapy. *Hum Reprod Update* 2004; **10**: 453–67.

PROBLEM

23 Premature Ovarian Failure

Case History

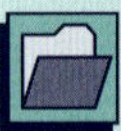

A 36-year-old woman has experienced a gradual decline in menstrual function over the past year. She has had no periods for the past 6 months and has noted frequent facial flushing and vaginal dryness. She previously had no problems with her periods and has had two children, with no difficulty in conceiving. There is no previous history of endocrine or autoimmune disease and no family history of note.

What investigations should be carried out?

Would you recommend that she have oestrogen replacement therapy?

If so, for how long should she be treated?

Background

Premature ovarian failure (POF) can be diagnosed when anovulation and amenorrhoea occur for more than 3 months and are associated with follicle-stimulating hormone (FSH) level greater than 30 U/l in a woman aged under 40 years.[1–3] It occurs in up to 1%

Table 23.1 Causes of premature ovarian failure

Cytogenetic abnormalities and X chromosome defects	Trisomy X (with or without mosaicism) *FMR1* (fragile X gene) premutations A variety of autosomal and X chromosome loci
Enzyme defects	17α-hydroxylase or 17,20-lyase deficiency Aromatase deficiency Galactosaemia
Other genetic defects	Bone morphogenetic protein-15 Inhibin-α gene Autoimmune regulator (*AIRE*) gene Forkhead transcription factor-2
Abnormalities in gonadotropin secretion and action	Mutations of the LH and FSH receptor genes Abnormalities of the β subunits of LH and FSH
Autoimmune	Autoantibodies to a variety of ovarian determinants Associated with other autoimmune diseases (particularly Addison's)
Destruction of ovarian tissue	Surgical damage/removal Pelvic irradiation Chemotherapy Virus (mumps) and toxins

FSH = follicle-stimulating hormone; LH = luteinizing hormone.

of women and, given its frequency, the aetiology of POF is surprisingly poorly understood. The definition does not necessarily imply permanent cessation of ovarian activity as up to 50% of women may continue to have intermittent ovarian activity and up to 25% may ovulate. It follows, therefore, that if the woman is sexually active and does not want to conceive, contraceptive measures should be considered. POF occurs in up to 25% of women with primary amenorrhoea and in up to 20% of women with secondary amenorrhoea. Around 4% of cases are familial, but the vast majority occur sporadically. The number of oocytes peaks at 20 weeks of gestation. Of 7 million potential eggs, only 500 are actually shed during a typical reproductive lifetime.

The cause of POF is not identified in the majority of cases. Potential causes are listed in Table 23.1. There has been extensive work to define underlying genetic causes. Abnormalities in a range of genes, located on the X chromosome and autosomal, have been identified.[3] None of these account for a large proportion of cases, and routine genetic screening is not recommended or available at present.[3] The contribution of genetic studies, thus, to management of patient with suspected POF is limited at present.

The role of autoimmunity is also controversial.[4] Autoantibodies to ovarian components have been described in 30–66% of women with POF. However, a clear role of these autoantibodies in the pathogenesis of ovarian failure remains to be established. They may be a secondary phenomenon in many cases, resulting from abnormal exposure of ovarian antigens during an underlying pathological process. Antibodies have been described to granulosa and theca cells, to zona pellucida, to oocyte cytoplasm, to corpus luteum, and to gonadotropins and their receptors. In some patients, presence of these antibodies is associated with recurrent reproductive failure in the absence of ovarian failure. There is a clearer role for autoimmunity in the ovarian failure associated with the autoimmune polyglandular

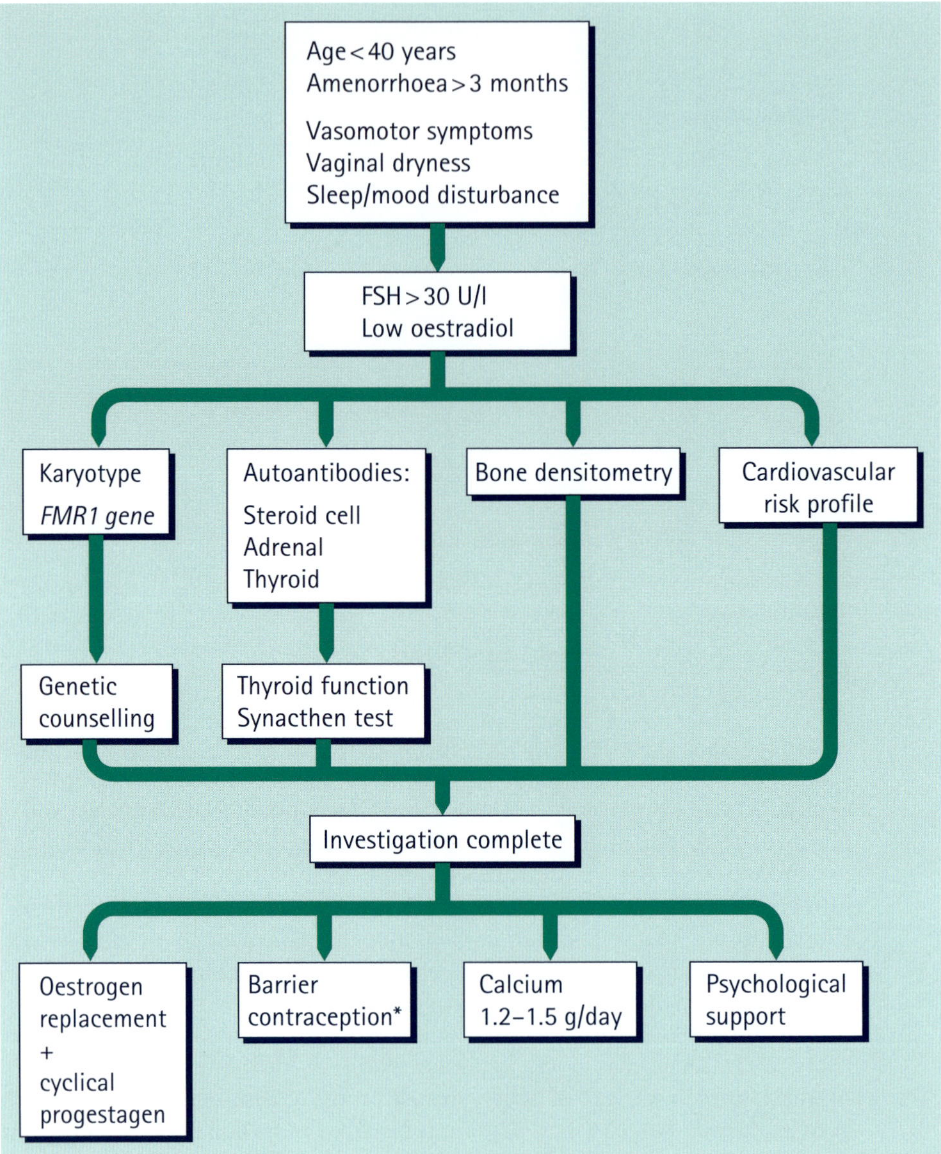

Fig. 23.1 Investigation and management of premature ovarian failure. Risks of osteoporosis and cardiovascular disease are increased in women with POF. Appropriate preventative measures should be taken once screening is complete. *Hormonal contraception is not reliable in the face of high gonadotropins. The correct approach depends upon whether pregnancy is desired. FSH = follicle-stimulating hormone.

syndromes. Antibodies to steroid-secreting cells in the adrenal, ovary (mainly theca interna), placenta, and testes are found in up to 20% of young patients with Addison's disease. The adrenal antibodies are most consistently directed at the 21-hydroxylase enzyme, whereas ovarian antibodies may be against determinants on other steroidogenic enzymes including 17α-hydroxylase and cytochrome P450-side chain cleavage.

The investigation of suspected POF is summarized in Figure 23.1. Diagnosis is made on the basis of increased gonadotropins (FSH $>$ 30 U/l) along with decreased oestradiol and oestrone. Ovarian ultrasound may be considered, but most gynaecologists would not carry out ovarian biopsy routinely. Karyotype should be requested, particularly in younger women and anti-ovarian antibodies, if present, may give a pointer to the underlying aetiology. A progestin challenge test is not routinely warranted. Thyroid function tests should be requested as up to 20% of women will have hypothyroidism. Investigations to exclude adrenal failure should be carried out in those with evidence of autoimmunity and should particularly be considered in younger women. Measurement of FSH on day 3 of the cycle is a useful indicator of incipient ovarian failure. Levels below 10 U/l indicate normal ovarian function, 10–15 U/l is associated with decreased likelihood of conceiving and with levels of 20 U/l and above the patient is unlikely to conceive.

The mainstay of treatment is replacement doses of oestrogen. Women with POF tend to require higher doses of oestrogen than do women who require oestrogen replacement following the menopause. Oestrogen should be administered with progestagen in a regimen that induces monthly bleeding. Other measures may be considered to control vasomotor symptoms. Since a proportion of women can conceive after a diagnosis of POF is made, patients should be counselled regarding contraception. In the face of high gonadotropin levels, hormonal contraception is not indicated as it may not be effective, and women who do not wish to become pregnant should use barrier contraception. There is a strong argument for screening for osteoporosis and patients should be advised to maintain a calcium intake of 1.2–1.5 g/day. This may require oral calcium supplementation. Symptoms such a low libido and general lack of energy may result from androgen deficiency. The role of androgen replacement remains controversial. Although up to 10% of women with POF can conceive spontaneously, there is no treatment known to increase this chance. For those who wish to have children, the major options are donor egg *in vitro* fertilization, embryo donation and adoption.

Recent Developments

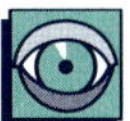

1. The prospects for fertility in women with developing POF are improving.[5] Improved understanding of the genetic or autoimmune basis may lead to earlier identification of patients while there is still a prospect of cryopreserving oocytes or ovarian tissue. It may be preferable to preserve tissue in younger women and preservation of tissue along with a vascular pedicle allows for later re-implantation either at the normal ovarian site (orthotopically) or in the forearm (heterotopically).

2. For patients who have to undergo chemotherapy, induction of hypogonadism with GnRH agonists or antagonists is a novel means of protecting the ovary from the effects of chemotherapeutic agents.[6] A high proportion of patients resume normal ovarian function once chemotherapy is over and the endocrine manipulation is reversed.

3. The notion that the oocyte complement may be supplemented from stem cells during adult life is an exciting, but controversial one.[7] Germline stem cells within the ovary may be induced to differentiate into mature oocytes. Bone-marrow-derived stem cells may also be induced to differentiate into oocytes.

4 For those who do not have autoimmune polyglandular syndrome, antibodies directed at the zona pellucida seem to be the most consistently detected of the ovarian auto-antibodies.[8] Insolubilized antigen may be used as the basis for an immunoassay. However, more precise measurement and screening methods will rely on precise identification of the antigen.

Conclusions

Using current definitions, premature ovarian failure occurs in up to 25% of women with primary amenorrhoea and in 20% with secondary amenorrhoea. The condition remains incompletely understood. Investigations will demonstrate high gonadotropin levels in the face of decreased oestrogen. Cyclical oestrogen therapy should be considered until the age of normal menopause. This may help to improve cardiovascular health and to protect against development of osteoporosis. The condition can cause considerable psychological distress, particularly if the patient desires to have children, and this aspect of management should not be neglected.

Further Reading

1 Rebar RW. Mechanisms of premature menopause. *Endocrinol Metab Clin North Am* 2005; **34**: 923–33.

2 Nelson LM, Covington SN, Rebar RW. An update: spontaneous premature ovarian failure is not an early menopause. *Fertil Steril* 2005; **83**: 1325–32.

3 Goswami D, Conway GS. Premature ovarian failure. *Hum Reprod Update* 2005; **11**: 391–410.

4 Monnier-Barbarino P, Forges T, Faure GC, Bene MC. Gonadal antibodies interfering with female reproduction. *Best Pract Res Clin Endocrinol Metab* 2005; **19**: 135–48.

5 Lobo RA. Potential options for preservation of fertility in women. *N Engl J Med* 2005; **353**: 64–73.

6 Franke HR, Smit WM, Vermes I. Gonadal protection by a gonadotropin-releasing hormone agonist depot in young women with Hodgkin's disease undergoing chemotherapy. *Gynecol Endocrinol* 2005; **20**: 274–8.

7 Bukovsky A. Can ovarian infertility be treated with bone marrow- or ovary-derived germ cells? *Reprod Biol Endocrinol* 2005; **3**: 36–9.

8 Kelkar RL, Meherji PK, Kadam SS, Gupta SK, Nandedkar TD. Circulating auto-antibodies against the zona pellucida and thyroid microsomal antigen in women with premature ovarian failure. *J Reprod Immunol* 2005; **66**: 53–67.

PROBLEM

24 Hirsutism

Case History

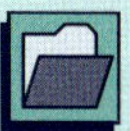

Miss HM is a 26-year-old woman who has been troubled with hirsutism since her late teens. She finds the problem so embarrassing that it interferes with her social functioning. Her periods are reasonably regular and she has no past medical history of note. She is not taking any medication at present and has not previously been investigated or treated for hirsutism.

What is the differential diagnosis?

What investigations are appropriate to screen for underlying pathology?

What treatment options are available, and what precautions should be taken with them?

Background

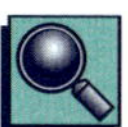

Hirsutism affects between 5 and 15% of women.[1] The condition frequently causes distress to patients, and care has to be taken that complex endocrine investigations do not unduly raise expectations about rapid improvement or even cure. Hirsutism is defined as excessive growth of terminal hairs in areas of the body normally associated with male-type hair distribution. It has to be distinguished from hypertrichosis, which is a more generalized overgrowth of hair and is most commonly drug induced.

The full adult complement of around 5 million hair follicles is present by 22 weeks of gestation. The differentiation of fine, pale vellus hair into course, dark terminal hair is androgen dependent. The androgen concentration threshold for this differentiation varies in different sites in the body, explaining the different hair distribution between men and women. Hirsutism arises because of increased production of androgens, increased bioavailability of androgens or because of increased sensitivity to androgens. The growth of hair takes place in three distinct phases:

- Anagen—this is the active growing phase of hair growth, occupying 70–85% of the life cycle of a hair.
- Catagen—in this phase there is no hair growth and a portion of the follicle regresses; this occupies about 3% of the hair cycle (the phase typically lasts a few weeks).
- Telogen—this is the resting phase of the hair cycle and typically occupies around 15% of the cycle (a period of up to 3 months).

The Ferriman–Gallwey score remains a very useful clinical tool. Nine areas of the body are considered and each is awarded a score of 0 (no hair) to 4 (very severe) depending on the degree of hirsutism.[1] A score of 8–15 is considered moderate hirsutism, above 15 is severe. All patients should have a thorough assessment, appropriate to the clinical setting—consider the family and racial background, and check for signs of virilization (deepening of the voice, frontal balding, increased musculature, enlargement of the clitoris). The presence of acne also points to a high androgen state. Polycystic ovarian syndrome (PCOS) is by far the commonest underlying cause of hirsutism—take a reproductive history, consider whether the patient is overweight, look for acanthosis nigricans. Consider other underlying causes: Cushing's, congenital adrenal hyperplasia, acromegaly, prolactinoma, hypothyroidism (increases hair growth by decreasing sex hormone-binding globulin [SHBG], and thus increasing free androgen).

Of women with moderate hirsutism (score 8–15), 50% have idiopathic hirsutism, and PCOS is by far the most common diagnosis in the remainder. There is considerable overlap in biochemical and clinical features between women with idiopathic hirsutism and those who are hyperandrogenaemic. In women with idiopathic hirsutism, subtle biochemical abnormalities may be apparent on dynamic testing. These include increased androgen response to Synacthen. Women with moderate hirsutism presenting to a medical practitioner should all be investigated. Serum testosterone, SHBG, and thyroid function is a suitable minimum battery of tests. Not all women with moderate hirsutism require referral to an endocrinologist (Figure 24.1).

SHBG levels are decreased in women with high androgens, as well as in patients with hypothyroidism. This increases free androgen levels. Direct measurement of free testosterone is not widely available. Free androgen index (FAI) is widely used, although the reference ranges vary from centre to centre. FAI is calculated as follows: testosterone (nmol/l)/SHBG (nmol/l) $\times$ 100. The normal range for women is 0–11 and for men is 25–190. Other methods to indirectly calculate free testosterone are available.

All women with severe hirsutism (score $>$ 15) should be thoroughly investigated (Figure 24.1). As baseline check the following: thyroid function; prolactin; androgens (testosterone, androstenedione, dehydroepiandrosterone sulphate); luteinizing hormone and follicle-stimulating hormone (taking note of the stage of the menstrual cycle); SHBG; 17-hydroxyprogesterone (17-OHP); and cortisol. A sinister cause should be excluded in all women with severe hirsutism, those with features of virilization, in which there are very high levels of androgens, and where the condition appears suddenly and advances rapidly. Investigation in the post-menopausal woman presents a particular problem. One condition that is frequently overlooked is ovarian hyperthecosis. It is a benign condition and may particularly occur in women who are insulin resistant and have a past history of PCOS.

Women with high androgens have either an adrenal or ovarian source, although local conversion also contributes to serum levels (Table 24.1). Improved hirsutism, acne, and menstrual function should result with hormonal therapy in at least 80% of cases. However, a large proportion of women experienced side effects with their treatment.

Most cases have predominantly ovarian pathology. The PCOS phenotype can be present in patients with adrenal androgen excess. Dehydroepiandrosterone is predominantly an adrenal androgen, and high levels suggest an adrenal pathology. In ovarian disorders, testosterone and androstenedione are predominantly elevated. Steroid suppression is useful in patients with classic and non-classic congenital adrenal hypoplasia, in many patients with high androgen levels without menstrual dysfunction, in a proportion of patients with idiopathic hirsutism, and in some with PCOS.

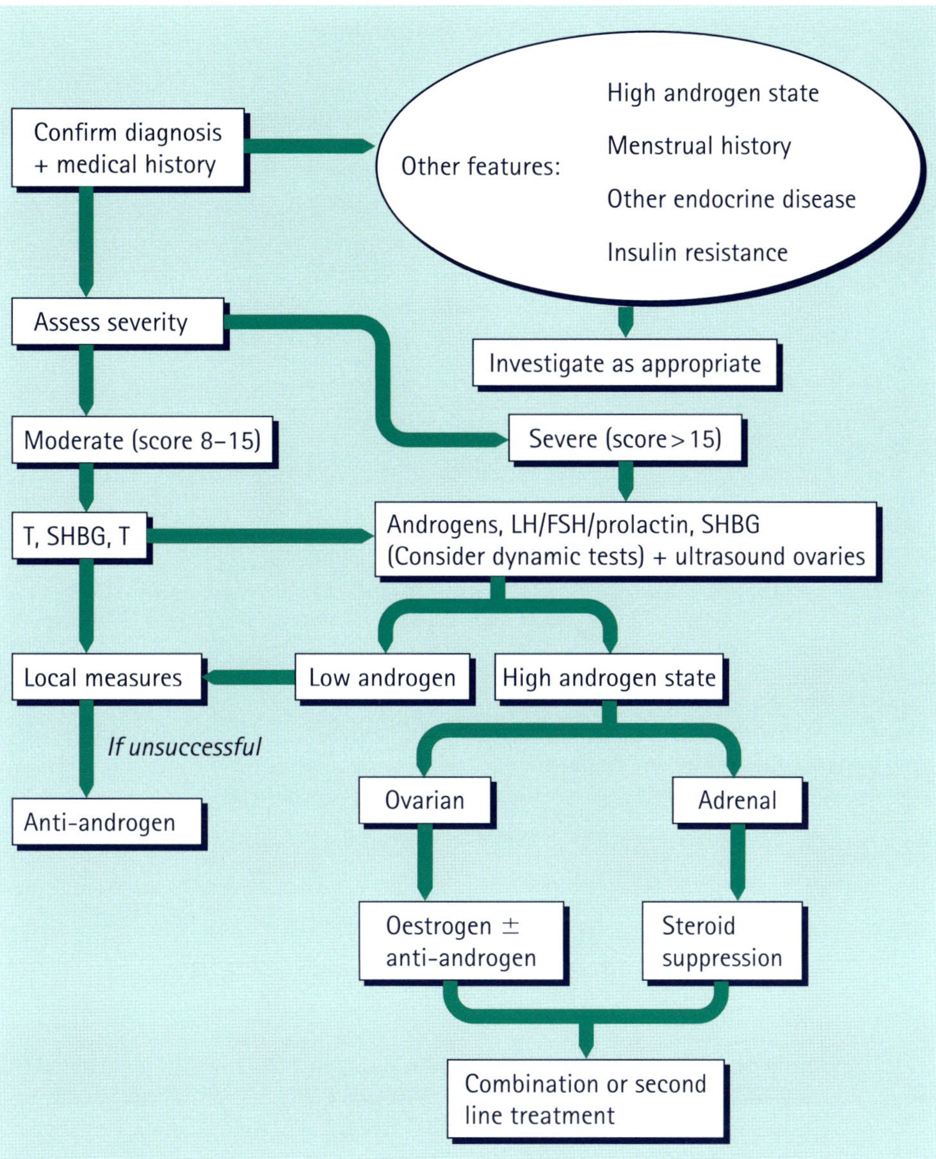

Fig. 24.1 Investigation and management of hirsutism. Full medical assessment should be undertaken from the outset in all cases. All women with high androgen states should be fully investigated, and referral to an endocrinologist should be considered. FSH = follicle-stimulating hormone; LH = luteinizing hormone; T = serum testosterone; SHBG = sex hormone-binding globulin.

Local and topical treatments

A detailed review of these is beyond the scope of this work but the reader is referred to two excellent recent reviews.[3,4] Local cosmetic treatments should always be considered as a first line, and as an adjunct in patients undergoing hormonal manipulation as the latter does not generally affect fully differentiated terminal hair. The available treatments are

Table 24.1 Differential diagnosis of high androgen states

Diagnosis	Per cent of patients
Polycystic ovarian syndrome	82.0
Increased androgen + hirsutism with normal menstruation	6.7
Idiopathic hirsutism	4.5
HAIR-AN syndrome	3.8
Non-classic 21-hydroxylase deficiency	2.1
Classic 21-hydroxylase deficiency	0.7
Androgen-secreting tumours	0.2

Adapted from Azziz *et al.*[2] HAIR-AN = HyperAndrogenism—Insulin Resistance—Acanthosis Nigricans.

Table 24.2 Local treatments for hirsutism

Cosmetic	Make-up Bleaching
Depilatory	Shaving Creams (thioglycolic acid)
Temporary epilation (remove hair from follicle)	Plucking Waxing Threading Mechanical devices
Permanent epilation (destroy hair + follicle)	Thermolysis (diathermy) Electrolysis Laser Intense pulsed light Photodynamic therapy (with aminolaevulinic acid)

summarized in Table 24.2. Shaving does not increase the rate of hair growth but, by producing shorter and coarser stubble, may make the patient more aware of the hair. Depilatory creams reduce the disulphide bonds in mature hair causing exfoliation. Epilation techniques require multiple treatments and may take up to 24 months to complete. Laser treatment is most effective and least likely to cause scarring in patients with dark hair and light skin. Those with dark skin require laser of longer wavelength.

Eflornithine 11.5% (Vaniqa) is an irreversible inhibitor of the enzyme ornithine decarboxylase, which converts ornithine to putrescine, a critical step in polyamine synthesis, and therefore hair growth. The cream is applied topically twice a day. Benefit may be apparent within 8 weeks, and up to 80% of women note significant benefit. It can be combined with other medical or topical treatment. Loss of benefit is apparent in many cases within 8 weeks of stopping treatment. Eflornithine inhibits growth of hair during the anagen phase. This is also the phase during which laser treatment is most effective. The two treatments, therefore, can be usefully combined.

Drugs to decrease ovarian androgen production

Since PCOS is by far the commonest diagnosis, the preferred approach in many patients with hirsutism is to decrease the production or limit the action of ovarian androgens, or a combination of both approaches. Combined oral contraceptives are commonly used. The oestrogen inhibits pituitary production of luteinizing hormone, thus greatly decreasing the stimulus to ovarian androgen production. A progestagen that either has low androgenic activity (medroxyprogesterone or dydrogesterone) or anti-androgenic activity (cyproterone) should be chosen.

Gonadotropin-releasing hormone (GnRH) agonists and antagonists have found wide usage in the treatment of men with prostate cancer, in precocious puberty, to lower oestrogen levels in patients with menorrhagia or endometriosis, and in *in vitro* fertilization. The agonists (leuprolide, buserelin, goserelin), after an initial flare on agonist activity, down-regulate GnRH receptors and profoundly inhibit gonadotropin release. Pure antagonists (cetrorelix and ganirelix) are now widely available. Short-term use of the latter may be tried as a diagnostic test if it is not certain that the ovary is the source of excess androgen.

Insulin-sensitizing drugs—metformin and the glitazones—decrease androgen production in women with PCOS, but their benefit in decreasing hirsutism is limited and not usually clinically apparent.

Drugs to decrease adrenal androgen production

This is achieved using slightly higher than physiological doses of glucocorticoid—for example, 5–7.5 mg prednisolone or 0.25–0.5 mg dexamethasone at night. The patient should understand that she is exposed to risks of steroid excess, and periodic measurements of adrenocorticotrophic hormone (ACTH) and adrenal steroids should be undertaken to ensure that suppression of ACTH drive is achieved with the minimum dose of steroid. Ketoconazole, used in the treatment of Cushing's, also blocks androgen production through its inhibitory effect on the 17α-hydroxylase and 17–20 desmolase enzymes.

Drugs to decrease delivery of androgen

SHBG (normal range: male 9–45 nmol/l, female 13–110 nmol/l) is decreased in high androgen states. Pharmacological doses of oestrogen increase SHBG, and thus decrease the levels of free bioavailable androgens. Finasteride is an inhibitor of the enzyme 5α-reductase, which converts testosterone to the more biologically active dihydrotestosterone. As with the anti-androgens, the drug should only be used with adequate contraception, as there would be a risk of feminizing a male foetus.

Anti-androgens

The steroid anti-androgen drugs, cyproterone and spironolactone, are widely used. Cyproterone is more commonly used in Europe, and spironolactone is the preferred drug in the USA and Australia. Cyproterone is most commonly used in combination with ethinyloestradiol at a dose of 2 mg and 35 μg, respectively. In resistant cases, 50 mg and 100 mg doses of cyproterone are sometimes used, but it is not clear if the higher doses are more beneficial than the low dose. Spironolactone is typically used at doses of 100–300 mg. Potent non-steroidal anti-androgens have become available for treatment of prostate cancer. Of these flutamide has been widely used in treatment of hirsutism. The newer drugs of this class, nilutamide and bicalutamide have not been widely used. Finally, the histamine-2 receptor antagonist cimetidine has appreciable anti-androgen activity and should certainly be considered in women who require concurrent therapy for gastric acid reduction.

Recent Developments

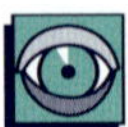

1 At best available treatments for hirsutism are only partially effective. Combinations of treatments to decrease androgen action, as have been used in prostatic carcinoma, may be of benefit. A recent trial[5] has confirmed the efficacy of combination treatment with spironolactone along with finasteride.

2 Drospirenone is an anti-mineralocorticoid progestogen that has recently become available. A recent limited trial[6] has confirmed that it is effective in decreasing hirsutism in women with PCOS. Other studies with the drug confirm that it is safe and probably has lower risk of side effects than spironolactone.

3 Insulin sensitizers have been widely used in women with PCOS, but they may be of wider use in women with hirsutism. Recently, the Pro12Ala polymorphism of the *PPAR-γ* gene has been studied in women with PCOS.[7] Compared with women with the wild-type Pro/Pro, those with at least one Ala allele were more insulin sensitive and less hirsute. This study lends further weight to the association between hirsutism and insulin resistance.

Conclusions

For women with moderate hirsutism (Ferriman–Gallwey score 8–15), a simple battery of tests consisting of serum testosterone, SHBG and thyroid function, is adequate. For those with proven high androgen and more severe hirsutism, full investigation is mandatory. PCOS is by far the commonest diagnosis and the management of this is governed not only by the hirsutism but also by other considerations including the need for fertility. Investigations of hirsutism should be directed at establishing whether a high androgen state exists, and if it does whether it is predominantly of ovarian or adrenal origin. Treatment approaches include cosmetic and topical approaches, decreasing androgen production (ovarian or adrenal), decreasing androgen delivery and blocking androgen action.

Further Reading

1 Rosenfield RL. Hirsutism. *N Engl J Med* 2005; **353**: 2578–88.

2 Azziz R, Sanchez LA, Knochenhauer ES, *et al.* Androgen excess in women: Experience with over 1000 consecutive patients. *J Clin Endocrinol Metab* 2004; **89**: 453–62.

3 Dawber RPR. Guidance for the management of hirsutism. *Curr Med Res Opin* 2005; **21**: 1227–34.

4 Lepselter J, Elman M. Biological and clinical aspects in laser hair removal. *J Dermatolog Treat* 2004; **15**: 72–83.

5 Kelestimur F, Everest H, Unluhizarci K, Bayram F, Sahin Y. A comparison between spironolactone and spironolactone plus finasteride in the treatment of hirsutism. *Eur J Endocrinol* 2004; **150**: 351–4.

6 Guido M, Romauldi D, Giuliani M, *et al*. Drosperinone for the treatment of hirsute women with the polycystic ovary syndrome: A clinical, endocrinological, metabolic pilot study. *J Clin Endocrinol Metab* 2004; **89**: 2817–23.

7 Hahn S, Fingerhut A, Khomtsiv U, *et al*. The peroxisome proliferator activated receptor gamma Pro12Ala polymorphism is associated with a lower hirsutism score and increased insulin sensitivity in women with polycystic ovary syndrome. *Clin Endocrinol (Oxf)* 2005; **62**: 573–9.

PROBLEM

25 Erectile Dysfunction

Case History

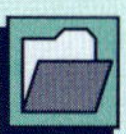

Mr AG is a 48-year-old man who complains of difficulty in sustaining an erection over the past 3 years. The problem is getting worse. He works as an insurance broker and enjoys good general health. He has had mild hypertension treated with bendrofluazide 2.5 mg/day for the past 2 years.

What features would suggest a possible endocrine cause for his problem?

What investigations should be carried out?

What are the chances of finding an underlying hormonal problem?

What treatment options are currently available to him?

Background

Erectile dysfunction (ED) is the persistent inability to achieve and/or maintain an erection sufficient for satisfactory sexual performance.[1] Erection is a neurovascular event, which at a biochemical level leads to release of nitric oxide from non-adrenergic, non-cholinergic (nitrergic) neurones (NANC) and vascular endothelial cells. These cells control contraction and relaxation of vascular smooth muscle mediated through cyclic GMP.

The true prevalence of ED is difficult to evaluate as previous studies have used different definitions for this condition. In addition sociocultural barriers have prevented affected men from coming forwards and therefore most estimates are likely to be conservative. A number of conditions can contribute to ED: androgen deficiency, hyperprolactinaemia, thyroid dysfunction. Diabetes and vascular disease remain the two main causes. In the Massachusetts Male Aging Study (MMAS)[2] the estimated combined prevalence of all grades of ED was 52% among 40–70-year-olds. ED was commoner with hypertension, hypotensive drugs, diabetes, ischaemic heart disease and depression.

ED can be the presenting symptom of a variety of conditions and therefore a detailed history including psychosocial history is important.[3] The aetiology is summarized in Box 25.1. A detailed history is likely to reveal evidence of any underlying systemic disease, endocrine problem or evidence of any problems with relationships. A complete physical examination should not only include assessment of secondary sex characteristics, but also palpation of the penis and assessment of testicular volume, and examination of the breast for gynaecomastia.

Box 25.1 Aetiology of ED

- Psychogenic: performance anxiety, relationship problems, psychological stress, and depression
- Neurogenic: cerebrovascular disease, spinal cord injury, autonomic neuropathy, radical pelvic surgery, pelvic injury
- Endocrine: hypogonadism, hyperprolactinaemia, acromegaly, diabetes mellitus
- Vascular disease: bilateral aorto-iliac atherosclerosis (Leriche's syndrome), coronary heart disease, Peyronie's disease
- Drug-induced: antihypertensive medications, anti-androgens, alcohol excess
- Systemic illness: chronic renal failure
- Old age

As well as full medical assessment, androgen status should be determined and prolactin measured. Magnetic resonance imaging (MRI) of the pituitary fossa and perimetry is indicated if a pituitary tumour is suspected. In the diabetic patient HbA1c and blood pressure are mandatory and formal assessment of vascular disease and autonomic neuropathy should be considered. Further evaluation including penile duplex ultrasonography, cavernosography and nocturnal penile monitoring in particular patients invariably involves referral to specialist urology clinics. Cavernosal artery peak systolic velocity (PSV) using penile duplex ultrasonography is a good indicator of the degree of penile arterial insufficiency and may be useful in diabetic men in whom a predominant vascular aetiology is being considered; a PSV of less than 25 cm/s suggests insufficiency in such cases.

Treatment of ED should focus on treatment of the underlying cause where possible. In men where a hormonal cause has been found and treated, and in most cases of ED due to diabetes, treatment with any of the phosphodiesterase-5 inhibitors (PDE-5) may be indicated. These agents act by inhibiting the action of PDE-5, the predominant phosphodiesterase in the cavernosal smooth muscle, thereby reinforcing and prolonging vasodilatation mediated by nitric oxide (Figure 25.1), which enhances tumescence resulting in a rigid penis for sexual intercourse. The drugs currently licensed for treatment of ED are sildenafil citrate, vardenafil and tadalafil. The drugs are similar in their mechanism of action but differ in their pharmacokinetics. Sildenafil and vardenafil have similar molecular configurations but tadalafil is an entirely different molecule, accounting

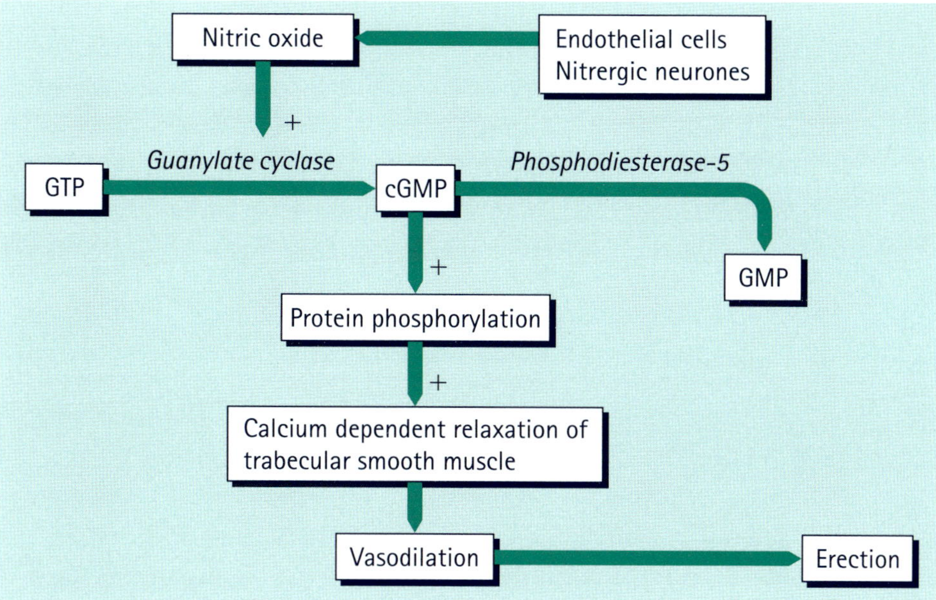

Fig. 25.1 Vasodilatation in the penis mediated by nitric oxide.

for its longer half-life compared to the other two agents. These agents enhance the quality of a stimulated erection and do not initiate an erection. The available PDE-5 inhibitors are compared in Table 25.1.

Oral PDE-5 inhibitors are effective in up to 70% of patients. Sildenafil and vardenafil should be taken 30–60 minutes before intercourse and not with a heavy meal or a large amount of alcohol. Tadalafil should be taken several hours before anticipated intercourse. These drugs may only work maximally after six to eight doses, and may lose their effect after prolonged usage (tachyphylaxis). Other medical treatments should be considered in cases where PDE-5 inhibitors are ineffective.[4,5] Intraurethral alprostadil is successful in up to 70% of cases. It is applied through an applicator applied to the tip of the penis. It may cause hypotension and the first dose should be given under supervision. Local pain may also result from the treatment. Priapism occurs in a small percentage, and patients should be instructed to seek advice if their erection lasts more than four hours. Intracavernosal injection of either papaverine or triple therapy (papaverine, phentolamine and alprostadil) is the most effective medical treatment. These agents work by relaxing cavernosal smooth muscle and dilating penile blood vessels. Scarring occurs in around 4%, local pain in a similar proportion, and priapism in less than 2%. Apomorphine is a centrally acting dopamine D_1 and D_2 agonist. Given sublingually it helps promote erection in 15–20 minutes, but is generally only effective in patients with mild ED. For resistant cases, PDE-5 inhibitors can be combined with alprostadil or intracavernosal injections. Vacuum tumescence devices are the most commonly used nonpharmacological treatment. In selected cases, referral for surgical management including inflatable penile implants should be considered.

Table 25.1 Comparison of the PDE-5 inhibitors

	Sildenafil	Vardenafil	Tadalafil
Pharmacokinetics			
T_{max} (median)	60 min	60 min	120 min
$T_{1/2}$	3–5 h	4 h	17.5 h
Food affecting absorption	Yes; especially fatty meal	Fatty meal	Not affected
Metabolism (CYP450 isoforms)	Plasma levels influenced by inducers and inhibitors	Plasma levels influenced by inducers and inhibitors	No clinically significant interactions
Selectivity against PDE-6 (retinal side effects)	Slight inhibitory activity; increased sensitivity to light	Minimal activity; no clinically significant effects	Minimal activity; no clinically significant effects
Contraindications to use			
Nitrates	Contraindicated	Contraindicated	Contraindicated
α-blockers	Contraindicated	Contraindicated	Contraindicated
Special groups			
Elderly men	Reduce dose	Reduce dose	No dose alteration necessary
Renal failure (moderate to severe)	Reduce dose	Reduce dose	Maximum recommended 10 mg
Liver cirrhosis	Reduce dose	Reduce dose	Maximum recommended 10 mg
Dosage	25–100 mg to be taken 1 hour before sexual activity	5–20 mg	10–20 mg

Recent Developments

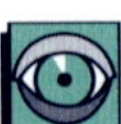

1 Endothelial dysfunction secondary to the insulin-resistant state may be an important causative factor in atherosclerotic disease and ED.[6] There is certainly an association between ED and vascular disease, although in many cases the ED results from poor blood supply to the penis.

2 There has been concern over the use of PDE-5 inhibitors in men with heart disease because of their potential to acutely lower blood pressure.[7] They are certainly contraindicated in men with severe heart disease and in those taking nitrates. However, with extensive experience in clinical trials, there is no systematic evidence that the group of drugs should not be used in men with well-controlled cardiac symptoms. Their potential to increase QTc prolongation has also been considered but, again, there is no suggestion that these drugs are dangerous in this regard.

3 There are many reports of a possible association between use of PDE-5 inhibitors and non-arteritic anterior ischaemic optic neuropathy (NAION). This condition causes sudden and irreversible loss of vision with optic disc oedema, nerve fibre layer haemorrhages,

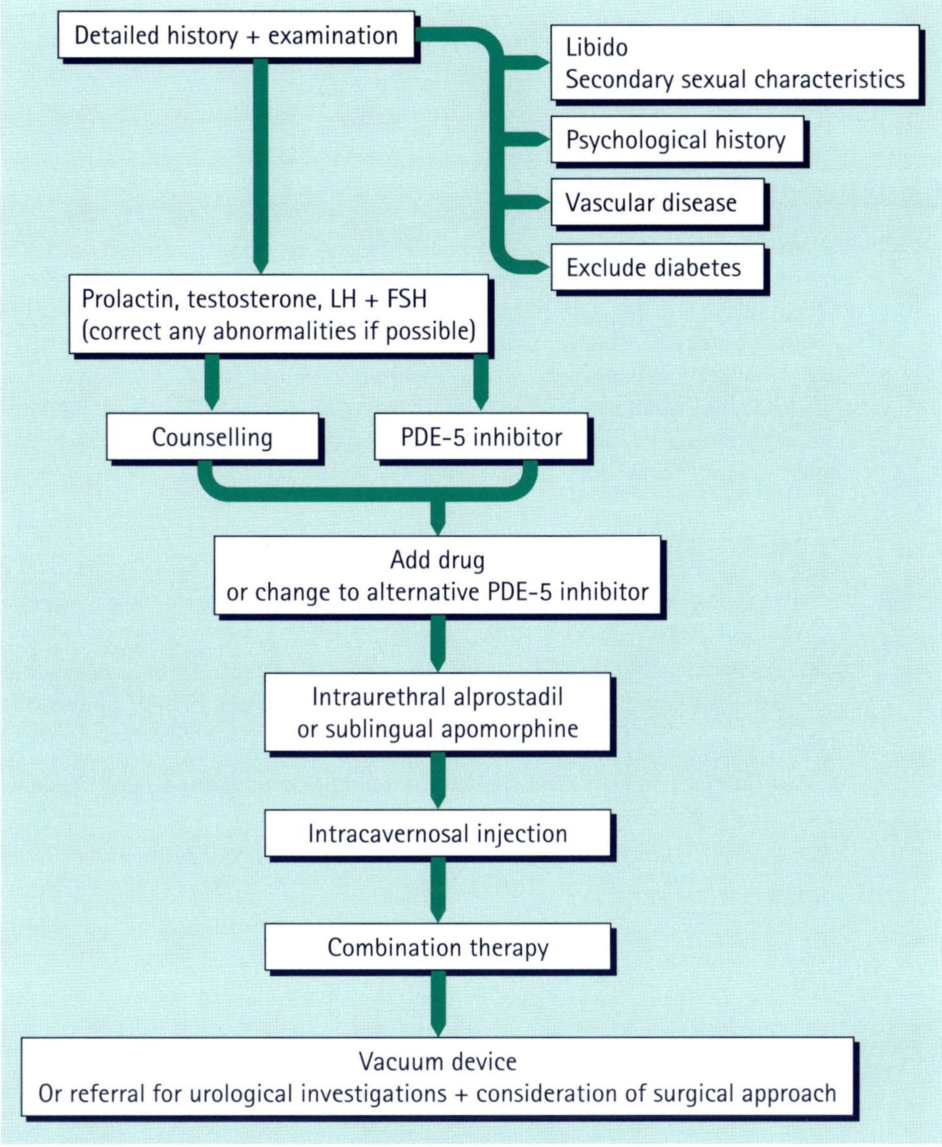

Fig. 25.2 Management of erectile dyfunction. FSH = follicle-stimulating hormone; LH = luteinizing hormone; PDE-5 = phosphodiesterase-5.

afferent pupillary defect and visual field defect. There is continuing uncertainty about the causative relation and the drugs should certainly not be used in patients with a history of NAION. A recent case–control study[8] comparing 38 patients with NAION with 38 age-matched normal men reported that use of drugs for ED was more common in the patient group.

4 In a recent meta-analysis[9] of 17 randomized controlled trials, administration of testosterone to men with borderline low testosterone improved erectile function.

Generally, androgen therapy is reserved for men with proven hypogonadism, but it may be time to lower the threshold for androgen treatment. The benefit of testosterone therapy in men with ED tends to decrease with time and is less marked in those with higher testosterone levels.

Conclusions

The progressive nature of the ED could suggest an endocrine cause in an otherwise healthy man. Thiazide diuretics may worsen impotence. Investigations should focus on checking complete pituitary hormone profile—follicle-stimulating hormone, luteinizing hormone, testosterone, prolactin, thyroid-stimulating hormone and free T_4. In the case of primary hypogonadism, testicular ultrasound, α-fetoprotein, and β-human chorionic gonadotropin should also be checked. An approach to the patient with erectile dysfunction is presented in Figure 25.2. Treatment should not be initiated until a thorough clinical evaluation has been carried out.

Further Reading

1 NIH Consensus Development Panel on Impotence. NIH Consensus Conference: impotence. *JAMA* 1993; **270**: 83–90.

2 Feldman HA, Goldstein I, Hatzichristou DG, Krane RJ, McKinley JB. Impotence and its medical psychosocial correlates: results of the Massachusetts Male Aging Study. *J Urol* 1994; **151**: 54–61.

3 Lue TF. Erectile dysfunction. *N Engl J Med* 2000; **342**: 1802–13.

4 McMahon CN, Smith CJ, Shabsigh R. Treating erectile dysfunction when PDE5 inhibitors fail. *BMJ* 2006; **332**: 589–92.

5 Beckman TJ, Haitham S, Mynderse LA. Evaluation and medical management of erectile dysfunction. *Mayo Clin Proc* 2006; **81**: 385–90.

6 Fonseca V, Jawa A. Endothelial and erectile dysfunction, diabetes mellitus, and the metabolic syndrome: common pathways and treatments? *Am J Cardiol* 2005; **96**(suppl): 13M–18M.

7 Carson CC. Cardiac safety in clinical trials of phosphodiesterase 5 inhibitors. *Am J Cardiol* 2005; **96**(suppl): 37M–41M.

8 McGwin G, Vaphiades MS, Hall TA, Owsley C. Non-arteritic anterior ischaemic optic neuropathy and the treatment of erectile dysfucntion. *Br J Ophthalmol* 2006; **90**: 154–7.

9 Isidori AM, Giannetta E, Gianfrilli D, *et al*. Effects of testosterone on sexual function in men; results of a meta-analysis. *Clin Endocrinol* 2005; **63**: 381–94.

PROBLEM

26 Male Hypogonadism

Case History

An 18-year-old man has previously been treated with low-dose testosterone to induce puberty. He has taken this treatment for 2 years and has reasonable secondary sex characteristics. He attends to review his therapy. You note that he has a very poor sense of smell and very small testes (2 ml). He would like to discuss his future management with you.

What is the differential diagnosis in this young man?

How would you approach investigation to establish a diagnosis?

Would you recommend ongoing androgen replacement?

What are the prospects of him fathering a child?

Background

Male hypogonadism is present when there is inadequate gonadal function to sustain spermatogenesis and/or physiological levels of testosterone secretion. It is hard to recognize before puberty unless there is concomitant growth failure. The following features are present when it occurs before puberty: small testes and penis; scant pubic and axillary hair; the arms and legs are disproportionately long due to delayed epiphyseal fusion; the voice is high pitched; and there may be gynaecomastia. After puberty there is loss of libido, failure to sustain an erection, decreased muscle mass and low sperm count, along with decreased wellbeing and cognitive function. Osteoporosis may occur in later life, and up to 20% of men with osteoporosis are hypogonadal.

Circulating testosterone is 2% free, 30% bound to sex hormone-binding globulin (SHBG), and up to 70% bound to albumin. There is a diurnal variation, with levels being highest in the morning. In most clinical centres, only total testosterone measurements are available. Free androgen index (see Chapter 24) or estimated free testosterone can be calculated. Total testosterone is not infrequently in the normal range, e.g. in Klinefelter's syndrome, since increased oestrogen leads to increased SHBG. The gold standard is measurement of free testosterone by equilibrium dialysis but this is only available as a research tool. Analogue displacement methods are not as reliable as they have become for the measurement of free thyroid hormones. For men with low luteinizing hormone (LH) and follicle-stimulating hormone (FSH) (secondary hypogonadism) it is not always possible to distinguish low from normal. In measuring gonadotropin levels, it should be remembered that secretion is pulsatile. FSH has a longer half-life in the circulation than LH, and may give a better index of pituitary status if the hormones are measured in a single sample. Consideration should be given to pooling samples taken 20–30 minutes apart. Serum prolactin should be measured in all cases of suspected hypogonadism. The following further investigations may be considered:

- *Gonadotropin-releasing hormone (GnRH) test.* GnRH 100 μg is administered intravenously. In normal people, LH will increase by threefold to sixfold in 30 minutes, and FSH will increase by 50%. For males who are pre-pubertal, the test may be carried out after repeated injections of GnRH to prime the pituitary.
- *Clomiphene stimulation test.* Clomiphene blocks the negative feedback of sex steroids on gonadotropin secretion. A dose of 100 mg is given daily for 5–7 days. In normal subjects, LH increases by at least twofold and FSH by at least 50%.
- *Human chorionic gonadotropin (hCG) stimulation test.* This is used when primary hypogonadism is suspected. Testosterone is measured at baseline and 72 hours after the intramuscular injection of 5000 units of hCG.
- *Semen analysis.* This should be carried out after 5–7 days' abstinence and the sample should be analysed within two hours of collection. Full investigation often requires three samples taken at 2–3-month intervals. A normal sample has volume of 1.5–6 ml, a sperm count >20 million per ml, and at least 50% of sperm will be mobile. Measurement of fructose in the semen of azoospermic men excludes obstruction or congenital absence of the ejaculatory ducts. Fructose is a normal component of the ejaculate. Very low levels suggest interruption to the normal flow of ejaculate.
- *Testicular examination* under anaesthetic and *biopsy* should be considered in those with normal or high FSH, and in men with azoospermia. This will exclude congenital abnormalities or obstruction of the ducts and abnormalities of the germinal cells.

The investigation of hypogonadism, and considerations regarding its treatment have been reviewed recently.[1,2]

Hypergonadotropic hypogonadism

See Table 26.1.

Hypogonadotropic hypogonadism

Prolactinoma should be excluded in all adult patients. A variety of tumours (pituitary, craniopharyngioma), granulomatous disorders (sarcoid, histoplasmosis), infiltrative and destructive processes (radiation therapy, haemochromatosis) can interfere with normal hypothalamic–pituitary function. Hypogonadism may also occur in the context of serious illness, and in patients with acquired immune deficiency syndrome (AIDS). Kallmann's syndrome is an X-linked recessive condition that occurs in 1:10 000 male births. The responsible gene on the X chromosome is required for development of the olfactory tracts and GnRH neurones. Features include anosmia, red–green colour blindness, cerebellar dysfunction, cleft palate and congenital deafness. Prader–Willi syndrome causes hypogonadism combined with short stature, mental retardation, and obesity due to a defect in appetite regulation. Laurence–Moon–Bardet–Biedl syndrome combines hypogonadism with mental retardation, retinitis pigmentosa and polydactyly. In the fertile eunuch syndrome, there is a selective deficiency of LH, but normal FSH and normal testicular response to hCG.

Table 26.1 **Differential diagnosis of hypergonadotropic hypogonadism**

Diagnosis	Comments
Trauma	
Mumps orchitis	30% of adults with mumps
Radiotherapy, chemotherapy	Consider storing sperm before treatment
Klinefelter's syndrome	See Chapter 30
Autoimmune	Antibodies directed against Leydig cells or sperm
Testicular feminization	Severe androgen resistance; female phenotype but blind vaginal pouch; no response to administered testosterone
Reifenstein's syndrome	Male phenotype but variable pseudohermaphroditism; hypospadias; abnormal testes should be removed
5α-reductase deficiency	Autosomal recessive; female genitalia until puberty; may need corrective surgery; increased ratio of testosterone to dihydrotestosterone
Dystrophia myotonica	Associated with frontal baldness and muscle weakness
Cryptorchidism, anorchia	
Haemochromatosis	
Sertoli cell only syndrome	Congenital absence of Leydig cells

With advancing age both LH and FSH tend to increase while androgen concentrations decrease, there are changes in the pulse frequency of gonadotropins, and a loss of the normal diurnal variation in the activity of the axis. Relative hypogonadism occurs in 15% of men over the age of 50, and in 30% of those aged over 70. Androgen treatment has the potential to increase lean body mass and to improve cardiovascular risk profile (particularly reversing dyslipidaemia), as well as improving sexual function and general well-being. The syndrome of partial androgen deficiency in ageing men (PADAM) continues to attract a great deal of attention in the literature, and it is likely that prescriptions for androgen replacement therapy will continue to increase with the ageing of the population. Investigation and management of PADAM is summarized in Figure 26.1.

Androgen treatment is contraindicated in men with prostate carcinoma, breast carcinoma, and in those with untreated prolactinoma. It is relatively contraindicated in men with obstructive sleep apnoea and in those with polycythaemia. It should not be given to men with an immediate desire for fertility as it will decrease testicular volume and sperm count. They should be treated with gonadotropins or GnRH. Table 26.2 summarizes the available androgen preparations. For many men, intramuscular injection of a mixture of testosterone esters (Sustanon) is the most convenient form of therapy. The patient should be reviewed at intervals with symptom assessment and measurement of hormones (testosterone, LH and FSH) to ensure the adequacy of treatment. It can be useful to time clinic visits to coincide with the estimated trough in testosterone concentration. Changes can be made either to the dose or to the timing to optimize treatment. Oral preparations have the disadvantage that absorption is variable and the tablets have to be taken two or

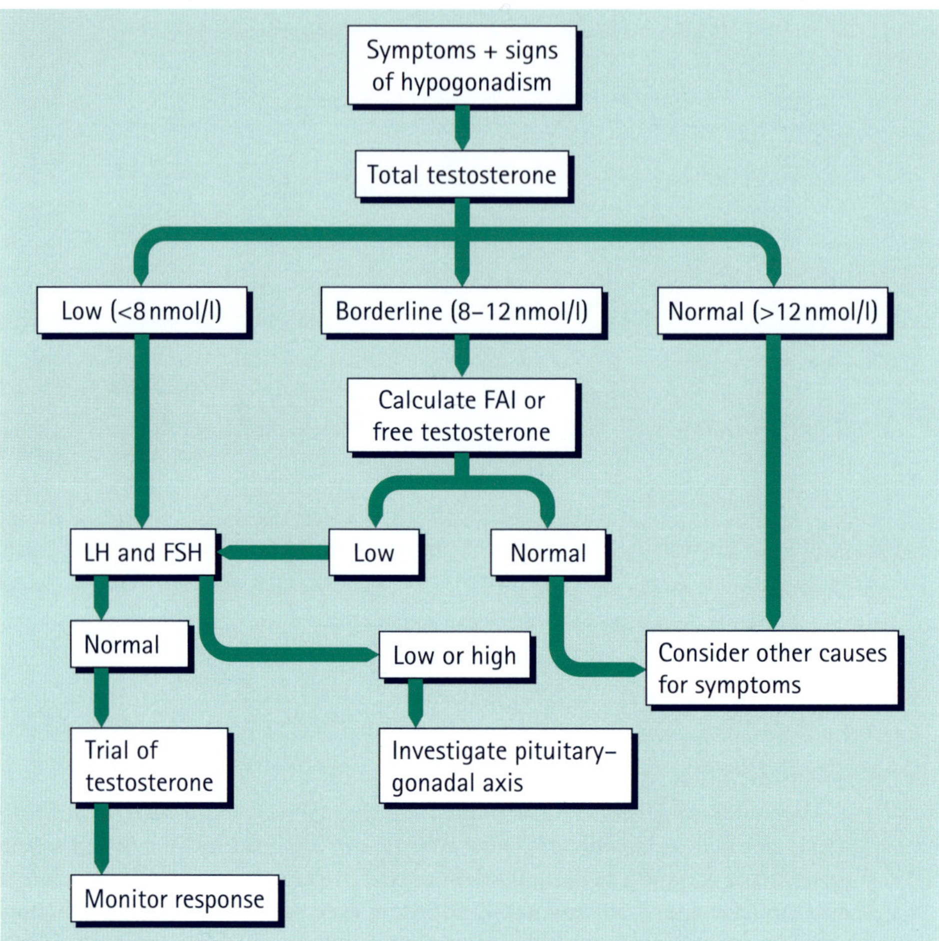

Fig. 26.1 Suggested management algorithm for the investigation and management of suspected hypogonadism in older men. FAI = free androgen index; FSH = follicle-stimulating hormone.; LH = luteinizing hormone.

three times per day. Older men should be asked about prostate symptoms regularly, an examination should be undertaken if there are symptoms, and prostate-specific antigen (PSA) should be measured annually.

For patients requiring fertility, hCG is the initial treatment of choice given by intramuscular or subcutaneous injection at a dose of 1000–2000 U two to three times per week. Testosterone should be measured monthly, testicular size monitored and sperm count checked when testosterone is at or near the normal range and testicular volume has increased. It is worth trying hCG alone for up to 6 months, particularly in men who have previously had satisfactory responses to hCG and those with partial gonadotropin deficiency. For those in whom spermatogenesis is not initiated, FSH given intramuscularly or subcutaneously at a dose of 75–150 U two to three times per week should be initiated. Another alternative for patients with intact pituitary, in specialist centres, is to use pump therapy with GnRH. Using 2-hourly pulses of GnRH, measuring hormone levels every 2 weeks and checking sperm count when LH, FSH and testosterone have increased.

Table 26.2 Available preparations for androgen replacement

Route	Preparation	Dose*
Oral	Testosterone undecanoate (Restandol) Mesterolon	40–120 mg daily 50–75 mg daily
Buccal	Striant SR Mucoadhesive buccal tablets	30 mg twice daily
Deep intramuscular	Sustanon 100 (mixed testosterone esters) Sustanon 250 Testosterone propionate	100 mg every 2 weeks 250 mg every 3 weeks 50 mg 2–3 times per week
Implant	100 or 200 mg pellets	Up to 600 mg every 4–5 weeks
Transcutaneous	Andropatch 2.5 or 5 mg patches Testoderm (scrotal patch) Testim (50 mg testosterone per 5 g tube) Testogel (50 mg testosterone per 5 g sachet)	One patch each day Scrotal area to be shaved. High local delivery of dihydrotestosterone Up to 100 mg per day 25–100 mg per day

Recent Developments

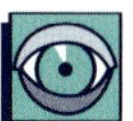

1 As with oestrogens, advances are taking place in the way androgens are administered and in the development of new agents.[3] Testosterone encapsulated in microspheres has been tried as a novel means of delivery. Dihydrotestosterone is probably underused clinically. Apart from being five times more potent than testosterone, it is non-aromatizable and is, therefore, theoretically preferable for use in delayed puberty and gynaecomastia. Aromatizable preparations may be better when brain, bone and cardiovascular health is a major consideration. Selective androgen receptor modulators have been developed in the laboratory. These are non-steroid drugs that are not aromatized and have the benefits of selective action on some androgen-responsive tissues but not on others.

2 There are many controversies surrounding the use of androgens in post-menopausal women;[4] 25% of circulating testosterone, and 40% of androstenedione, is of ovarian origin. Levels of all four major androgens decrease after menopause by up to 50%. Trials to date have clearly shown that these, and other, symptoms are related to androgen deficiency and improved by treatment. Trials have used a number of preparations: tibolone 2.5 mg/day; methyltestosterone 1.25–2.5 mg four times daily; dehydro-3-epiandrosterone 30–50 mg/day. Other forms of testosterone have also been used, and androstenedione has also been considered as a useful agent being the most abundant ovarian androgen in the pre-menopausal woman. Caution should be exercised with androgen therapy in post-menopausal women as increased androgen levels after menopause are considered to be a risk factor for breast cancer.[5]

3 Care should be exercised when giving androgen replacement to men with prolactinoma.[6] Increased prolactin and tumour bulk have been documented with androgen therapy. Problems could be avoided by using non-aromatizable androgens or by the concurrent use of aromatase inhibitors.

4 Decreased levels of testosterone are seen in men with visceral obesity, type 2 diabetes, and those who are at high risk of cardiovascular disease. Testosterone is considered to have an important role in regulating insulin sensitivity. Short-term intervention trials[7] have shown that administering testosterone to men with PADAM improves insulin sensitivity and cardiovascular risk profile.

Conclusions

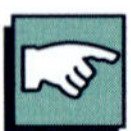

With his history of poor sense of smell it is possible that the above patient has Kallmann's syndrome. Initial investigations will readily establish whether he has primary or secondary hypogonadism. Care should be exercised when introducing androgen to a patient who has not been exposed for some time or who has never been exposed as major mood changes may occur. Patients should be monitored at intervals to ensure adequacy of replacement, to consider the choice of preparation, and to screen for complications including prostatic disease. The prospects for fertility with gonadotropin therapy are very good in men with secondary hypogonadism, particularly if this has developed in later life. There is no general agreement on what to do with androgen replacement in later life when androgen levels generally decrease.

Further Reading

1 Petak SM, Nankin HR, Spark RF, Swerdloff RS, Rodriguez-Rigau LJ. American Association of Clinical Endocrinologists medical guidelines for clinical practice for the evaluation and treatment of hypogonadism in adult male patients—2002 update. *Endocr Pract* 2002; **8**: 439–56.

2 Jockenhovel F. Testosterone therapy—what, when and to whom? *Aging Male* 2004; **7**: 319–24.

3 Gooren LJG, Bunck MCM. Androgen replacement therapy: past, present and future. *Drugs* 2004; **64**: 1861–91.

4 Cameron DR, Braunstein GD. Androgen replacement therapy in women. *Fertil Steril* 2004; **82**: 273–89.

5 Kaaks R, Rinaldi S, Key TJ, *et al.* Postmenopausal serum androgens and breast cancer risk: the European prospective investigation into cancer and nutrition. *Endocr Relat Cancer* 2005; **12**: 1071–82.

6 Sodi R, Fikri R, Diver M, Ranganath L, Vora J. Testosterone replacement-induced hyperprolactinaemia: case report and review of the literature. *Ann Clin Biochem* 2005; **42**: 153–9.

7 Kapoor D, Malkin CJ, Channer KS, Jones TH. Androgens, insulin resistance and vascular disease in men. *Clin Endocrinol* 2005; **63**: 239–50.

SECTION FIVE 05

Growth

PROBLEM

27 Delayed Puberty

Case History

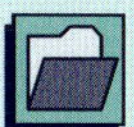

A 17-year-old boy attends with his guardian. He is concerned because he is of short stature—by far the shortest in his class. Also, his voice has not broken and he has an infantile appearance. Apart from the social discomfort, he is troubled as he is about to start applying for jobs and feels that his appearance might hamper his chances of gaining suitable employment.

Outline how he should be assessed and investigated.

What is the differential diagnosis?

Assuming this is delayed puberty, how should he be managed?

Background

Delayed puberty is the absence or incomplete development of secondary sex characteristics by any age at which 95% of the children of that sex and ethnic background have initiated sexual maturation.

Puberty is the process of acquiring normal sexual maturation and reproductive capability. The process begins with adrenarche at around the age of 8 years. Maturation of the zona glomerulosa leads to increased adrenal androgen secretion and thus the beginning of the development of secondary sexual characteristics. The process is also part of priming the hypothalamic–pituitary axis for puberty. The latter begins with the secretion of

Table 27.1 Causes of delayed puberty

Cause	Per cent of cases
Constitutional delay	53
Functional hypogonadotropic hypogonadism Growth hormone deficiency Hypothyroidism Coeliac disease Inflammatory bowel disease Anorexia nervosa Intense exercise Under-nutrition Asthma Other chronic diseases	19
Permanent hypogonadotropic hypogonadism Kallmann's syndrome Isolated gonadotropin deficiency Hypophysitis Rathke's pouch cyst or cleft CNS tumours—craniopharyngioma, glioma, etc. Congenital syndromes—Prader-Willi, etc.	12
Hypergonadotropic hypogonadism Ovarian failure Chemotherapy or gonadal irradiation Genetic or congenital syndromes: Klinefelter's Turner's Galactosaemia Androgen insensitivity syndromes	13
Other syndromes not fitting into the above classification	3

The percentages and differential diagnoses in this table are adapted from those of Sedlmeyer and Palmert.[3]

gonadotropins from the pituitary (gonadarche). Following this, normal patterns of gonadotropin and growth hormone secretion are gradually established. A number of hormones are involved in this process including testosterone, oestradiol, inhibin, activin and follistatin.

Delayed puberty results from defective gonadotropin-releasing hormone (GnRH) secretion. This, in turn, leads to low levels of gonadotropins. A careful history is very important and should focus on the growth pattern up to the time of evaluation. In constitutional delay there is a temporal association with declining growth velocity and delayed skeletal maturation. High exercise intensity or underlying metabolic problems may delay growth and also lead to delayed puberty. A positive family history of delayed puberty may be present. Patients are usually of a short stature. In those with congenital GnRH deficiency, associated abnormalities or midline defects may be present. A positive family history may also be present. Differential diagnosis of delayed puberty is shown in Table 27.1.[1–3] In a recent large retrospective series,[3] constitutional delay was present in over half. This condition is not generally associated with underlying pathology and tends to run in families. It is commoner in males.

Physical examination may reveal a eunuchoidal body habitus (arm span exceeding height by more than 5 cm). The height should be plotted on growth charts that include

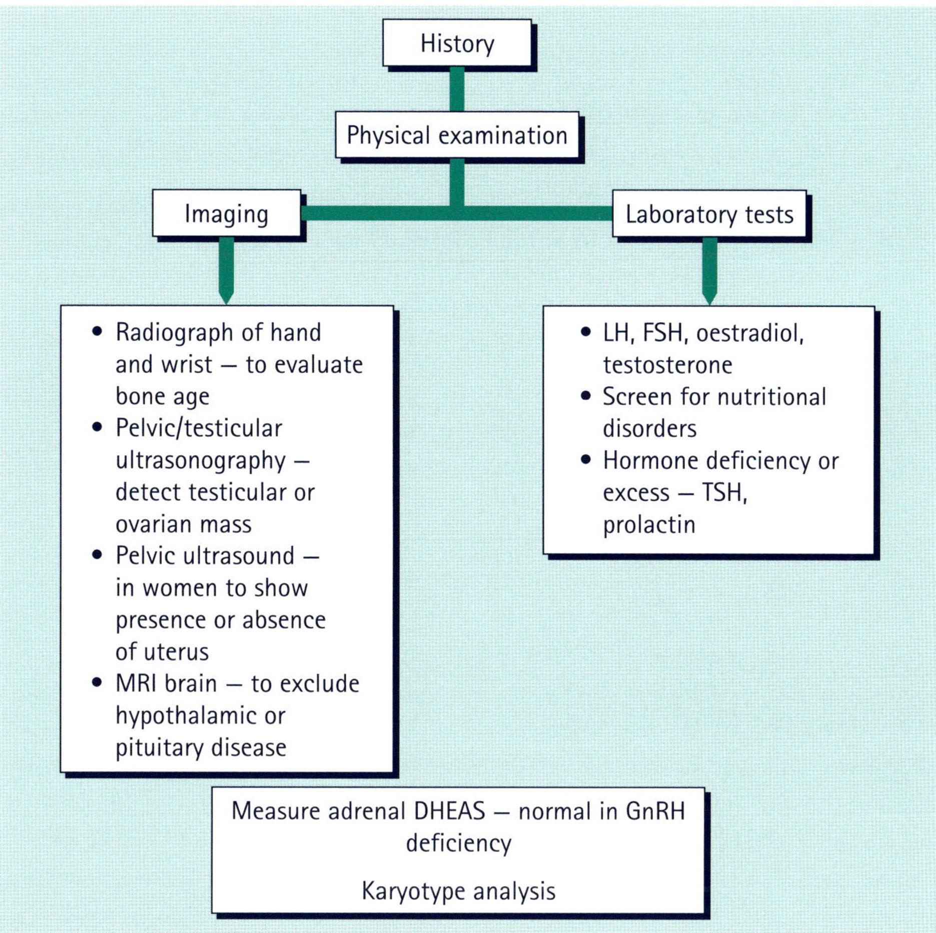

Fig. 27.1 Investigations for delayed puberty. DHEAS = dehydro-3-epiandrosterone sulphate; FSH = follicle-stimulating hormone; GnRH = gonadotropin-releasing hormone; LH = luteinizing hormone; TSH = thyrotropin (thyroid-stimulating hormone).

normal growth pattern with centiles to allow comparison from previous readings and evaluate growth velocity and be able to relate that with bone age. Secondary sexual characteristics should be staged using the Tanner scale. Investigation of delayed puberty is summarized in Figure 27.1. An X-ray of the left wrist is compared with standard films compiled by Greulich and Pyle to assess bone age. The epiphyses of the phalanges and carpal bones are compared with standards, the presence or absence of the sesamoid bone of the thumb is noted. Growth is considered to be delayed if the bone age is more than two standard deviations below the chronological age. Investigations should include blood count, liver function tests, glucose and electrolytes. Up to 8% of adolescent patients with short stature have coeliac disease and anti-endomysial antibody measurement should be requested. Thyroid function and prolactin levels should be measured. Insulin-like growth factor (IGF)-1 level may give an indication of the growth hormone status. It is difficult to reliably distinguish constitutional delay from isolated growth hormone or gonadotropin deficiency: growth hormone stimulation tests can be carried out after priming with sex steroids—carry out the stimulation test 72 hours after 50 mg intramuscular testosterone propanoate in boys or after 3 days of 25 μg ethinyloestradiol in girls. The GnRH test is of limited use in distinguishing constitutional delay from isolated gonadotropin deficiency.

The aims of treatment in constitutional delay are to initiate normal puberty, to promote the development of normal secondary sex characteristics and reproductive function. In the absence of an identified underlying cause, watchful waiting with reassurance to patient or family is the usual approach. Sex steroid treatment is indicated if constitutional delay causes concern to the patient. Treatment in boys can be initiated with 50 mg of testosterone ester per month given intramuscularly, or with low doses of oral testosterone. Patches or gels could be used, but commercially available preparations deliver too high a dose for initiating puberty. There is also a choice of therapies for girls with constitutional delay. The most convenient is usually 1–3 μg/day of ethinyloestradiol. Co-treatment of boys with aromatase inhibitors has been proposed. Decreased local generation of oestrogen may delay epiphyseal maturation and thus the patient may achieve a greater height. Anabolic steroids have also been used to promote growth without hastening sexual maturation.

Recent Developments

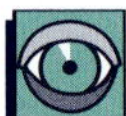

1. The age at which puberty is initiated is falling in developed countries.[4,5] This is particularly important in girls, in whom the timing of puberty is more apparent because of the onset of menstruation. Endocrinologists need to be aware of this trend since patients with pubertal delay may seek advice at an earlier stage.

2. Regulation of puberty is under both environmental and genetic control.[5,6] Environmental influences may be acquired *in utero*. The trend towards increasing body weight in children and teenagers is one of the major factors governing the earlier onset of puberty. The regulation of luteinizing hormone (LH) and follicle-stimulating hormone (FSH) secretion through neuronal activation and inhibitory pathways in the forebrain is now quite well understood.[6]

3. The response to injected human chorionic gonadotropin (hCG) has been used to discriminate between constitutional delay and hypogonadotropic hypogonadism. Testosterone responses to hCG are considerably higher in patients with constitutional delay.[7] GnRh agonists may also be useful in dynamic testing.[8] Short-term administration of a GnRH agonist leads to a brisk increase in LH in patients with constitutional delay, while FSH levels may be less discriminatory.

4. There are important nutritional influences on growth, and a variety of nutritional supplements have been shown to accelerate growth in children with constitutional delay. In a recent study by Zadik *et al.*[9] vitamin A (6000 IU/week) and iron (12 mg/day) were compared with hormone treatment. Growth in the group treated with nutritional supplements was higher than in controls, and comparable with that of boys treated either with testosterone or with anabolic steroid.

Conclusions

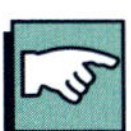

Most cases of delayed puberty are constitutional and not, therefore, associated with underlying pathology. The degree to which a patient is investigated depends on how much the patient or guardian(s) are concerned, the age of the patient, and the degree to which growth or maturation is compromised. For most patients, initially simple endocrine investigations should be carried out followed by regular surveillance to assess growth and development. For those who do not progress as expected, underlying hypogonadism, hypopituitarism or a genetic syndrome should be considered. For patients with constitutional delay who are concerned about their progress, initiating pubertal changes with low doses of sex steroids is usually straightforward.

Further Reading

1. Israel EJ, Levitsky LL, Anupindi SA, Pitman MB. Case 3-2005: a 14-year old boy with recent slowing of growth and delayed puberty. *N Engl J Med* 2005; **352**: 393–403.
2. Nathan BM, Palmert MR. Regulation and disorders of pubertal timing. *Endocrinol Metab Clin North Am* 2005; **34**: 617–41.
3. Sedlmeyer IL, Palmert MR. Delayed puberty: analysis of a large case series from an academic center. *J Clin Endocrinol Metab* 2002; **87**: 1613–20.
4. Herman-Giddens ME. Recent data on pubertal milestones in US children: the secular trend toward earlier development. *Int J Androl* 2005; **29**: 24–6.
5. Gluckman PD, Hanson MA. Evolution, development and timing of puberty. *Trends Endocrinol Metab* 2006; **17**: 7–12.
6. Ojeda SR, Roth C, Mungenast A, *et al*. Neuroendocrine mechanisms controlling female puberty: new approaches, new concepts. *Int J Androl* 2006; **29**: 256–63.
7. Degros V, Cortet-Rudelli C, Soudan B, Dewailly D. The human chorionic gonadotropin test is more powerful than the gonadotropin-releasing hormone agonist test to discriminate male isolated hypogonadotropic hypogonadism from constitutional delayed puberty. *Eur J Endocrinol* 2003; **149**: 23–9.
8. Wilson DA, Hofman PL, Miles HL, Unwin KE, McGrail CE, Cutfield WS. Evaluation of the buserelin stimulation test in diagnosing gonadotropin deficiency in males with delayed puberty. *J Pediatr* 2006; **148**: 89–94.
9. Zadik Z, Sinai T, Zung A, Reifen R. Vitamin A and iron supplementation is as efficient as hormonal therapy in constitutionally delayed children. *Clin Endocrinol* 2004; **60**: 682–7.

PROBLEM

28 Gynaecomastia

Case History

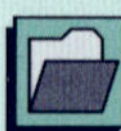

A 19-year-old boy finally plucks up the courage to seek medical help. He has noted enlargement of both breasts since the age of 15 years. The problem is getting worse and he finds it difficult to conceal the breast enlargement. He does not have a girlfriend and has not felt able to swim or participate in sporting activities for some time.

Is he likely to have an endocrine disorder?

What investigations should be carried out?

What treatment is available?

Background

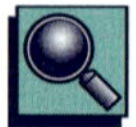

Gynaecomastia is visible or palpable enlargement of the male breast. It is by far the most common disorder of the male breast,[1] occurring in 30% of men under the age of 30 and 50% of those over the age of 45. It is unilateral in about a third of cases, and arises because of an imbalance between oestrogenic stimulation and androgenic inhibition of breast growth. Hyperprolactinaemia *per se* does not appear to be a direct cause, except through producing secondary hypogonadism. An approach to the differential diagnosis of gynaecomastia is shown in Figure 28.1.

Pubertal enlargement of the breast affects up to 60% of boys, and can begin as early as the age of 10 years. Typically, there is subareolar swelling which is firm and often tender, extending up to 5 cm in diameter. It usually disappears within 12–18 months of puberty. The neonatal period and old age are other times when oestrogenic action predominates and the male breast may enlarge. In ageing men, testosterone and other androgen levels decline whereas, particularly in those who are obese, peripheral aromatization to produce oestrogen is increased. Serious causes of gynaecomastia relatively rare.

Thyrotoxicosis and liver disease can both be associated with increased sex hormone-binding globulin (SHBG), leading to a decrease in free androgens. Peripheral aromatization to oestrogen is increased in patients with liver disease. Renal failure is associated with increased oestrogen and prolactin, along with decreased androgen levels. Production of human chorionic gonadotropin (hCG) by germ cell tumours of the testes or by other solid tumours, leads to excessive stimulation of steroid-secreting cells in the testes, with a relative predominance of oestrogen. Leydig cell tumours are small tumours of the testes, 90% of which are benign. Many are impalpable, and investigation with testicular ultrasound or thermography is warranted. Oestrogen-secreting adrenal tumours are usually

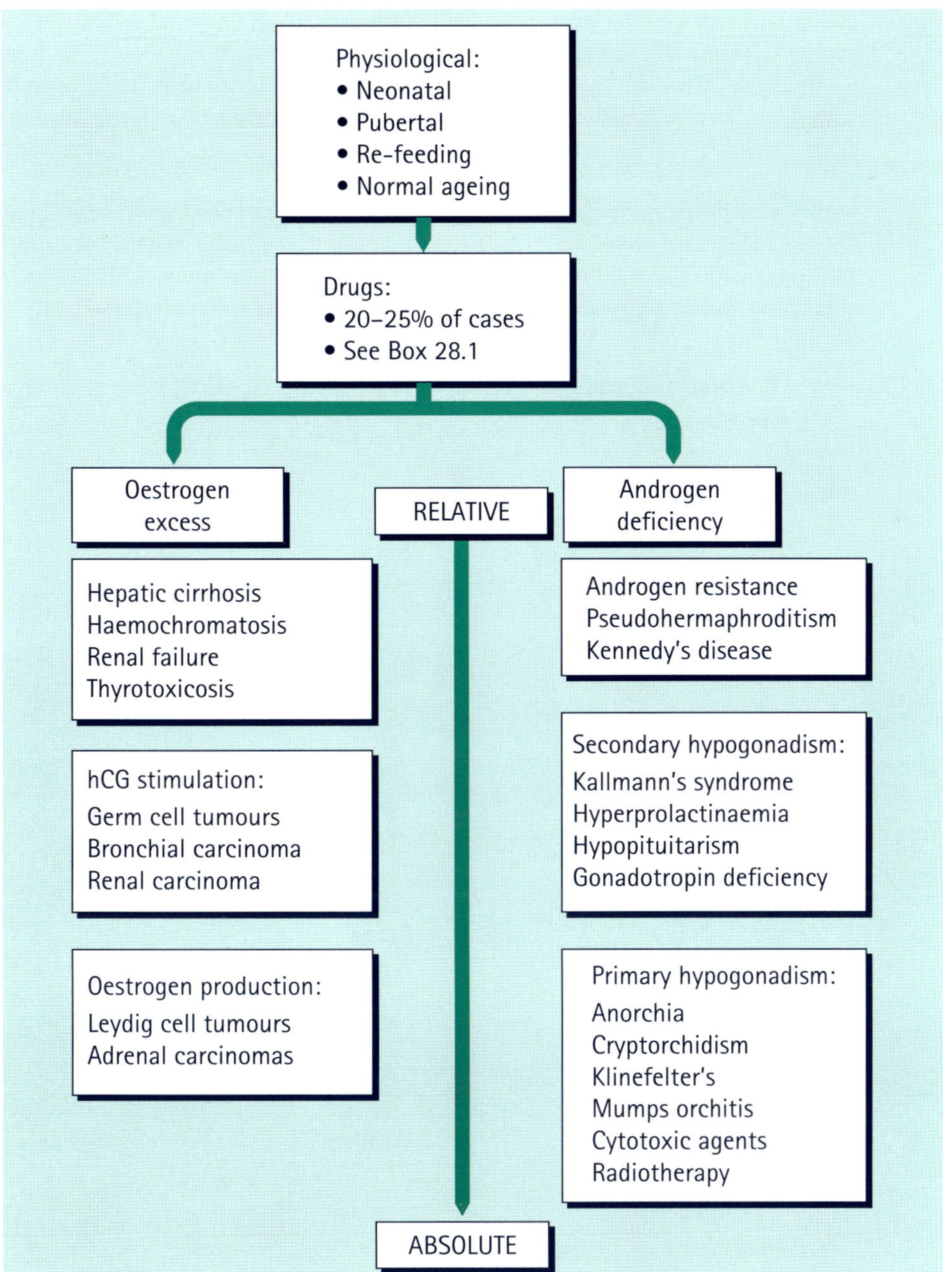

Fig. 28.1 Differential diagnosis of gynaecomastia. Gynaecomastia is very common around the time of puberty and in later life. The major thrust of investigation is to determine whether the patient is hypogonadal and, if so, whether this is due to primary (testicular) or secondary causes. Tumours secreting oestrogen or human chorionic gonadotropin (hCG) are quite rare but should be borne in mind in all cases.

malignant and carry a poor prognosis. Other markers, such as dehydro-3-epiandrosterone (DHEA) and its sulphate are also generally increased.

Insensitivity to androgens can lead to gynaecomastia, as can primary or secondary hypogonadism. Low testosterone levels with increased gonadotropin levels suggest primary hypogonadism, and low testosterone with low gonadotropin suggests pituitary or hypothalamic disease. Around 20–25% of cases of gynaecomastia are drug induced (Box 28.1). In some cases, the drugs interfere with the normal oestrogen/androgen balance. In other cases the mechanism is not known. Gynaecomastia caused by testosterone may not simply be due to aromatization of the hormone to oestrogen, since non-aromatizable androgens such as methyltestosterone and dihydrotestosterone can also cause gynaecomastia.

Box 28.1 **Drug-induced gynaecomastia**

Hormone treatments

- Testosterone, DHEAS
- Oestrogen
- Corticosteroids
- Anabolic steroids
- Anti-androgens
- Finasteride
- Cimetidine

Anti-infectives

- Isoniazid
- Ketoconazole
- Metronidazole

Cardiovascular drugs

- Furosemide, bumetanide
- Calcium-channel blockers
- Methyldopa
- Digoxin

Social drugs

- Alcohol
- Amphetamines
- Narcotics
- Marijuana

Centrally acting drugs

- Tricyclics
- Phenothiazines
- Diazepam

Other drugs

- Cytotoxic agents
- Theophylline
- Penicillamine

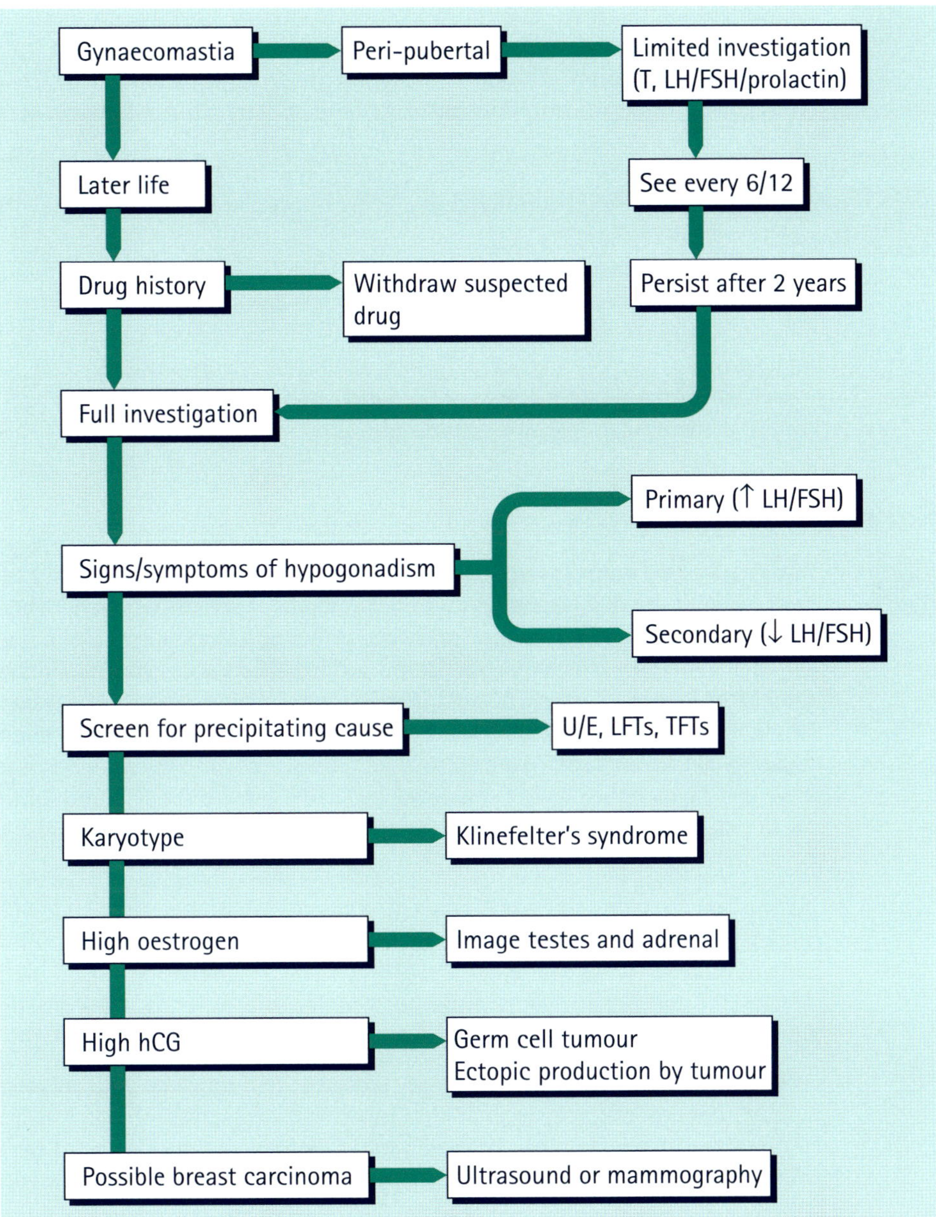

Fig. 28.2 Investigation of gynaecomastia. The approach to investigation is, to some degree, determined by the patient's anxiety about the condition. It is clearly essential not to miss a sinister underlying diagnosis, but important to recognize that excessive investigation may increase the patient's anxiety.
FSH = follicle-stimulating hormone; hCG = human chorionic gonadotropin; LFT = liver function test; LH = luteinizing hormone; T = testosterone; TFT = thyroid function test; U/E = urea and electrolytes.

A protocol for the investigation of gynaecomastia is suggested in Figure 28.2. Not all cases require investigation, and most cases do not require extensive investigation at the initial presentation. Around the time of puberty, measurement of serum testosterone yields limited information but may help to determine whether the patient is entering, or has entered, puberty. In later life, gynaecomastia should be investigated when there is no apparent precipitating cause such as drugs, and where the condition is of recent onset, associated with hypogonadism, or possible features of other underlying disease.

Surgery is the mainstay of treatment for those patients who require it. Subcutaneous mastectomy using a circumareolar incision is widely employed. There is a variety of plastic surgical approaches, including liposuction (with or without ultrasound guidance). Complications of surgery include haematoma and infection, unsightly scar formation, asymmetrical breast tissue, necrosis of the nipple or areola, and sensory changes. Medical treatment to manipulate hormonal status has, at present, a limited role.

Recent Developments

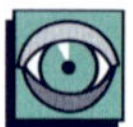

1 Breast cancer accounts for only 0.2% of malignancies in males. It should be suspected in gynaecomastia that is painful, asymmetrical and of recent onset, and where there is fixation to surrounding tissues or regional lymphadenopathy. It remains unclear whether gynaecomastia is a risk factor for breast cancer, except in patients with Klinefelter's where there is a 50-fold increase in risk compared with the general population.[2] The increased risk associated with Klinefelter's syndrome may extend to other causes of hypogonadism.[3] An extensive follow-up study in Sweden has suggested that there may be increased risk of squamous cell carcinoma of the skin and testicular cancer in patients with gynaecomastia, but there was no overall increased risk of malignancy in the study.[4]

2 The evidence relating to drug treatment of gynaecomastia is surprisingly limited. In small series, tamoxifen and the selective oestrogen receptor modulator (SERM) raloxifene have been shown to be of benefit.[5,6] Other drugs that have been used include clomiphene and the aromatase inhibitor testolactone. Recently, there has been some published experience with another aromatize inhibitor, anastrazole.[7]

3 Gynaecomastia is also being increasingly recognized among men who are infected with human immunodeficiency virus (HIV). In a recent series,[8] hormonal measurements in HIV-positive men with gynaecomastia were compared with those in controls with HIV who did not have breast enlargement. The presence of gynaecomastia was correlated with hypogonadism but not with the use of particular antiretroviral drugs.

Conclusions

The likelihood is that this patient does not have an underlying endocrine disturbance. Pubertal gynaecomastia does not always require investigation. It may be best to simply reassure the patient and review at 6-monthly intervals. Breast enlargement that persists for more than 2 years after the completion of puberty, or where there is pain or the breasts continue to grow, should be investigated. Initial investigations should include levels of testosterone, luteinizing hormone, follicle-stimulating hormone and prolactin. An ultrasound scan to confirm the presence of breast tissue should also be carried out. For those who require treatment, surgery is usually recommended. For those who do not wish operative treatment, particularly if the breasts are tender, a 6-month trial of drug treatment (e.g. tamoxifen) may be considered.

Further Reading

1 Wise GJ, Roorda AK, Kalter R. Male breast disease. *J Am Coll Surg* 2005; **200**: 255–69.

2 Giordano SH. A review of the diagnosis and management of male breast cancer. *Oncologist* 2005; **10**: 471–9.

3 Weiss JR, Moysich KB, Swede H. Epidemiology of male breast cancer. *Cancer Epidemiol Biomarkers Prev* 2005; **14**: 20–6.

4 Olsson H, Bladstrom A, Alm P. Male gynecomastia and risk for malignant tumours—a cohort study. *BMC Cancer* 2002; **2**: 26–32.

5 Khan HN, Blamey RW. Endocrine treatment of physiological gynaecomastia. *BMJ* 2003; **327**: 301–2.

6 Lawrence SE, Faught KA, Jethamuthu J, Lawson ML. Beneficial effects of raloxifene and tamoxifen in the treatment of pubertal gynaecomastia. *J Pediatr* 2004; **145**: 71–6.

7 Riepe FG, Baus I, Wiest S, Krone N, Sippell WG, Pertsch CJ. Treatment of pubertal gynaecomastia with the specific aromatise inhibitor anastrazole. *Horm Res* 2004; **62**: 113–18.

8 Biglia A, Blanco JL, Martinez E, *et al*. Gynaecomastia among HIV-infected patients is associated with hypogonadism: a case control study. *Clin Infect Dis* 2004; **39**: 1514–19.

PROBLEM

29 Turner's Syndrome

Case History

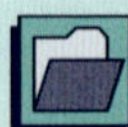

The mother of a 15-year-old girl with Turner's syndrome consults you because she is concerned about her daughter's development. She is poorly developed and of short stature. The girl and her mother would like to know if there is any hormonal treatment that might improve the situation.

How would you approach sex steroid replacement in this patient?

Is growth hormone therapy an option?

What are the long-term implications of this diagnosis?

Background

Turner's syndrome – 45,X occurs in 1:2500 female births. In fact, only about half of patients have the pure 45,X genotype. Ten per cent have duplication (isochromosome) usually of the long arm of X – 46,X,i(X_q). The remainder have mosaicism, with some cells having the 45,X genotype and other cells having normal, or a variety of other abnormal, genotypes.[1,2] To diagnose mosaicism, up to 100 cells may need to be counted. Also, it may not be possible in some cases to diagnose mosaicism from peripheral blood lymphocytes. In these cases, skin biopsy and karyotyping of fibroblasts can be used.

The major features of the syndrome are summarized in Table 29.1. Other features include—obesity, insulin resistance and hypertension; cataracts; scoliosis; inflammatory bowel disease; autoimmune thyroid disease; keloid scar formation.

Short stature and ovarian failure are virtually universal in Turner's syndrome. Up to a third are diagnosed in childhood or early adolescence because of growth failure. The number of germ cells in the ovary degenerates from mid-gestation onwards. Spontaneous fertility is rare but can occur in girls who are 46,XX or 47,XXX mosaics, or in those who have distal X_p deletions. In the minority, there is sufficient endocrine function to initiate breast development and other changes of puberty. Indeed, up to 40% of girls with Turner's syndrome who are left untreated will develop spontaneous menarche. However, complete ovarian failure ensues in almost all cases. Swollen hands and feet are due to congenital lymphoedema, and susceptibility locus for this has been identified on the short arm of the X chromosome. This feature is often responsible for the diagnosis of Turner's syndrome in the pre-natal or early neonatal period.

The skeletal features include widening of the chest, often described as shield chest, which leads to widely spaced nipples. The nipples are sometimes inverted. Increased carrying angle of the elbow (cubitus valgus), and webbing of the neck (pterygium colli) are also

Table 29.1 Clinical features of Turner's syndrome

Feature	Per cent of cases
Short stature	100
Ovarian failure	95
Broad chest	80
Low posterior hairline	80
Swollen hands and feet	80
Increased carrying angle	70
Inner canthal folds	70
Small lower jaw	70
Soft upturned nails	70
Renal abnormalities	60
Cardiac abnormalities	50
Webbed neck	50
Short fourth digit	50
Pigmented naevi	50
Hearing loss	50

characteristic skeletal features. Small lower jaw is due to hypoplasia of the mandibular bone. Of the other major congenital defects, those affecting the kidney and heart are the most significant. Renal abnormalities are more common but frequently asymptomatic, although they may cause problems through hydronephrosis or urinary tract infections. The most common renal abnormalities are horseshoe kidney and duplication of the collecting systems (renal pelvis or ureters). Cardiac problems include coarctation of the aorta and bicuspid aortic valve, with hypoplastic left heart occurring in a minority of cases. Dilatation of the ascending aorta and aortic aneurysm have also been described. Essential hypertension is common and may lead to secondary cardiovascular problems in later life.

There is increased incidence of strabismus and premature cataract. Anatomical changes associated with Turner's syndrome make recurrent otitis media a common problem in childhood. The cause for the reported increase in inflammatory bowel disease (both Crohn's and ulcerative colitis) is not known. Coeliac disease may also be more common in Turner's syndrome. Autoimmune thyroid disease occurs in up to 30%, and warrants regular screening from the age of 10. The effects of Turner's syndrome on psychological, psychomotor and cognitive development are complex—sometimes subtle, sometimes of major clinical significance. These include delayed motor or visual–spatial development, and problems with gender identity and socialization. Overall, there is increased morbidity associated with Turner's syndrome, but a major effect of the syndrome on life expectancy has not been documented. Girls who have mosaicism that includes Y-chromosomal material have increased risk of gonadoblastoma.

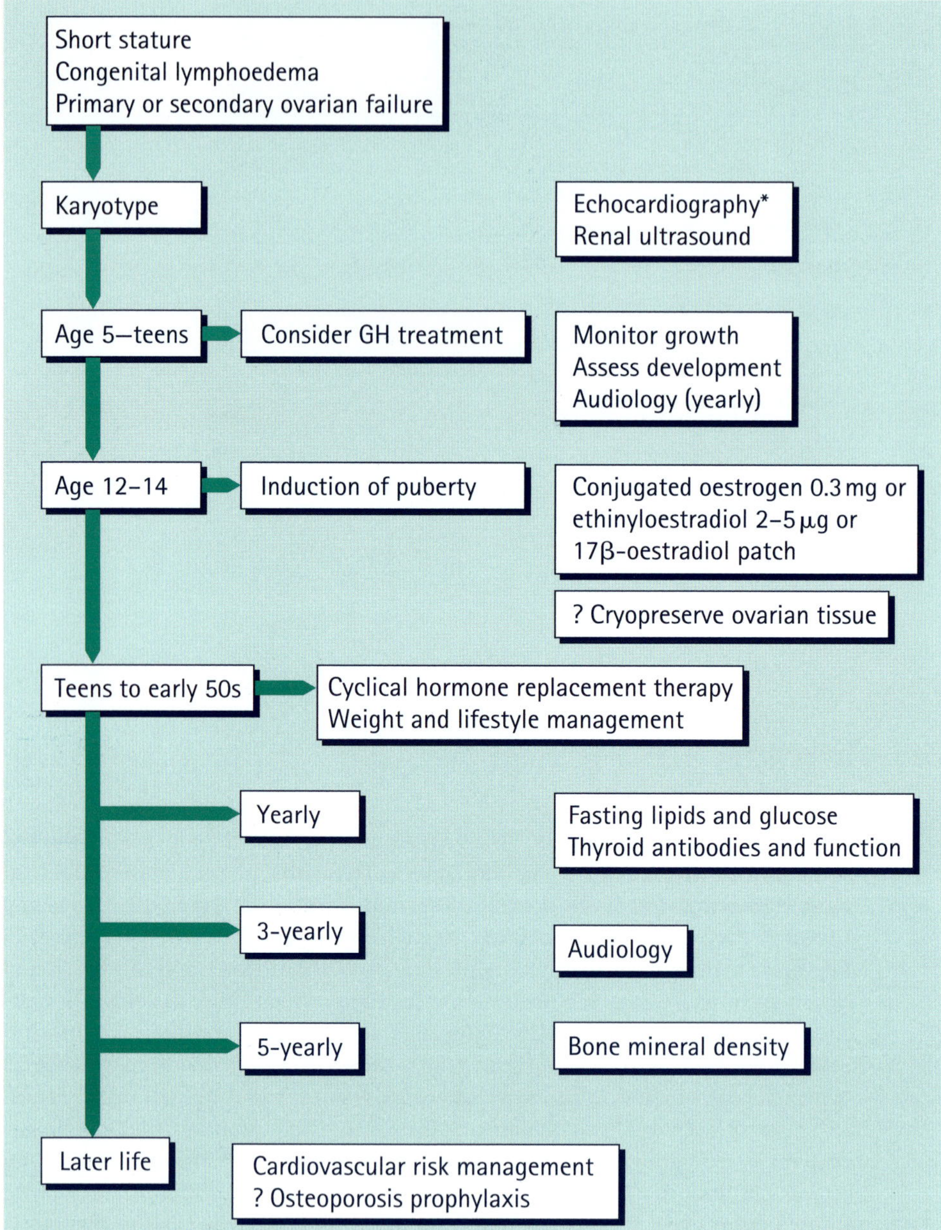

Fig. 29.1 Management of Turner's syndrome. *Screening for cardiac and renal anomalies should take place whenever the diagnosis is made. The suggested management flow may need to be amended according to the presence of specific associated conditions.

At diagnosis, patients should be screened for cardiac and renal abnormalities. Around a quarter of cases are now diagnosed at birth, largely because of puffy skin and redundant nuchal skin. These girls need to be carefully screened for associated congenital abnormalities and undergo periodic thorough developmental assessment. About a third are identified because of short stature during childhood. Growth hormone therapy is now routinely used. Although it may increase risk of insulin resistance and hypertension with prolonged use, no real safety issues have been identified. Ninety per cent of girls with Turner's syndrome will require hormone treatment to initiate puberty. Oestrogen treatment can be started at the age of 12 in girls who are receiving growth hormone, and at 14 years in those who are not. Initial treatment should be with conjugated oestrogen (Premarin) 0.3 mg, ethinyloestradiol 2–5 μg, or a 17β-oestradiol patch at night. The dose of oestrogen should be increased at 6 months in those who show no, or limited, response. After 1 year of unopposed oestrogen, combined cyclical therapy should be initiated. A recent qualitative study[3] has confirmed that lack of fertility is the major issue concerning women with Turner's syndrome throughout their life. Management of this remains difficult. For some, it may be possible to cryopreserve viable ovarian tissue from a young age. Oocyte donation techniques now have an outcome in women with Turner's syndrome that is comparable with that of other patient groups. A scheme for the management of Turner's syndrome is proposed in Figure 29.1.

Recent Developments

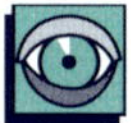

1. Ovarian transplantation from tissue type matched donors is a novel approach to treating fertility in patients with Turner's syndrome.[3] Various grafting methods and both vascular and avascular approaches have been described. This treatment is still experimental, and has the disadvantages of requiring both surgery and immunosuppression.
2. Up to half of women with Turner's syndrome have impaired glucose tolerance, and the prevalence of type 2 diabetes is two to four times that of the background population. Decreased insulin sensitivity is present from an early age, and may temporarily worsen during treatment with growth hormone.[4] In a recent study,[5] Turner's syndrome patients had some increased markers for metabolic syndrome (C-reactive protein and interleukin-6), although fasting levels of insulin and leptin were lower than for a comparable group with premature ovarian failure.
3. Women with Turner's syndrome have an annual incidence of hypothyroidism of around 3%.[6] Thus, routine testing of thyroid function is warranted. Thyroid antibodies do not appear to be invariably detected and may not thus be a useful guide to identifying patients who are at risk of thyroid dysfunction.
4. Although long-term effects of growth hormone in patients with Turner's syndrome are not known, it seems reasonable with available evidence to offer treatment from the age of about 5 years.[7] Patients should be periodically screened for conditions that might decrease growth rate, including coeliac disease and hypothyroidism.

Conclusions

Most girls with Turner's syndrome will require induction of puberty with oestrogen therapy. The timing of this should take into account the clinical condition and wishes of the patient, and should involve careful discussion with the parents. When puberty has been induced, ongoing treatment with a cyclic oestrogen/progestagen regimen is indicated—probably until the estimated age of normal menopause. The use of growth hormone in girls with Turner's syndrome is widespread and does safely increase final height with no apparent major risks. Growth hormone should be employed preferably before puberty is induced. Of the many associated problems and disorders, the issue of fertility is the one that causes the patient most anguish in many cases. Ongoing problems include screening for and managing: obesity, glucose intolerance and cardiovascular risk; hearing loss due to sensorineural changes; osteoporosis.

Further Reading

1. Sybert VP, McCauley E. Turner's syndrome. *N Engl J Med* 2004; **351**: 1227–38.
2. Gravholt CH. Epidemiological, endocrine and metabolic features in Turner syndrome. *Eur J Endocrinol* 2004; **151**: 657–87.
3. Mhatre P, Mhatre J, Magotra R. Ovarian transplant: a new frontier. *Transplant Proc* 2005; **37**: 1396–8.
4. Mazzanti L, Bergamaschi R, Castiglioni L, Zapulla F, Pirazzoli P, Cicognani A. Turner syndrome, insulin sensitivity and growth hormone treatment. *Hormone Res* 2005; **64**(suppl 3): 51–7.
5. Ostberg JE, Attar MJ, Javad H, Mohamed AV, Conway GS. Adipokine dysregulation in Turner syndrome: comparison of circulating interleukin-6 and leptin concentrations with measures of adiposity and C-reactive protein. *J Clin Endocrinol Metab* 2005; **90**: 2948–53.
6. El Mansoury M, Bryman I, Berntop K, Hanson C, Wilhelmsen L, Landin-Wilhelmsen K. Hypothyroidism is common in Turner syndrome: results of a five year follow up. *J Clin Endocrinol Metab* 2005; **90**: 2131–5.
7. Pasquino AM. Turner syndrome and GH treatment: the state of the art. *J Endocrinol Invest* 2004; **27**: 1072–5.

PROBLEM

30 Klinefelter's Syndrome

Case History

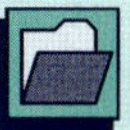

TB is a 27-year-old man who is concerned that his wife is not becoming pregnant. He is tall, with poor secondary sex characteristics and small testicles. You note gynaecomastia, which the patient says has been present since puberty. Investigations demonstrate low testosterone and his karyotype demonstrates that he has Klinefelter's syndrome.

What does he need to know about the implications of this diagnosis?

Does he require any treatment and, if so, for how long?

What are the prospects of him fathering a child?

How should he be followed up?

Background

The 47,XXY karyotype confers the phenotypic features of Klinefelter's syndrome, and occurs in 1:1000 male births.[1] Mosaicism occurs in 15% of cases, and is usually associated with milder phenotypic features. In these cases, a normal karyotype is present in some cells but the Klinefelter karyotype is found in others. Patients may have three or four X chromosomes, and rarely there is an additional Y chromosome (XXYY). These forms tend to be associated with severe phenotypic features. It is not clear whether increased paternal or maternal age is a risk factor.

Klinefelter's syndrome is commonly diagnosed in adolescence or in early adulthood. Features include increased height with limbs that are disproportionately long in relation to the torso, small testes, and gynaecomastia. Increased leg length is related to the chromosome abnormality *per se*, and not only to hypogonadism—unlike in eunuchoid individuals, arm span does not exceed body height in Klinefelter's. Hypergonadotropic hypogonadism in adult life causes decreased libido, decreased muscle bulk and diminished bone mineral density compared with normal men. Learning and psychological difficulties may be apparent in childhood. These include cognitive impairment, delayed development of motor skills as well as speech and language, and attention deficit. These developmental defects are usually relatively mild. There is probably no increase in the risk of severe psychiatric disorders. Patients with Klinefelter's syndrome are also at increased risk of thromboembolism, diabetes and cardiovascular disease. Up to 30% have varicose veins, venous stasis ulcers or thromboembolism (androgen deficiency leading to decreased fibrinolysis). Obesity and glucose intolerance are relatively common, and there is a disproportionate increase in the risk of death from diabetic vascular complications. An increased risk of midline germ cell tumours, leukaemia and lymphoma has been reported.

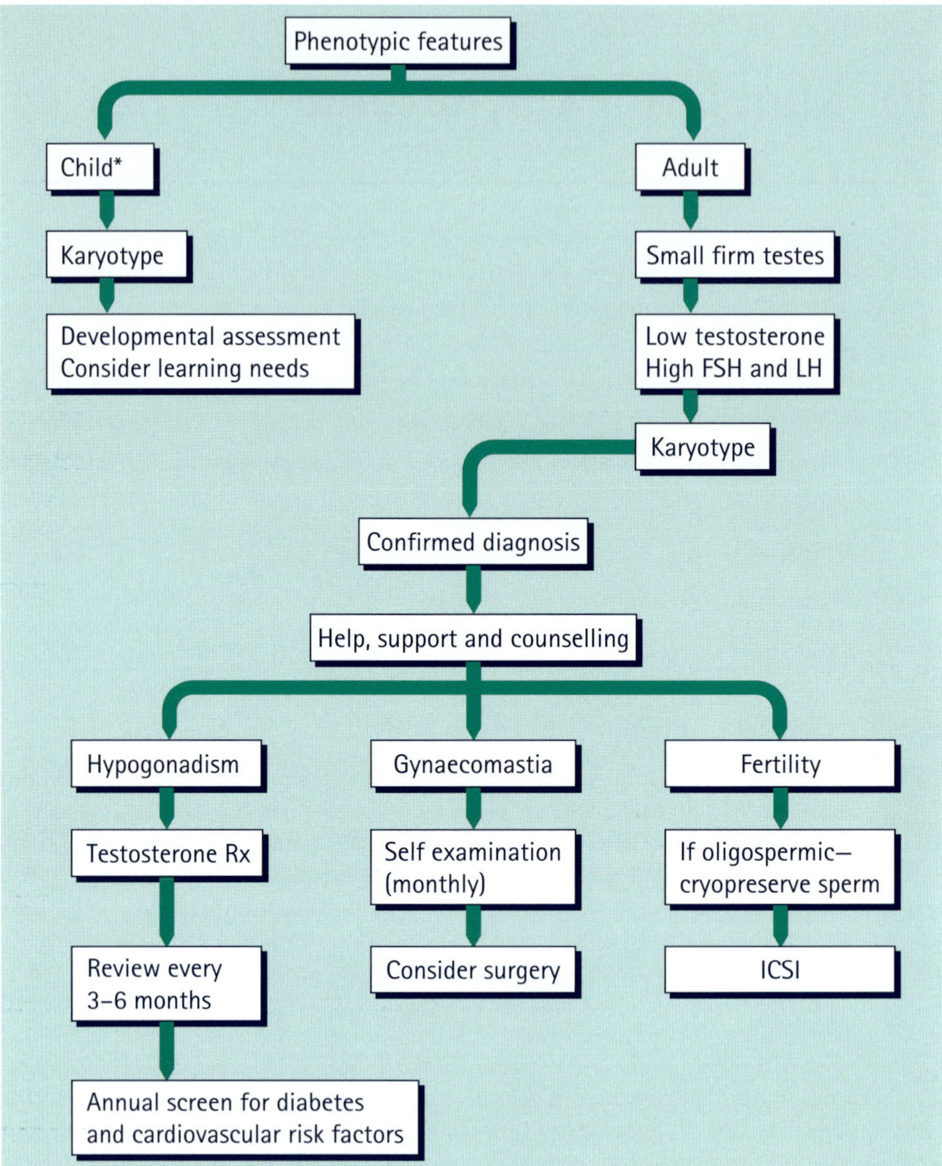

Fig. 30.1 Diagnosis and management. *Phenotypic features do not usually become apparent until puberty. Childhood diagnosis is usually made when karyotype is requested because of a family history of chromosomal disorders, or where there are developmental or learning problems. FSH = follicle-stimulating hormone; ICSI = intracytoplasmic sperm injection; LH = luteinizing hormone.

The patient will have features of hypogonadism with high gonadotropin (luteinizing hormone [LH] and follicle-stimulating hormone [FSH]) levels and low testosterone. Testicular volume should be assessed using a Prader orchidometer or with ultrasound. Typically, the man with Klinefelter's syndrome has small (around 5 ml) and firm testes. The average normal European man has testicular volume of 18 ml (range 12–30 ml). The mechanism for testosterone deficiency is not known, and Leydig function is variable. Testosterone may increase to a variable degree in response to human chorionic gonadotropin (hCG). This has been suggested as a therapy but there are no randomized trials at this stage. Because of the variable Leydig cell function, FSH is more discriminating for diagnosis than is LH measurement. Sex hormone-binding globulin (SHBG) levels are generally increased, and this further decreases the free androgen index. Because of the high LH, the androgen sensitivity index, which is the product of LH and testosterone concentration, is increased markedly. Karyotyping should be requested at an early stage in the investigation of all hypogonadal men. In some cases of mosaicism the 47,XXY karyotype may be present in the testes but not in peripheral blood lymphocytes. A testicular biopsy should be considered in cases where the diagnosis is suspected but not confirmed with standard karyotyping.

Diagnosis and management of Klinefelter's syndrome is summarized in Figure 30.1. Careful explanation and counselling is required to avoid undue psychological distress related to the diagnosis. In most cases, it is appropriate to initiate androgen replacement from an early stage. It usually does not improve gynaecomastia, and certainly has no bearing on fertility. Surgery for gynaecomastia may be considered for cosmetic and psychological reasons, and also because of the increased risk of breast cancer. Almost all men with Klinefelter's syndrome are infertile. Less than 10% of men with Klinefelter's syndrome have sperm in their ejaculate. As the number of sperm, and the chance of having sperm, diminishes rapidly after puberty, early recovery and cryopreservation should be considered in those men who have sperm in their ejaculate. In many cases, sperm can be recovered from a testicular biopsy, even if there is no sperm in the ejaculate.

The technique of intracytoplasmic sperm injection (ICSI) has recently transformed the outlook for men who are infertile through oligospermia, including those with Klinefelter's syndrome. In this technique, a recovered sperm is injected into an egg through the zona pellucida and the wall of the egg. After the embryo is cultured, as for standard *in vitro* fertilization, it is implanted into the female partner. Most infants with a Klinefelter's father born by this technique have normal karyotype. There is, however, increased risk of sex and somatic chromosomal abnormalities, as well as of imprinting disorders. Genetic counselling should be undertaken in all cases, and pre-implantation genetic diagnosis is now available in some centres.

Recent Developments

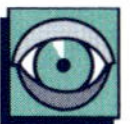

1 The $(CAG)_n$ repeat polymorphism in the androgen receptor gene, the length of which is inversely proportional to androgen action, may have a significant role in determining how the hypogonadal features develop.[2] Diabetes has usually been ascribed to obesity and insulin resistance, but men with Klinefelter's are more prone to autoimmune disease making it important that type 1 diabetes is considered in a man who becomes hyperglycaemic.

2 Overall, risk of premature death is increased in Klinefelter's syndrome. A recent study from UK[3] assessed standard mortality ratios (SMRs) for 3518 men diagnosed since 1959. SMR was 1.5 (95% confidence interval [CI] 1.4 to 1.7) overall with increased deaths from cardiovascular, respiratory and central nervous system causes. Deaths from diabetes, epilepsy, pulmonary embolism, peripheral vascular disease, renal disorders and hip fracture were

particularly increased. Surprisingly, deaths from ischaemic heart disease were decreased (SMR 0.7). The latter may reflect protection from increased oestrogen levels.

3 The authors of the above cohort study have published a further study examining SMRs of various cancers.[4] They found only a minimal overall increase in cancer incidence. Mortality from lung cancer was increased (SMR 1.5), whereas that for breast cancer was markedly increased (SMR 57.8), and SMR for non-Hodgkin's lymphoma was also increased (SMR 3.5). There was a remarkably low mortality from prostate cancer. These differences to the normal population obviously largely reflect the hypogonadal state but other hormonal changes including increased activity of the growth hormone/insulin-like growth factor-1 axis due to decreased negative feedback from androgens may also play a role.[5]

4 There has been a remarkable improvement in the prognosis for the man with Klinefelter's who wishes to father a child. In a recent series of 42 men with Klinefelter's syndrome,[6] pre-treatment with aromatase inhibitors both increased testosterone level and sperm recovery. Sperm was recovered in 39 of 54 (72%) biopsies and dissections, and 18 pregnancies achieved with ICSI resulted in birth of 21 healthy children, all of whom had a normal karyotype.

Conclusions

It seems prudent, in Klinefelter's syndrome, to treat the hypogonadal state from the time of normal puberty. There is even an argument for starting androgen replacement sooner. A variety of androgen replacement treatments is now available and we usually monitor patients every 3–6 months clinically and with measurement of serum testosterone, LH and FSH. Annual screening for diabetes and for cardiovascular risk factors is also indicated. The prognosis for fertility has improved immensely in recent years. If there is sperm in the ejaculate around the time of puberty (less than 10% of cases), consideration should be given to cryopreservation. Sperm can be recovered from testicular biopsies of many men who do not have sperm in their ejaculate. ICSI now has a high rate of success and most offspring are chromosomally normal, although careful genetic counselling should be undertaken prior to fertility treatment in each case.

Further Reading

1 Lanfranco F, Kamischke A, Nieschlag E. Klinefelter's syndrome. *Lancet* 2004; **364**: 273–83.

2 Zunn AR, Ramos P, Elder FF, Kowal K, Samango-Sprouse C, Ross JL. Androgen receptor CAGn repeat length influences phenotype of 47, XXY (Klinefelter) syndrome. *J Clin Endocrinol Metab* 2005; **90**: 5041–6.

3 Swerdlow AJ, Higgins CD, Schoemaker MJ, Wright AF, Jacobs PA. Mortality in patients with Klinefelter syndrome in Britain: a cohort study. *J Clin Endocrinol Metab* 2005; **90**: 6516–22.

4 Swerdlow AJ, Schoemaker MJ, Higgins CD, Wright AF, Jacobs PA. Cancer incidence and mortality in men with Klinefelter syndrome: a cohort study. *J Natl Cancer Inst* 2005; **97**: 1204–10.

5 Scheithauer BW, Moschopulos M, Kovaks K, Jhaveri BS, Percek T, Lloyd RV. The pituitary in Klinefelter syndrome. *Endocrine Pathol* 2005; **16**: 133–8.

6 Schiff JD, Palermo GD, Veeck LL, Goldstein M, Rosenwaks Z, Schlegel PN. Success of testicular sperm injection and intracytoplasmic sperm injection in men with Klinefelter syndrome. *J Clin Endocrinol Metab* 2005; **90**: 6263–7.

SECTION SIX **06**

Calcium

PROBLEM

31 Primary Hyperparathyroidism

Case History

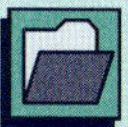

Mrs LD is a 72-year-old woman who enjoys reasonably good health but consults you because she has recently noticed increased thirst, constipation, and that her memory is not as good as she would like it to be. She takes a small dose of atenolol (50 mg) for hypertension but no other medications. Clinical examination is unremarkable. Among the investigations you request is plasma calcium which is elevated at 2.9 mmol/l (normal 2.2–2.6 mmol/l).

Consider the differential diagnosis, bearing in mind her age.

What investigations should be carried out?

What are the factors that would make you consider referring her for surgery?

Background

The majority of calcium in the body is in the bone. Plasma calcium exists as free ionized calcium (50%), as a protein-bound fraction chiefly bound to albumin (40%) and a small amount is complexed with anions such as phosphate and citrate. To avoid artefactual elevations in plasma calcium, a fasting sample of blood should be collected with the patient supine and without the aid of a tourniquet. The commonest cause of hypercalcaemia in ambulatory patients is hyperparathyroidism (>90%). Malignancy is the most important cause in hospitalized patients (65%). The causes of hypercalcaemia are listed in Table 31.1.

In the usual situation hypercalcaemia causes suppression of parathyroid hormone (PTH). The approach to a patient with hypercalcaemia must include a careful history with particular care to understand the rapidity of evolution of the hypercalcaemia, weight loss and associated symptoms. Clinical examination may suggest underlying malignancy

Table 31.1 Causes of hypercalcaemia

Primary hyperparathyroidism	Sporadic Associated with MEN1 or MEN2A familial After renal transplantation
Secondary hyperparathyroidism	Vitamin D deficiency Chronic renal failure
Malignancies	Humoral hypercalcaemia caused by PTHrP, 1,25(OH)$_2$ D or rarely ectopic PTH Local osteolytic hypercalcaemia as in multiple myeloma
Sarcoidosis and other granulomatous diseases	
Endocrinopathies	Thyrotoxicosis Hypoadrenalism Phaeochromocytomas VIPoma
Familial benign hypercalciuric hypercalcaemia	
Drug induced	Milk-alkali syndrome Vitamin A intoxication Vitamin D intoxication Lithium therapy Thiazide diuretics

MEN = multiple endocrine neoplasia; PTH = parathyroid hormone; PTHrP = parathyroid related protein.

supported by a history of rapid weight loss, very high calcium levels and rapid evolution of hypercalcaemia. Initial biochemical tests should include plasma calcium, phosphate, PTH, vitamin D, alkaline phosphatase and 24-hour urinary calcium output.

Primary hyperparathyroidism

The majority (85%) of cases of primary hyperparathyroidism are due to solitary parathyroid adenomas.[1] Parathyroid hyperplasia accounts for most of the remainder, including those with multiple endocrine neoplasia (MEN) 1 or MEN2A. Parathyroid carcinoma is rare. About 75% cases of individuals with primary hyperparathyroidism are women; mean age at diagnosis is 55 years. Clinically overt primary hyperparathyroidism may present with anorexia, nausea, vomiting and constipation if the serum calcium is high. Polyuria and polydipsia are common. Weakness, tiredness and lassitude, lack of concentration and mood changes are also seen. Complications of primary hyperparathyroidism include nephrolithiasis (20%), nephrocalcinosis and rarely distal renal tubular acidosis due to prolonged effects of hypercalcaemia on the renal tubules. Chondrocalcinosis resulting from deposition of crystals of calcium pyrophosphate typically affects the menisci of the knees and may present as attacks of pseudogout and lead to degenerative arthritis. Other features include corneal calcification, hypertension, peptic ulceration, pruritus and myopathy. Peptic ulceration may be the result of increased gastrin release due to hypercalcaemia, although Zollinger–Ellison syndrome as a part of the MEN1 syndrome may need to be excluded if ulcerations are severe or intractable.

Differential diagnosis is from other causes of hypercalcaemia, most often malignancy (Figure 31.1). In primary hyperparathyroidism, both plasma calcium and PTH are elevated.

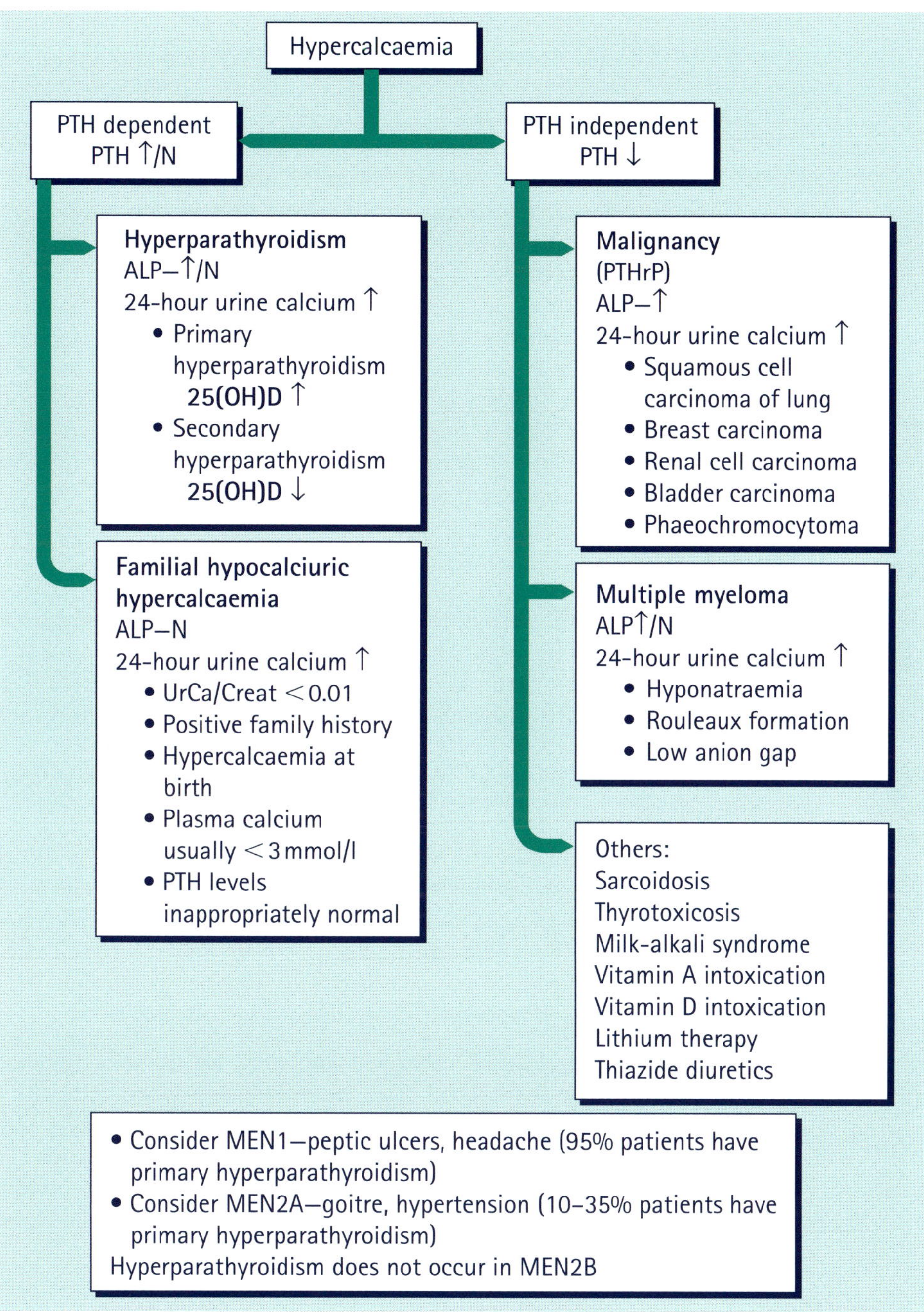

Fig. 31.1 Differential diagnosis of hypercalcaemia. ALP = alkaline phosphatase; MEN = multiple endocrine neoplasia; N = normal; PTH = parathyroid hormone; PTHrP = parathyroid-related protein.

It is also associated with a state of hyperchloraemic acidosis and hypercalciuria. In humoral hypercalcaemia of malignancy, PTH is suppressed as the hypercalcaemia is maintained by the parathyroid-related protein (PTHrP) which has structural homology with PTH but is not detected by the sensitive two-site assays for PTH currently used by most laboratories. Localization of the parathyroid tumour is by ultrasonography and ^{99}Tc Sestamibi scanning. Computed tomography (CT) and magnetic resonance imaging (MRI) may provide additional information but are not routinely necessary.

In the case of clinically overt hyperparathyroidism, surgery should be offered to all patients where there is no contraindication. In the asymptomatic patient, surgery is recommended when the plasma calcium is 0.26 mmol/l (1 mg/dl) above the upper limit of normal, urinary calcium excretion is greater than 400 mg over 24 hours, there is a 30% reduction in creatinine clearance or bone mass density T-score is greater than −2.5 at any site in an individual under 50 years of age. In patients who undergo parathyroidectomy, biochemical aberrations return to normal and are associated with an increase in bone mineral density. However, the majority (75%) of asymptomatic patients who do not undergo surgery, do not show evidence of disease progression.

Recent Developments

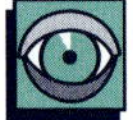

1. Isolation of the calcium-sensing receptor has led to possible new approaches in the treatment of primary hyperparathyroidism in the future. Cinacalcet is a drug that binds to the calcium-sensing receptor and inhibits the release of PTH. Preliminary studies with this drug have shown promising results both in primary hyperparathyroidism and that secondary to chronic renal failure. In a recent trial,[2] the drug was shown to decrease PTH and to normalize calcium in patients with primary hyperparathyroidism.

2. Bisphosphonates should be considered for short-term management in the emergency situation. However, the decrease in serum calcium is only temporary and levels of PTH increase. The latter may give rise to secondary bone changes if bisphosphonates are used for the long-term. For the present, the only definitive treatment with proven long-term benefit is surgery.[3] Surgery may be considered for a greater proportion of patients as minimally invasive parathyroidectomy becomes more widely available.[4]

3. Primary hyperparathyroidism is associated with increased risk for cardiovascular disease. The precise reason for this is not clear, nor is it known whether the risk decreases with successful treatment. N-terminal pro-B-type natriuretic peptide is increased in patients with cardiac failure. A recent study[5] has shown that this peptide is increased in hyperparathyroid patients. Levels of the inflammatory markers C-reactive protein and tumour necrosis factor α were also increased. Another study[6] has demonstrated increased levels of circulating markers of endothelial activation.

Conclusions

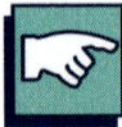

Primary hyperparathyroidism, malignancies including lymphoproliferative disorders, and multiple myeloma should be considered in the differential diagnosis. A careful history including previous smoking habits will be necessary. However, due to the mild elevations in calcium concentration, primary hyperparathyroidism is the likely cause. The investigations should confirm the diagnosis biochemically followed by localization of the tumour. Given that this patient is symptomatic, surgery is the preferred mode of treatment.

Further Reading

1 Bilezikian J, Silverberg S. Asymptomatic primary hyperparathyroidism. *N Engl J Med* 2004; **350**: 1746–51.

2 Peacock M, Bilezikian JP, Klassen PS, Guo MD, Turner SA, Shoback D. Cinacalcet hydrochloride maintains long-term normocalcemia in patients with primary hyperparathyroidism. *J Clin Endocrinol Metab* 2005; **90**: 135–41.

3 Jansson S, Morgan E. Biochemical effects from treatment with bisphosphonate and surgery in patients with primary hyperpaprathyroidism. *World J Surg* 2004; **28**: 1293–7.

4 Ollila DW, Caudle AS, Cance WG, *et al.* Successful minimally invasive parathyroidectomy for primary hyperparathyroidism without using intraoperative parathyroid hormone assays. *Am J Surg* 2006; **191**: 52–6.

5 Ogard CG, Engelman MD, Kistorp C, Nielsen SL, Vestergaard H. Increased plasma N-terminal pro-B-type natriuretic peptide and markers of inflammation related to atherosclerosis in patients with primary hyperparathyroidism. *Clin Endocrinol* 2005; **63**: 493–8.

6 Fallo F, Cella G, Casonanto A, *et al.* Biochemical markers of endothelial activation in primary hyperparathyroidism. *Horm Metab Res* 2006; **38**: 125–9.

PROBLEM

32 Hypocalcaemia

Case History

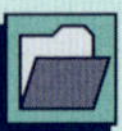

A 36-year-old woman presents having had her first ever fit. She has recently delivered a child who is healthy and thriving. She has been treated for hypothyroidism with 100 μg thyroxine per day over the past 8 years. There is no history of head injury and no family history of epilepsy. Routine investigations reveal plasma calcium of 1.4 mmol/l (normal 2.2–2.6 mmol/l).

What are the likely causes of her hypocalcaemia?

Is her recent pregnancy relevant?

How should replacement therapy be approached?

Discuss the management should she present again with a fit as an emergency?

Are there any special precautions to take if she was to become pregnant again?

Background

The majority (99%) of calcium in the body resides in the bone, and 99% of calcium in the bone exists in the crystalline mineral phase whereas the remainder is in equilibrium with extracellular calcium. Of the plasma calcium, 45–50% is bound to protein, chiefly albumin. The remaining calcium is the free or ionized form and is biologically available. True hypocalcaemia occurs when the level of ionized calcium decreases. In hospitals where ionized calcium is not routinely measured, corrected total calcium may be used. The correction used is:

$$\frac{[(40\text{-albumin})\times 0.2]}{10} \quad \text{measured [Ca]} = \text{actual calcium concentration}$$

The most common causes of hypocalcaemia are primary hypoparathyroidism and vitamin D deficiency (see Table 32.1). Primary hypoparathyroidism commonly results from autoimmunity or occurs following neck surgery. Autoimmune hypoparathyroidism may occur as part of an autoimmune polyendocrinopathy syndrome. Hypomagnesaemia

Table 32.1 Causes of hypocalcaemia

PTH-related causes	
Impaired secretion or lack of PTH	Congenital absence of parathyroid glands Autoimmune polyendocrinopathy syndrome type1 Post-operative Infiltrative disorders Idiopathic Following radioiodine ablation Respiratory alkalosis Hypomagnesaemia Autosomal dominant hypocalcaemia Pseudohypoparathyroidism
Resistance to the action of PTH	Hypomagnesaemia Chronic renal failure
Vitamin D-related causes	
Vitamin D deficiency	Dietary absence Reduced exposure to sunlight Malabsorption syndrome
Loss of vitamin D	Impaired enterohepatic circulation Anticonvulsant therapy
Impaired 25-hydroxylation	Liver disease Isoniazid
Impaired 1α-hydroxylation	Vitamin D resistant rickets type 1 Isoniazid Chronic renal failure
Oncogenic osteomalacia	
Tissue resistance to vitamin D	Vitamin D resistant rickets type 2
Other causes	
Excessive deposition in the skeleton	Osteoblastic metastases 'Hungry bone' syndrome
Chelation	Infusion of citrated blood or EDTA-containing products Phosphate infusion Foscarnet
Neonatal hypocalcaemia	Prematurity Asphyxia
HIV infection	Drug therapy Vitamin D deficiency Hypomagnesaemia PTH resistance
Critical illness	Intensive care patients Acute pancreatitis Toxic shock syndrome Erythroderma

HIV = human immunodeficiecy virus; PTH = parathyroid hormone.

impairs secretion of PTH and also induces a state of PTH resistance. Both these factors lead to hypocalcaemia that is seen more often in chronic alcoholics.

The symptoms and signs of low ionized calcium in adults include paraesthesiae of the hands, feet and around the mouth. Carpopedal spasm is less common in adults and fits and stridor are rare. Children, in addition to carpopedal spasm, may experience stridor and convulsions. These features result from a decrease in ionized calcium that leads to increased excitability in the peripheral nerves. Trousseau's sign of latent tetany is elicited by inflating the sphygmomanometer cuff above the systolic blood pressure when carpal spasm appears within 3 minutes. Chvostek's sign, a less specific sign of hypocalcaemia, is seen when twitching of the facial muscles occurs in response to a gentle tap over the branches of the facial nerve as they emerge from the parotid gland. In more severe hypocalcaemia, bradycardia, hypotension, seizures, and prolongation of the QT interval on the electrocardiogram occur.

Investigations to find the underlying cause of hypocalcaemia should initially include ionized calcium, plasma inorganic phosphate, 25(OH) D, parathyroid hormone and albumin. Investigations should reveal the underlying diagnosis in the majority of cases. Primary hypoparathyroidism is relatively uncommon. More often the patient has vitamin D deficiency with secondary hyperparathyroidism. In patients with primary hypoparathyroidism, other autoimmune conditions need to be excluded. In the alcoholic patient, hypomagnesaemia may be the cause of hypocalcaemia in which correction of the magnesium defect will lead to correction of the hypocalcaemia. In individuals with another autoimmune condition, Addison's disease should be excluded by plasma adrenocorticotrophic hormone (ACTH) and rapid ACTH stimulation test (the short Synacthen test).

Treatment of hypocalcaemia depends on the rapidity of onset and should initially focus on correcting the biochemical abnormality which often involves calcium supplementation, followed by treatment of the underlying cause. In mild acute hypocalcaemia (total calcium 2.0 mmol/l; ionized calcium 0.8 mmol/l) oral calcium supplementation at a dose of 1000 mg/day is all that is necessary (Figure 32.1). In acute symptomatic hypocalcaemia (total calcium 1.8 mmol/l and ionized calcium 0.7 mmol/l), treatment is urgently needed, and 10–20 ml of a 10% solution of calcium gluconate should be given intravenously over 10–20 minutes. The calcium should be diluted in dextrose or saline as concentrated calcium is irritant to the veins. It should not be administered more rapidly, because of the risk of cardiac arrhythmias and even systolic arrest. A bolus of calcium will raise the calcium concentration for not more that 2–3 hours and should be followed by a slow infusion at 0.5–1.5 mg/kg per hour. Where hypomagnesaemia is suspected, 16 mmol of magnesium as magnesium sulphate should be given over 10 minutes followed by 8 mmol in 100 ml over 1 hour. Subsequent management will depend on the underlying cause. Calcium supplementation is contraindicated in autosomal dominant hypocalcaemia.

In pregnancy, special precaution is needed and calcium supplementation should be started early. Additional $1,25(OH)_2$ vitamin D replacement will be needed and the dose should be reduced to pre-pregnancy levels after delivery. If the woman wishes to breastfeed, the dose is reduced to one-half the pre-pregnancy dose as prolactin increases $1,25(OH)_2$ vitamin D production and also increases secretion of parathyroid hormone-related protein.

Recent Developments

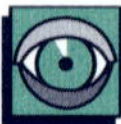

1. Novel genetic abnormalities causing inherited forms of hypoparathyroidism are being identified. These include abnormalities in the genome near the gene for the SOX3 transcription factor causing the X-linked recessive form of hypoparathyroidism.[1] A mutation in the *GATA3* gene has been identified as the cause of the HDR syndrome (hypoparathyroidism, sensorineural deafness and renal abnormality).[2] Mutations of the parathyroid hormone gene at chromosome 11p15 have been identified in autosomal forms of inherited hypoparathyroidism.

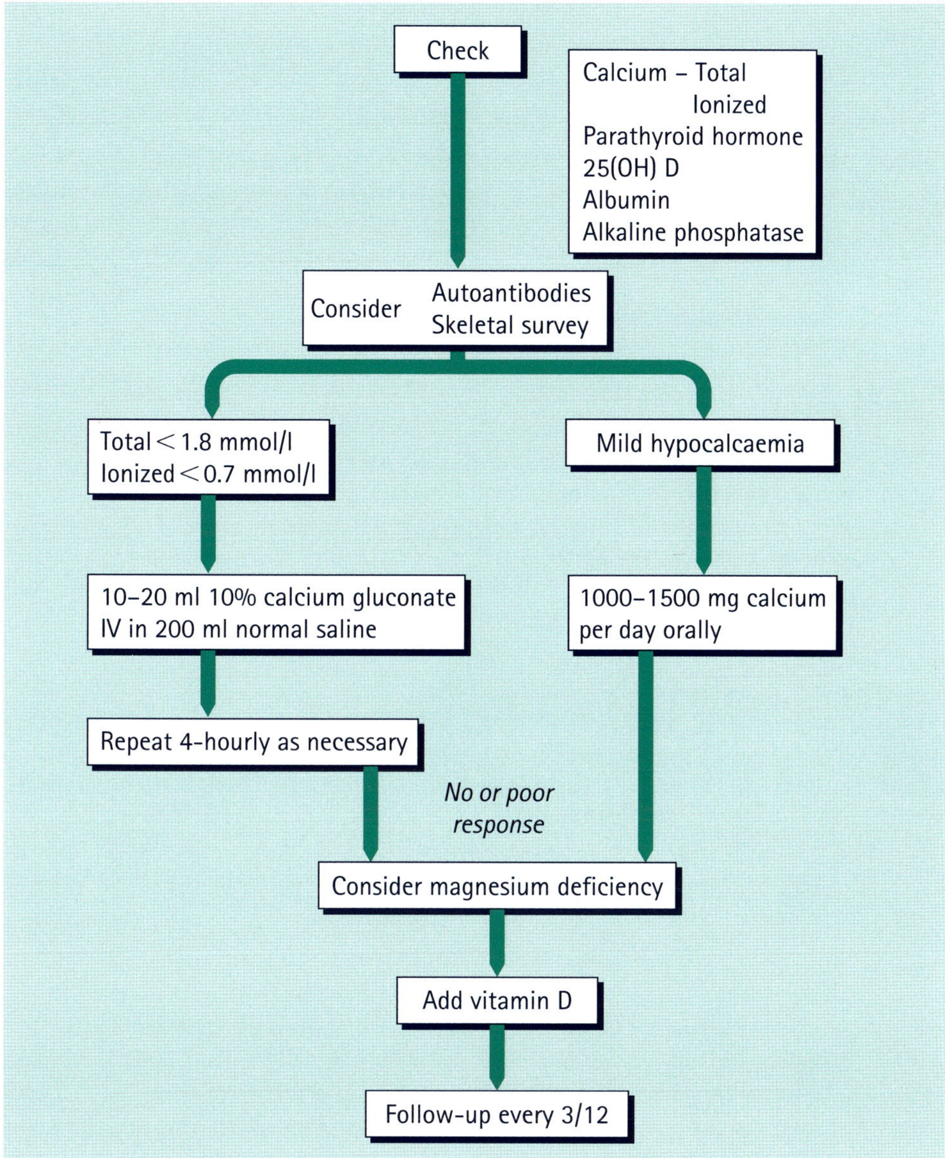

Fig. 32.1 Management of hypocalcaemia.

2 Abnormalities of the calcium sensing receptor gene located at chromosome 3q21.3 have been linked to disorders of calcium metabolism.[3] Loss of function mutations are responsible for familial benign hypocalciuric hypercalcaemia, which may occur in up to 1:16 000 of the population. Rare cases of neonatal severe hyperparathyroidism have been described. Activating mutations of the gene cause autosomal dominant hypocalcaemia with hypercalciuria. This condition, which occurs in about 1:70 000, is often asymptomatic but some patients require treatment with vitamin D analogues.

3 It is not always easy for the surgeon to preserve parathyroid function during thyroidectomy as the blood supply to the glands is often damaged or affected by thrombosis. Long-term management of hypercalcaemia with calcium and vitamin D is not always straightforward. Increasingly, parathyroid autotransplantation is being used as an alternative to trying to preserve the glands *in situ*.[4]

4 An intriguing and novel treatment for hypoparathyroidism has been proposed by Tiffany *et al.*,[5] who have developed PTH-loaded, biodegradable microspheres to be implanted as a controlled-release form of PTH therapy. Use of this system could obviate the need for complex calcium and vitamin D therapy and may simplify management of patients with disorders of the parathyroid glands.

Conclusions

In this woman, the most likely cause for her hypocalcaemia is autoimmune hypoparathyroidism as a part of autoimmune polyendocrinopathy syndrome. Pregnancy is likely to have worsened the hypocalcaemia and the rapid deterioration in calcium levels led to a seizure. Treatment would necessitate rapid correction of the hypocalcaemia with intravenous calcium followed by oral calcium and Vitamin D. In the future, the dose of vitamin D should be increased when she becomes pregnant.

Further Reading

1 Bowl MR, Nesbit MA, Harding B, *et al.* An interstitial deletion–insertion involving chromosomes 2p25.3 and Xq27.1, near SOX3 causes X-linked recessive hypoparathyroidism. *J Clin Invest* 2005; **115**: 2822–31.

2 Masanori A, Katsihuko T, Yumi A, Takayoshi T. A novel mutation in the *GATA*3 gene in a family with HDR syndrome (hypoparathyroidism, sensorineural deafness and renal anomaly syndrome). *J Pediat Endocrinol Metab* 2006; **19**: 87–92.

3 Gunn IR, Gaffney D. Clinical and laboratory features of calcium-sensing receptor disorders: a systematic review. *Ann Clin Biochem* 2004; **41**: 441–58.

4 Palazzo FF, Sywak MS, Sidhu SB, Barraclough BH, Delbridge LW. Parathyroid autotransplantation during total thyroidectomy—does the number of glands transplanted affect outcome? *World J Surg* 2005; **29**: 629–31.

5 Tiffany A, Fong P, Goyal A, Saltzman WM, Moss RL, Breuer C. Development of a parathyroid hormone controlled release system as potential surgical treatment for hypoparathyroidism. *J Pediatr Surg* 2005; **40**: 81–5.

SECTION SEVEN 07

Hypertension

PROBLEM

33 Hypertension – is it Endocrine?

Case History

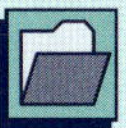

A 28-year-old sales executive has a routine medical in relation to an application for a mortgage. His past medical history is unremarkable and he is not taking any medications. He drinks around 50 units of alcohol per week but is a non-smoker. His mother had hypertension and his father died at the age of 62 from a myocardial infarction. On examination, his blood pressure is 190/100 mmHg and he has arteriovenous nicking in his retina.

How would you further assess his risk from hypertension?

What underlying causes would you consider?

How likely are you to find an underlying cause?

How would you approach his treatment and follow-up?

Background

It is important to consider secondary causes of hypertension as they may be:

- an indication for specific treatments
- curable by surgery
- familial
- associated with other clinical features as part of a recognized syndrome.

Secondary hypertension should be considered in younger patients, those with associated electrolyte abnormalities (particularly hypokalaemia), in patients with adrenal

Table 33.1 Causes of secondary hypertension

Renal	Primary renal disease Polycystic kidney disease Renovascular
Endocrine	Primary hyperaldosteronism Cushing's syndrome Phaeochromocytoma 17α-hydroxylase deficiency 11β-hydroxylase deficiency Syndrome of apparent mineralocorticoid excess Glucocorticoid remediable hyperaldosteronism
Vascular	Coarctation of the aorta
Sleep apnoea syndrome	Vasculitis

nodules, and in whon an adrenal nodule is discovered. The common causes of secondary hypertension are summarized in Table 33.1.

The following should be undertaken in all patients with suspected hypertension:

- *Detect and confirm hypertension.* Out of office confirmation is recommended—this may involve patients monitoring their blood pressure or the use of ambulatory monitors.
- *Detect target organ damage.* Examination of the retina and heart, electrocardiogram (ECG), renal functions and measurement of urine protein content should be carried out.
- *Identify other cardiovascular risk factors.* Calculating the 10-year risk of a cardiovascular event is useful when planning treatment and follow-up.
- *Detect secondary cause of hypertension.* See Table 33.1.

The general approach to the patient with hypertension is summarized in Figure 33.1. Treatment for hypertension must include non-pharmacological measures such as regular exercise, reduced salt intake and weight loss. Alcohol consumed in moderation (one to two drinks per day) may be less harmful. Based on the recent recommendations of the Joint National Committee 7 (JNC 7), initial drug therapy should be with a thiazide. β-blockers such as atenolol are no longer recommended as first line agents. The next agent may be an angiotensin-converting enzyme inhibitor, angiotensin-receptor blocker or a calcium-channel blocker. When a specific cause for hypertension has been isolated, treatment should be directed to correct the underlying abnormality. In many cases of secondary hypertension, long-standing high blood pressure may cause medial hypertrophy of the arterial wall and lead to perpetuation of the hypertension even after the primary problem has been corrected.

Various endocrine causes of hypertension

Renal artery stenosis accounts for less than 1% of all patients with hypertension. Levels of both renin and aldosterone are increased. Sixty-five per cent of cases are due to atherosclerotic disease. In patients under the age of 50, who represent 35% of the total, fibromuscular

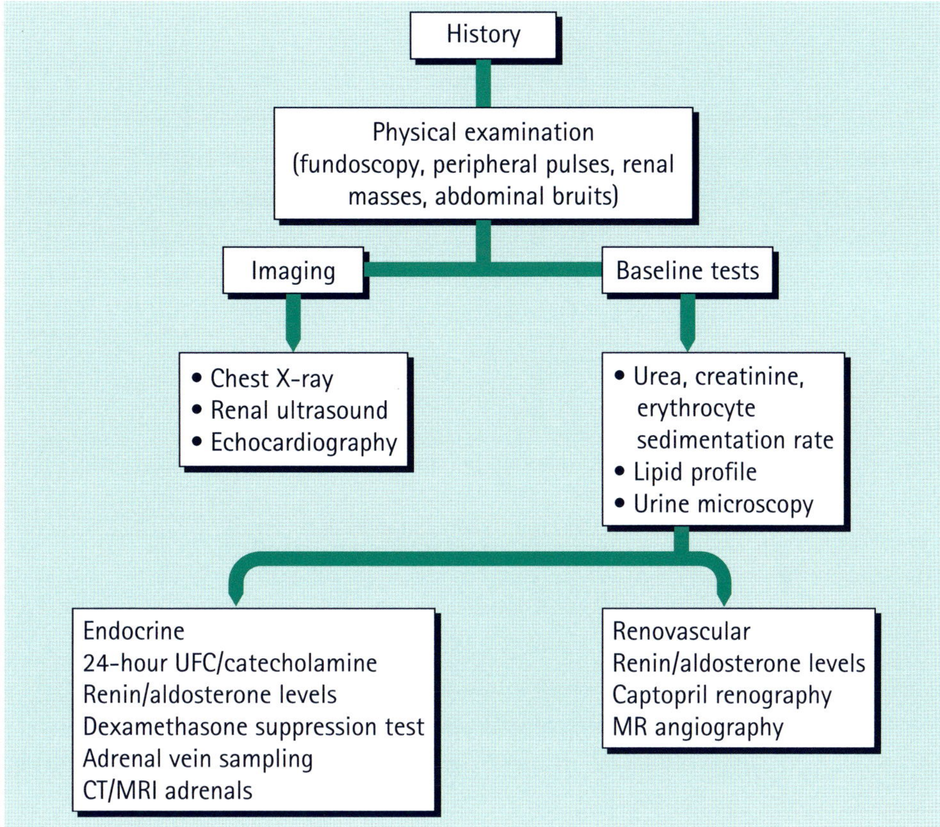

Fig. 33.1 Diagnostic evaluation of the hypertensive patient. UFC = urine free cortisol.

dysplasia is the usual underlying cause. Magnetic resonance angiography is a useful screening tool, being both non-invasive and highly sensitive. Duplex ultrasound may also be used as a screening tool. Renal angiography remains the gold standard for diagnosing renal artery stenosis. The captopril isotope renogram is still used in some centres—uptake of isotope into the affected kidney is decreased or delayed following captopril administration. Management of renal artery stenosis is surgical in patients in whom this is possible.

The general approach to endocrine-related hypertension is presented in Figure 33.2. Hypertension is common among patients with thyrotoxicosis and diastolic blood pressure, in particular, may be increased in patients with hypothyroidism. Blood pressure is often increased in patients with acromegaly, although other features of the syndrome are usually present. An increasing number of patients with subclinical Cushing's syndrome are being diagnosed, often in association with an adrenal adenoma. Single cortisol estimation late in the evening may be useful, although 24-hour urine free cortisol and overnight dexamethasone suppression test are the screening methods of choice.

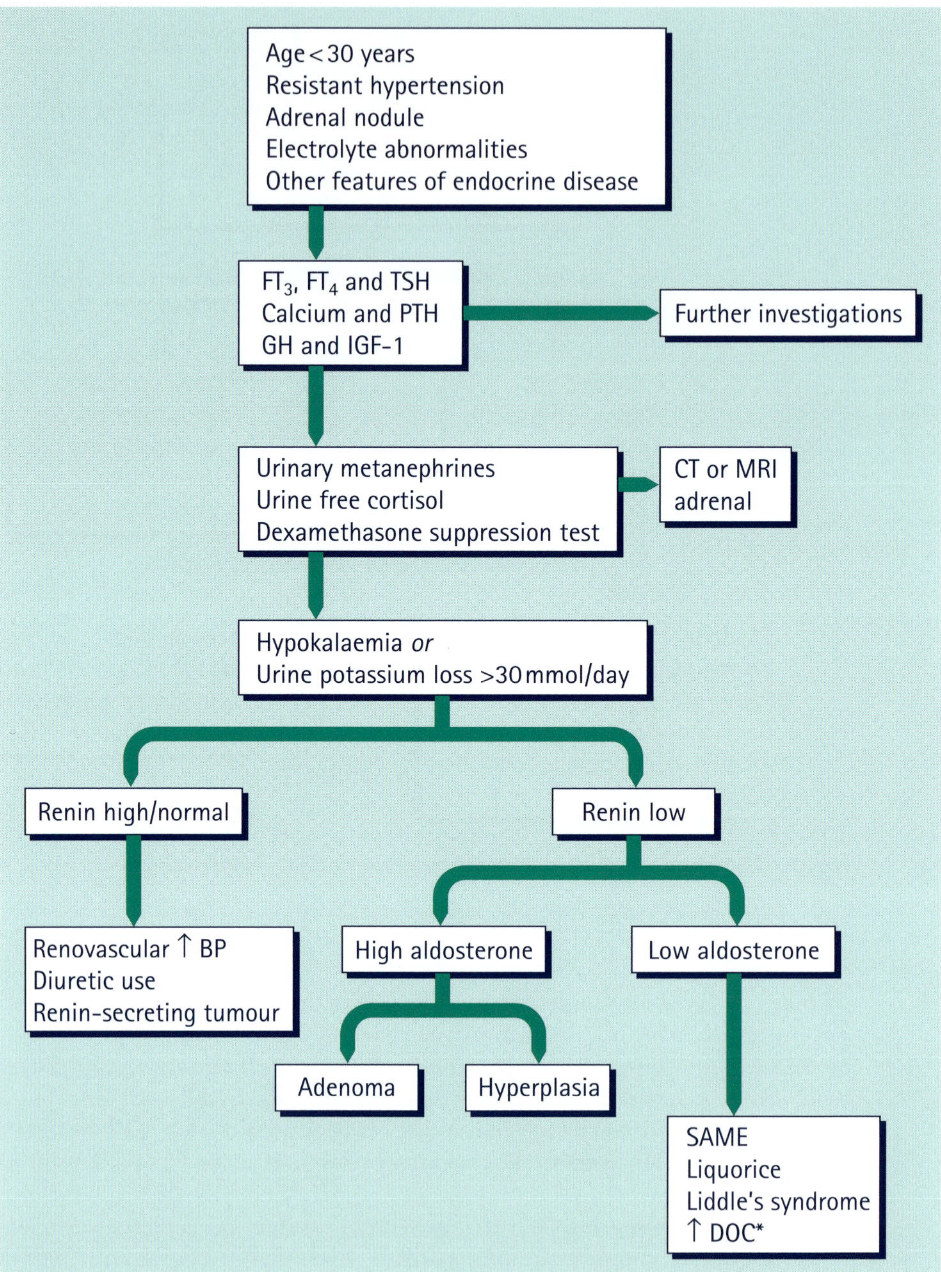

Fig. 33.2 Differential diagnosis of endocrine hypertension. *Deoxycorticosterone (DOC) is increased in some patients with adrenal tumours and in certain forms of congenital adrenal hypoplasia. BP = blood pressure; GH = growth hormone; IGF = insulin-like growth factor; PTH = parathyroid hormone; SAME = syndrome of apparent mineralocorticoid excess; TSH = thyroid-stimulating hormone.

Phaeochromocytoma

This accounts for less than 0.1% of all cases of hypertension. It should be considered when hypertension is paroxysmal and associated with symptoms such as palpitations, sweating and anxiety, or where blood pressure control deteriorates after β-blocker therapy is instituted. Up to a quarter of phaeochromocytomas are now recognized to occur as part of a familial syndrome and a careful family history is, therefore, mandatory in all cases. The tumours occur in multiple endocrine neoplasia type 2, in von Hippel–Lindau disease, and in families with mutation in the genes of the succinate dehydrogenase complex. The tumours usually secrete predominantly noradrenaline. Some secrete significant amounts of adrenaline. The clinical significance of dopamine-secreting lesions remains to be established. The tumours also secrete peptides including neuropeptide Y and endothelins. Initial investigation should be measurement of urinary metanephrines, followed by plasma catecholamines or metanephrines. Localization of the tumour with computed tomography or magnetic resonance imaging followed by metaiodobenzylguanidine (MIBG) scanning should be undertaken once biochemical diagnosis has been confirmed.

Mineralocorticoid hypertension

This group of disorders represents the commonest endocrine cause for hypertension. The commonest form of mineralocorticoid hypertension is primary hyperaldosteronism (Conn's syndrome), which is most commonly due to an adrenal adenoma. This is often suspected in patients with persistent hypokalaemia, but it is important to recognize that as many as half of the patients will have normal potassium levels. The ratio of circulating aldosterone to renin is the best screening tool for Conn's. Whenever possible, antihypertensive therapy should be stopped 2–3 weeks before the test is carried out. Patients who require antihypertensive treatment should be given an α-blocker which will affect neither aldosterone nor renin levels. The response to posture change after overnight recumbency is useful—normal people or those with essential hypertension will have increased renin and aldosterone after standing up whereas patients with Conn's will have no change in renin and may have a decrease in aldosterone because of the common diurnal variation of the hormone in Conn's patients. Once biochemical diagnosis is confirmed, computed tomography or magnetic resonance imaging of the adrenals should be carried out followed, if necessary, by adrenal vein sampling. Surgery is the treatment of choice for patients with a solitary functioning adenoma.

A severe form of hypertension exacerbated during pregnancy is due to an activating mutation of the mineralocorticoid receptor, leaving it with enhanced responsiveness to non-mineralocorticoid steroids, including progesterone.[1] The mutant receptor also binds cortisone, which is the major metabolite of cortisol, and because of the relative abundance of cortisone, this may account for early onset hypertension in patients with the mutation.

Deoxycorticosterone (DOC) is a relatively weak mineralocorticoid compared with aldosterone. The metabolite is produced in excess in some patients with adrenal carcinoma, and in certain forms of congenital adrenal hypoplasia (CAH). 11β-hydroxylase deficiency leads to accumulation of DOC as well as androgen metabolites. 17β-hydroxylase deficiency also leads to DOC accumulation but with decreased androgen production leading to a failure of normal male development. Both of these forms of CAH cause mineralocorticoid hypertension with suppression of renin.

The syndrome of apparent mineralocorticoid excess (SAME) is due to a deficiency in the enzyme 11β-hydroxysteroid dehydrogenase. This enzyme is responsible for conversion of cortisol to its metabolite cortisone. When the enzyme is deficient, cortisol accumulates locally in target tissues and is able to activate the mineralocorticoid receptor. The syndrome is inherited in an autosomal recessive manner, and causes severe hypertension. It can be treated either by mineralocorticoid receptor blockade or by using the pure glucocorticoid dexamethasone to decrease cortisol production. An acquired form of this condition is seen with excessive liquorice ingestion, which inhibits the enzyme.

Liddle's syndrome is due to mutations in the β or γ subunits of the epithelial sodium channel, leading to its constitutive activation and excessive sodium reabsorption in the distal renal tubule. Blockade of the channel with amiloride both decreases sodium reabsorption and improves hypertension. The syndrome has an autosomal dominant form of inheritance.

Glucocorticoid-remediable aldosteronism is also an autosomal dominant condition due to a recombination event between the 11β-hydroxylase and aldosterone synthase genes. This event renders the latter gene responsive to adrenocorticotrophic hormone (ACTH), and activity of the chimeric gene can be decreased by suppressing ACTH with glucocorticoids.

Recent Developments

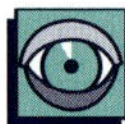

1. In a recent Japanese study[2] of 1020 hypertensive patients attending a general outpatient clinic, 61 patients were diagnosed as having primary hyperaldosteronism, 5 renovascular hypertension, 11 Cushing's and 10 subclinical Cushing's, and there were six cases of phaeochromocytoma. The overall prevalence of secondary hypertension was 9.1%.
2. Diurnal variation (night-time blood pressure lower) is lost in patients with endocrine hypertension,[3] particularly those with phaeochromocytoma. Successful removal of the underlying endocrine tumour restores the diurnal variation to something approaching normal in many cases.
3. High alcohol intake should not be neglected as a cause of hypertension. The relation between alcohol and risk of vascular disease is complex since, in spite of increasing blood pressure, modest amounts of alcohol appear to be protective.[4] Even alcoholic beverages that have been associated with vascular protection have a tendency to elevate blood pressure.[5]

Conclusions

Although the vast majority of patients with hypertension have no single identifiable underlying cause, investigation is warranted in young patients with severe hypertension. Even so, less than 10% will have secondary hypertension. The range of possible diagnoses is wide, but primary hyperaldosteronism is by far the most common. The potential effect of excess alcohol intake in the above patient should be borne in mind. The identification of an underlying cause is important as it may lead to more specific treatment, including surgical removal of adrenal tumours. Examination of the retina and heart (including ECG), along with checking renal function and the presence of proteinuria will help to identify patients who have end-organ damage and who may, therefore, require more vigorous treatment for their hypertension.

Further Reading

1 Rafestin-Oblin ME, Souque A, Bocchi B, Pinon G, Fagart J, Vandewalle A. The severe form of hypertension caused by the activating S810l mutation in the mineralocorticoid receptor is cortisone related. *Endocrinology* 2003; **144**: 528–33.

2 Omura M, Saito J, Yamaguchi Y, Kakuta Y, Nishikawa T. Prospective study on the prevalence of secondary hypertension among hypertensive patients visiting a general outpatient clinic in Japan. *Hypertens Res* 2004; **27**: 193–202.

3 Zelinka T, Strauch B, Pecen L, Widimsky J. Diurnal blood pressure variation in phaeochromocytoma, primary aldosteronism and Cushing's syndrome. *J Hum Hypertens* 2004; **18**: 107–11.

4 Kammersgaard LP, Skyhoj OT. Cardiovascular risk factors and 5-year mortality in the Copenhagen Stroke Study. *Cerebrovasc Dis* 2006; **21**: 187–93.

5 Zilkens RR, Burke V, Hodgson JM, Barden A, Beilin LJ, Puddey IB. Red wine and beer elevate blood pressure in normotensive men. *Hypertension* 2005; **45**: 874–9.

PROBLEM

34 Phaeochromocytoma

Case History

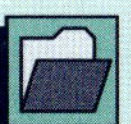

Mr MP is a 38-year-old man who recently presented with a transient speech disturbance (dysphasia). He has been intermittently hypertensive for 6 years and describes episodes of feeling afraid and panic stricken. Currently he takes atenolol 500 mg/day, enalapril 20 mg/day, and furosemide 40 mg/day. He attends for review and his blood pressure is recorded at 170/95 mmHg.

How would you investigate him for possible phaeochromocytoma?

What would be the best approach to his medical treatment?

Describe the approach to surgery, assuming that he has phaeochromocytoma?

Background

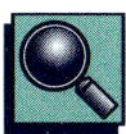

Catecholamine-secreting tumours arise from the chromaffin cells of the adrenal medulla in 80–85% of cases and from extra-adrenal sympathetic tissue in 15–20% (paraganglioma).[1,2] The condition is relatively rare, occurring in up to 0.5% of hypertensive patients in hospital clinics, but less than 0.05% of total hypertensive patients. The symptoms are variable, and it is not uncommon for years to elapse before the diagnosis is made. Adrenal phaeochromocytomas secrete mainly noradrenaline. Dopamine-secreting tumours are increasingly being recognized. The latter are often clinically silent, sometimes large by the time they are diagnosed, and frequently not associated with high blood pressure.

Episodes of increased catecholamine secretion cause hypertension, palpitation, headache and sweating. Patients often describe a sensation of fear or impending doom. The hypertension may be severe enough to precipitate hypertensive crisis or vascular events, including stroke. Precipitating factors include food, exercise, or drugs (commonly tricyclic antidepressants or metoclopramide). Episodes may last from seconds to up to an hour. Other symptoms include panic, anxiety and postural hypotension (due to hypovolaemia). Fever and flushing are less common symptoms. Hyperglycaemia, which is present not just during episodes of catecholamine surge, lactic acidosis and weight loss may also occur. Around 40–50% of phaeochromocytomas arise sporadically. Many cases are familial or genetic. Screening should be undertaken in the following genetic syndromes:

- Multiple endocrine neoplasia type 2—may be diagnosed through screening for mutations of the receptor tyrosine kinase (RET) proto-oncogene.
- Neurofibromatosis type 1—the major features are multiple fibromas of the skin and mucosa and 'café au lait' skin lesions.
- von Hippel–Lindau syndrome. Occurs in 1:36 000 live births—pancreatic and renal cysts and neoplasms; retinal and central nervous system haemangioblastomas; epidydimal cystadenoma.
- Mutations of the mitochondrial succinate dehydrogenase (*SDH*) gene. *SDHB* (1p 36.13) and *SDHD* (11q 23) mutations are associated with risk of phaeochromocytoma which is frequently extra-adrenal, often metabolically silent, and which may present at later stage with large tumour or malignant disease.

Less than 5% of adrenal adenomas are phaeochromocytomas, but up to 25% of phaeochromocytomas are picked up as incidentally discovered adrenal adenomas. The most widely used screening test is urinary metanephrines. Measurement of fractionated metanephrines (metadrenaline and normetadrenaline) has a sensitivity of 97% and a specificity of 69% for the diagnosis of phaeochromocytoma. Measurement of urinary vanillylmandelic acid is much less sensitive but just as specific. Plasma free metaphrine and normetanephrine measurement has a sensitivity approaching 100% and specificity of 90%. Plasma catecholamine measurements should be undertaken in the resting state through an indwelling cannula. Tricyclics, metoclopramide and phenoxybenzamine, paracetamol, labetalol, L-dopa and methyldopa may all produce false-positive results, whereas β-blockers and calcium-channel blockers may increase catecholamine values.

Chromogranin A can be a useful marker for chromaffin tumours although, with more widespread availability of accurate catecholamine measurements, the place of this test is less important than it once was. Similarly, the clonidine suppression test is not used as often as it once was. Within 3 hours of administration of 0.3 mg clonidine, plasma catecholamines should suppress by more than 50% or into the normal range. The test has a positive predictive value of 97%.

Computed tomography (CT) and magnetic resonance imaging (MRI) scanning are equally useful in detecting adrenal phaeochromocytomas, although MRI is more likely to detect tumours less than 1 cm in diameter. T2-weighted MRI with gadolinium enhancement is more sensitive for detection of extra-adrenal tumours. ^{131}I-metaiodobenzylguanidine (^{131}I-MIBG) is widely available for use as a radiopharmaceutical for functional scanning. It is 75–90% sensitive but fairly specific. Positive scans may also be obtained in patients with small cell lung tumour, medullary carcinoma of the thyroid, carcinoid tumour, or neuroblastoma. A number of drugs interfere with uptake of the agent including adrenergic agents, tricyclics, calcium-channel blockers, labetalol, and cocaine. These drugs should not be used in the week before the scan is done. ^{123}I-MIBG performs slightly better but is not yet widely available. Other scans that may be useful include an isotope bone scan to detect metastases, positron emission tomography with ^{18}F-fluorodopamine or ^{18}F-fluorodeoxyglucose, and scanning with ^{111}Indium-labelled octreotide. The latter is, of course, not specific and only binds to 25% of phaeochromocytomas but it may be useful in cases where tumour localization is proving difficult.

The initial medical treatment of choice is the selective, non-competitive α_2-blocker phenoxybenzamine. This is started at a dose of 10 mg twice daily, and can be increased every few days up to a maximum of 1 mg/kg. Alternatives are doxazosin or prazosin. β-blockade should not be started before the patient is fully alpha blocked as it may cause the blood pressure to increase. Cardioselective β_1-blockers such as metoprolol or calcium-channel blockers are the second line of therapy.

Once blood pressure is well controlled and there is no orthostatic hypotension, the patient should be ready for surgery, which requires a surgeon and an anaesthetist with specific experience of dealing with the condition. Surgery is now generally carried out laparoscopically for both intra- and extra-adrenal tumours. This has decreased length of hospital stay, rate of complications and cost. Patients with bilateral disease may undergo selective removal of tumours to spare functioning adrenal cortex. All patients require careful follow-up as the recurrence rate for intra-adrenal tumours is 14% and for extra-adrenal tumours it is as high as 33%.

Malignancy is particularly likely in tumours that are large (>5 cm), those that are extra-adrenal, and in patients with *SDH* mutations. Malignant phaeochromocytoma has a 5-year survival rate of 50%. The tumours metastasize to bone, lung, liver and lymph nodes. Treatment is with radical surgery, therapeutic doses of ^{131}I-MIBG, and with chemotherapy.

Recent Developments

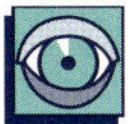

1 Sawka *et al.*[3] used data from the Mayo clinic to compare three algorithms for screening for phaeochromocytoma. None was entirely cost-effective, but an algorithm based on screening fractions of plasma metanephrines with defined cut-offs appeared to be the most affordable.

2 Tumours that produce predominantly dopamine are rare but may be missed because plasma and urinary metanephrines are typically not increased.[4,5] Dopamine-producing tumours are typically paraganglionomas, and do not produce the classic clinical picture of phaeochromocytoma. Because they are clinically silent, they may be large when detected and more frequently malignant. They do not take up MIBG. α-blockade is contraindicated as it may produce hypotension and circulatory collapse.

3 More than a quarter of patients with head and neck paragangliomas carry mutations of one of the *SDH* genes. Recent data from an international registry[6] identified *SDHC*

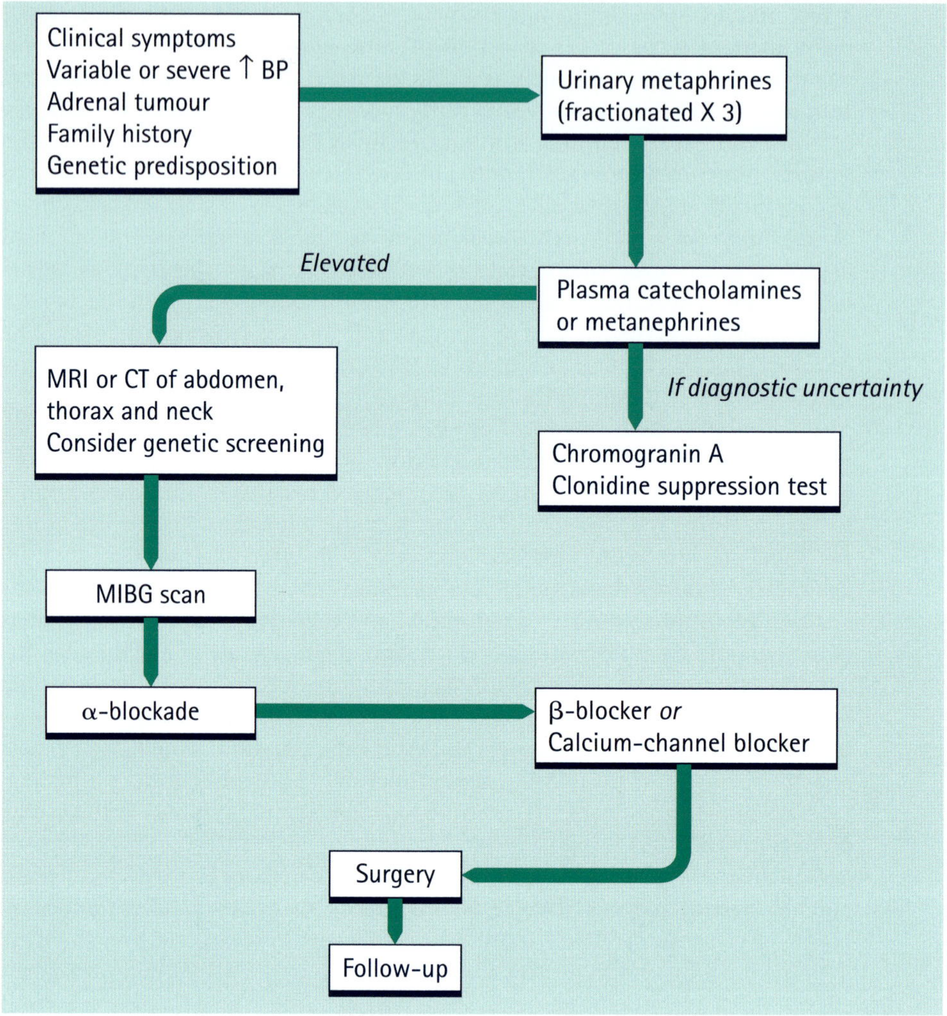

Clinical symptoms
Variable or severe ↑ BP
Adrenal tumour
Family history
Genetic predisposition

Urinary metaphrines
(fractionated X 3)

Plasma catecholamines
or metanephrines

Elevated

MRI or CT of abdomen,
thorax and neck
Consider genetic screening

If diagnostic uncertainty

Chromogranin A
Clonidine suppression test

MIBG scan

α-blockade

β-blocker *or*
Calcium-channel blocker

Surgery

Follow-up

Fig. 34.1 Diagnosis and management of phaeochromocytoma. The figure shows flow of investigations for patients with suspected phaeochromocytoma. Imaging tests are generally best carried out once biochemical diagnosis is established.

mutations in 4% of patients with paragangliomas but not in patients with phaeochromocytoma. The authors recommended screening for *SDH* mutations in all cases of paraganglioma so that the patients can receive appropriate genetic counselling.

Conclusions

The above patient has symptoms suggestive of phaeochromocytoma and should be investigated for the condition. A suggested algorithm for diagnosis and management of phaeochromocytoma is presented in Figure 34.1. Fractionated urinary metanephrines is still the initial screening test of choice in most centres. This should be followed by plasma measurements in patients suspected of having the condition. Imaging studies (CT/MRI followed by MIBG scan) should generally only be undertaken once the biochemical diagnosis is made. Initial treatment is with α-blockade, followed by β-blocker or calcium-channel blocker to control blood pressure before and during surgery. A laparoscopic approach to surgery is now favoured for most patients.

Further Reading

1 Manger WM, Eisenhofer G. Pheochromocytoma: diagnosis and management update. *Curr Hypertens Rep* 2004; **6**: 477–84.

2 Lenders WM, Eisenhofer G, Mannelli M, Pacak K. Phaeochromocytoma. *Lancet* 2005; **366**: 665–74.

3 Sawka AM, Gafni A, Thabane L, Young WF. The economic implications of three biochemical screening algorithms for pheochromocytoma. *J Clin Endocrinol Metab* 2004; **89**: 2859–66.

4 Dubois LA, Gray DK. Dopamine secreting pheochromocytomas: in search of a syndrome. *World J Surg* 2005; **29**: 909–13.

5 Eisenhofer G, Goldstein DS, Sullivan P, *et al*. Biochemical and clinical manifestations of dopamine-producing paraganglionomas: utility of plasma methoxytyramine. *J Clin Endocrinol Metab* 2005; **90**: 2068–75.

6 Schiavi F, Boedeker CC, Bausch B, *et al*; European-American Paraganglioma Study Group. Predictors and prevalence of paraganglioma syndrome associated with mutations of the SDHC gene. *JAMA* 2005; **294**: 2057–63.

PROBLEM

35 Conn's Syndrome

Case History

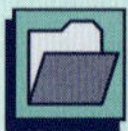

Mrs PS is 47 years old and has been treated by a general practitioner for hypertension over the past 8 years. She has also been noted to be hypokalaemic on a number of occasions. This has been attributed to diuretic therapy. She often feels weak and easily fatigued. Her current medication is amlodipine 10 mg/day, lisinopril 10 mg/day, bendrofluazide 2.5 mg/day.

What test would you do to decide whether or not she has Conn's syndrome?

Describe the approach to her medical therapy?

Should she be considered for surgery if the diagnosis is substantiated?

What is the prognosis following surgery?

Background

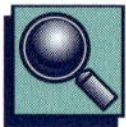

The syndrome of hypertension, hypokalaemia, increased urinary potassium loss and metabolic alkalosis is the commonest remediable form of hypertension. Conn's syndrome is diagnosed typically in the fourth to seventh decades of life, and is twice as common in men. It is due to excess aldosterone secretion or primary aldosteronism. Aldosterone, produced in the zona glomerulosa, acts at the mineralocorticoid receptor in the distal convoluted tubule to increase sodium reabsorption, while potassium and hydrogen ions are lost in exchange. Magnesium is also lost in the urine. Primary aldosteronism is caused by:

- Aldosterone-producing adenoma (APA)—60% of cases
- Bilateral adrenal hyperplasia (BAH)—30% of cases
- Multiple adrenal nodules (usually bilateral)—10% of cases
- Adrenal carcinoma—rarely.

Secondary hyperaldosteronism occurs in patients with cirrhosis, cardiac failure or nephrotic syndrome. High circulating aldosterone is associated with increased risk of left ventricular hypertrophy, cardiac fibrosis and impaired diastolic function, microalbuminuria and proteinuria, abnormal vascular remodelling, and stroke. The prevalence of primary aldosteronism is not known. Estimates range from <1% to 20% of patients with hypertension. Such variation arises because of the different screening tests and diagnostic criteria used, and because of differences in the populations screened. There is a strong selection bias in patients referred to specialist centres for management of their hypertension. Primary aldosteronism is definitely under-diagnosed. In a recent study[1] involving five centres across the world, the use of the ratio of plasma aldosterone to plasma renin (ARR) increased detection of primary aldosteronism by up to 15-fold. In the different centres, 9–33% of patients were hypokalaemic at presentation. As the numbers of patients detected increased, so too did the proportion who were not hypokalaemic, and the proportion with BAH.

Investigations

Investigation of suspected Conn's syndrome is summarized in Figure 35.1. The first step is to confirm the presence of primary aldosteronism. Renin and aldosterone should be measured when the patient has been recumbent overnight, and then when they have been upright for 4 hours.

Normal ranges for aldosterone

- Supine—140–400 pmol/l
- Upright—340–800 pmol/l

Plasma cortisol should be checked concurrently. This will fall during the morning of the test and as ACTH stimulates aldosterone secretion there will be a high basal level with some decrease during the morning in many patients with APA. If the patient is stressed, both cortisol and aldosterone will increase during the morning. Patients with BAH will show an increase on assuming the upright posture.

There is now widespread acceptance that ARR is the best available screening test. The cut-off used (to separate those with primary aldosteronism from controls) varies from 13.5 to 35 ng/dl per ng/ml/h, with different timing and posture. Renin is still generally quantified as enzyme activity. Standardization between different laboratories has been a problem, and samples need to be very carefully transported to preserve enzyme activity. The recent availability of immunoassays to measure plasma renin concentration should prove advantageous. Using such an assay, and a cut-off of 71 pmol/mU, Perschel *et al.*[2] have recently been able to reliably separate patients with primary aldosteronism from controls.

The failure of aldosterone to suppress following administration of sodium chloride or exogenous mineralocorticoid is a useful feature in diagnosis. Measurement of ARR after 2 l of intravenous 0.9% saline over 4 hours is a simple test readily applied to ambulant patients. Alternatively, the patient may be loaded with oral sodium chloride for 4 days prior to measurement of ARR. The fludrocortisone suppression test involves administering 0.1 mg fludrocortisone every 6 hours of 4 days. At the end of this, and after 2 hours upright, the ARR should be measured. Suppressed renin with increased aldosterone is consistent with the diagnosis of primary aldosteronism. In patients with proven primary aldosteronism, the captopril suppression test may be useful in differential diagnosis if imaging studies are inconclusive. The patient is given 25 mg captopril by mouth. Normally, aldosterone is completely suppressed at 60 and 120 minutes. Patients with APA fail to suppress, whereas those with BAH may suppress substantially.

Hypokalaemia is associated with decreased aldosterone secretion and, if not corrected, false-negative results may be obtained. It is always easier to interpret results of biochemical

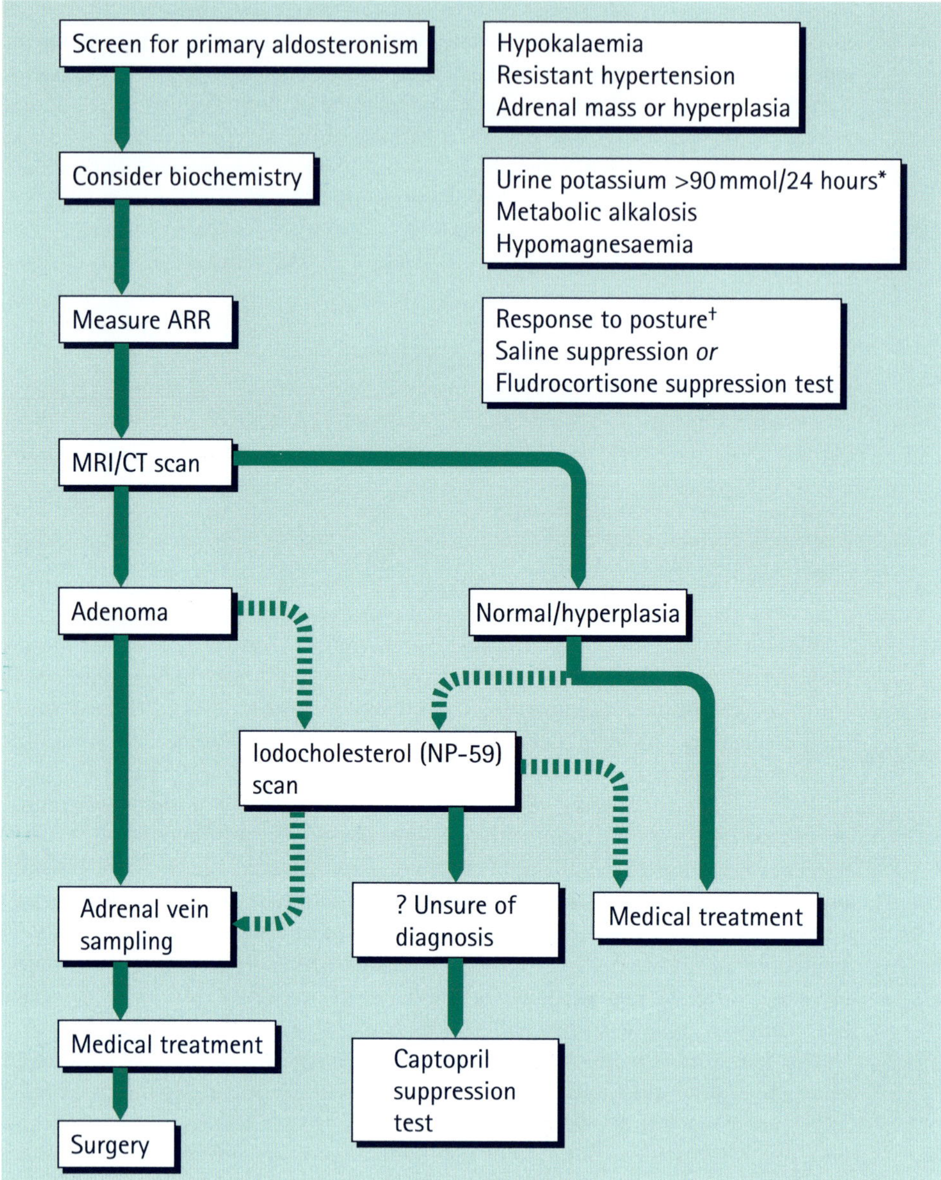

Fig. 35.1 Investigation of primary hyperaldosteronism. *Potassium status depends on intake and concurrent medications. †Measure the ratio of plasma aldosterone to plasma renin (ARR) lying and after 4 hours of being upright. Cortisol should be measured at the same time.

tests if the patient is not on medications. However, it is not always safe to stop antihypertensive medication in patients with primary aldosteronism, but the effect of drugs should be borne in mind. In particular β-blocking drugs should be stopped (or substituted) as they lower renin, and thus increase ARR, leading to potential false-positive results. Similar effects may be seen with clonidine, methyldopa and non-steroidal anti-inflammatory drugs. On the other hand diuretic therapy, dihydropyridine calcium-channel blockers, angiotensin-converting enzyme inhibitors, and angiotensin-receptor blockers may lower ARR, leading to false-negative results. If antihypertensive medication is required during investigation for suspected primary aldosteronism then drugs with relatively little effect on the renin–angiotensin system are preferred, e.g. hydralazine, prazosin or slow-release verapamil.

Both computed tomography (CT) and magnetic resonance imaging (MRI) detect adrenal nodules with a high degree of sensitivity. It must be remembered, however, that non-functioning adrenal nodules are not uncommon in the general population (Chapter 13) and that APAs account for only 2% of adrenal nodules. Functional scanning with ^{131}I-6-β-iodomethylnorcholesterol (NP-59) is useful in the diagnosis of APA, and there will also be increased, generalized uptake in patients with BAH. Finally, selective venous catheterization should be considered prior to surgery in patients with suspected APA. There is increased aldosterone in the adrenal vein on the side of the adenoma, whereas the adrenal on the other side is suppressed—adrenal venous aldosterone concentration is similar to that of the peripheral circulation.

Management

Surgery is the treatment of choice for patients with proven APA. This will lead to normalization, or at least substantial improvement, of hypertension in at least 70% of cases. Pretreatment with spironolactone in doses of up to 400 mg/day will help control blood pressure and restore electrolyte balance. It may also help restore mineralocorticoid production in the non-adenomatous adrenal tissue, obviating the need for post-operative mineralocorticoid. Medical treatment is indicated in patients with BAH, and those not suitable for surgery. Spironolactone is often not sufficient alone to control blood pressure. Addition of an angiotensin-converting enzyme inhibitor, or other agent, is indicated and electrolyte balance should be carefully monitored.

Recent Developments

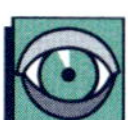

1 In a study involving the Framingham Offspring Study cohort,[3] patients with plasma aldosterone in the highest quartile were at 1.60-fold (95% confidence interval [CI] 1.19 to 2.14) risk of an increase in blood pressure and a 1.61-fold (95% CI 1.05 to 2.46) risk of developing hypertension compared with those in the lowest quartile. Thus, plasma aldosterone level within the normal physiological range appears to be a significant risk factor for hypertension.

2 Aldosterone antagonists have clear potential to improve outcome for patients with cardiovascular disease.[4] This has been clearly demonstrated in the recent Randomised Aldactone Evaluation Study (RALES) and in the Epleronone Neurohormonal Efficacy and Survival Study (EPHESUS). The endocrine side effects of spironolactone relate mainly to its anti-androgenic and progestagenic properties and may include increased risk of breast cancer. Its active metabolite is canrenone. Potassium canrenoate has been used with minimal anti-androgenic effects. Eplerenone is the first of a new group of drugs—selective aldosterone receptor antagonists—to become available.

3 Two distinct familial hyperaldosteronism (FH) syndromes are now recognized. FH-I is dexamethasone-suppressible hyperaldosteronism, and FH-II is a distinct syndrome

recently described and linked to a locus around 7p22.[5] Polymorphisms in the gene *CYP11B2*, and other steroidogenic enzymes, may relate to the risk of developing hyperaldosteronism, and such markers may prove to be of clinical use in the future.

Conclusions

With modern diagnostic tests and imaging techniques, primary aldosteronism is being diagnosed in an increasing number of patients with hypertension. The ratio of plasma aldosterone to plasma renin is the most sensitive test at present. We would initially measure this recumbent and after 4 hours of being upright. An intravenous saline suppression test is easy to carry out, and can be done as an outpatient if the patient is fit. Medical treatment to normalize blood pressure and correct hypokalaemia should be offered for up to 2 months before surgery. Spironolactone is currently the only widely available aldosterone antagonist. Additional therapy may be required to control the blood pressure. Long-term medical treatment is required for patients who have BAH, or those patients with APA who are not suitable for surgery. Prognosis is excellent after surgery, although some patients remain hypertensive.

Further Reading

1 Mulatero P, Stowaser M, Loh KC, *et al.* Increased diagnosis of primary aldosteronism, including surgically correctable forms, in centers from five continents. *J Clin Endocrinol Metab* 2004; **89**: 1045–50.

2 Perschel FH, Shemer R, Seiler L, *et al.* Rapid screening test for primary hyperaldosteronism: ratio of plasma aldosterone to renin concentration determined by fully automated chemiluminescence immunoassays. *Clin Chem* 2004; **50**: 1650–5.

3 Vasan RS, Evans JC, Larson MG, *et al.* Serum aldosterone and the incidence of hypertension in nonhypertensive persons. *N Engl J Med* 2004; **351**: 33–41.

4 Magni P, Motta M. Aldosterone receptor antagonists: biology and novel therapeutic applications. *Curr Hypertens Rep* 2005; **7**: 206–11.

5 So A, Duffy DL, Gordon RD, *et al.* Familial hyperaldosteronism type II is linked to the chromosome 7p22 region but also shows predicted heterogeneity. *J Hypertens* 2005; **23**: 1477–84.

Electrolytes

PROBLEM

36 Hyponatraemia

Case History

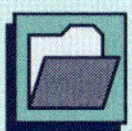

A 75-year-old man presents acutely unwell with a chest infection. He has mild chronic obstructive airways disease and takes regular inhaler therapy. He stopped smoking 3 years ago. Among the routine investigations you request, his white cell count is increased at 14×10^9/l and his serum sodium is low at 128 mmol/l (normal 135–145 mmol/l).

Discuss the differential diagnosis of his hyponatraemia.

What further investigations might be helpful?

How would you manage this situation?

Background

Sodium is the most abundant extracellular cation.[1,2] Sodium and the anions chloride and bicarbonate are the major electrolytes in extracellular fluid. Decrease in plasma sodium, blood pressure or extracellular volume stimulates the renin–angiotensin system, increasing the secretion of aldosterone, which increases sodium reabsorption in the distal convoluted tubule. If arginine vasopressin (AVP [antidiuretic hormone]) is present, water will also be reabsorbed. AVP acts through V_2 receptors in the collecting ducts, increasing cyclic AMP (cAMP), and leading to the phosphorylation of aquaporin-2. Volume depletion and high plasma sodium are the main stimuli for AVP secretion, which is inhibited by alcohol and caffeine.

Table 36.1 **Clinical features of hyponatraemia.**

Plasma sodium (mmol/l)	Symptoms
130–134	Generally asymptomatic
125–130	Nausea General malaise Headache Lethargy
120–125	Disorientation Weakness
Below 120	Seizures Coma Respiratory depression/arrest

With a plasma sodium concentration of 135 mmol/l and a glomerular filtration rate (GFR) of 120 ml/min, the kidneys filter about 170 l/day, equating to 22 moles of sodium. Less than 1% of this is excreted in the urine, and 99% is reabsorbed in the renal tubules and collecting ducts. Sodium intake varies widely but a typical intake of 100–200 mmol/day is roughly equivalent to renal losses. The amount lost from sweat or from the gastrointestinal tract is normally small but can increase to 50 mmol/day for sweat and higher than that from the gastrointestinal tract in disease states. Under normal circumstances, the kidney is the major regulator, and diuretic therapy is the most common cause of altered renal sodium handling. Sixty per cent of filtered sodium is reabsorbed in the proximal tubule and is not influenced by diuretic therapy, and 30% is reabsorbed in the loop of Henle. Loop diuretics block the Na-K-2Cl co-transporter and can increase sodium loss up to about 25% of total filtered sodium, i.e. 5 moles/ day. Seven per cent of filtered sodium is reabsorbed in the distal convoluted tubule. Thiazide diuretics block the Na-Cl co-transporter (mutations of which cause Gitelman's syndrome) and can increase sodium loss to about 5% of the total filtered, i.e. about 1 mole/day. Two per cent of filtered sodium is reabsorbed in the collecting ducts. Amiloride and triamterene act at this site and have limited potency as diuretics but, of course, have additional major effects on potassium balance.

Mild hyponatraemia (130–134 mmol/l) is present in up to 30% of hospital admissions, and more severe disturbance (<130 mmol/l) occurs in 1–4%. Plasma sodium concentration less than 120 mmol/l is associated with severe symptoms and can be life-threatening. The symptoms of hyponatraemia are detailed in Table 36.1.

Alcoholism and other chronic disease states can lead to resetting of the osmostat. When this occurs, antidiuretic hormone (ADH) is released at a lower plasma osmolality than normal and the patient has chronic low, but stable, sodium levels and no symptoms of hyponatraemia. This may partly explain the low sodium in many elderly people. Ageing is also associated with decreased total body water—typically around 50% compared with 60% in younger adults—and this makes elderly people more vulnerable to fluid and electrolyte problems. Around 10–15% of residents of elderly care homes have hyponatraemia.

The common causes of hyponatraemia are shown in Table 36.2, and an algorithm for diagnosis and management is shown in Figure 36.1. Pseudohyponatraemia, in which

Table 36.2 **Causes of hyponatraemia**

Plasma volume	Urine sodium (mmol/l)	Cause	Pathology
Low	<20	Non-renal loss	Burns Vomiting Diarrhoea Gastrointestinal fistula Malabsorption
	>20	Renal loss	Diuretics Salt-wasting nephropathy Cerebral salt wasting Aldosterone deficiency
Normal	<20	Water excess	Psychogenic polydipsia Hypotonic fluids
	>20	SIADH	Drugs Lung tumours Other malignancies Pneumonia Tuberculosis Empyema HIV infection Meningitis Encephalitis Cerebrovascular accident Subarachnoid bleed Cerebral abscess Guillain–Barré Porphyria
		Hypothyroidism Adrenal failure Hypopituitarism	
High	<20	Renal failure	
	>20	Nephrotic syndrome Cirrhosis Cardiac failure	

HIV = human immunodeficiency virus; SIADH = syndrome of inappropriate antidiuretic hormone secretion.

high levels of lipids or plasma proteins increased the apparent volume within which sodium was distributed, should no longer occur since most laboratories use sodium electrodes. High levels of mannitol or glucose in the blood lead to osmotic shifts, and thus a decrease in circulating glucose concentration. The approach to determining the diagnosis, and therefore the most appropriate treatment, is deciding on the patient's volume status and the likely speed of onset of the hyponatraemia. Urine sodium concentration is extremely helpful but this measurement is often omitted in clinical practice.

In low-volume states, sodium loss exceeds water loss and there is often a non-osmotic stimulus to AVP secretion. Euvolaemic hyponatraemia is most commonly associated with the syndrome of inappropriate ADH secretion (SIADH), where there is a stimulus to water retention but no true loss of sodium. About

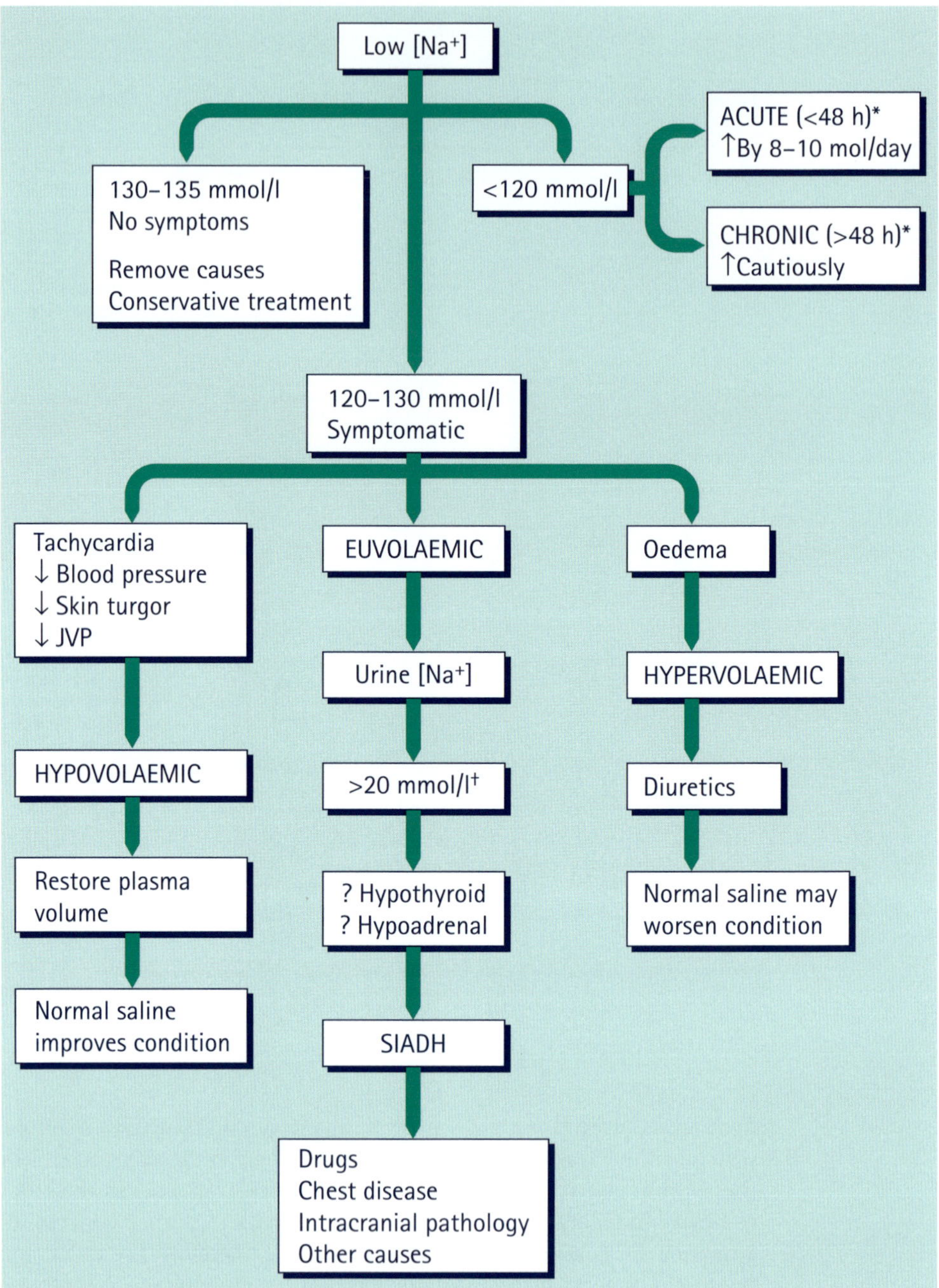

Fig. 36.1 Management of hyponatraemia. *In the emergency situation, when a patient has seizures or impaired consciousness, consider the use of low-volume hypertonic saline. †In patients who are euvolaemic but have low urine osmolality and low urine sodium, consider psychogenic polydipsia or other overload with hypotonic fluids. JVP = jugular venous pressure; SIADH = syndrome of inappropriate antidiuretic hormone secretion.

10% of patients with untreated hypothyroidism are hyponatraemic, partly due to associated SIADH. Volume overload states are characterized by oedema because of sodium loss in excess of water loss.

Treatment

Management of hyponatraemia is summarized in Figure 36.1. Aim to correct the sodium at roughly the same rate at which it was lost. If sodium is only modestly decreased (>125 mmol/l), the patient is relatively asymptomatic, and if they are able to eat and drink normally, conservative management is appropriate. Remove any underlying cause (such as diuretics) and restrict fluid intake initially to 1–1.25 l/day depending on body mass, the patient's and ambient temperature, and assessment of the patient's daily fluid losses. Normal saline should be administered if the patient is hypovolaemic or unable to drink. This may further decrease the plasma sodium in patients with SIADH. Initial rate of correction should be no more than 0.5 mmol/l per hour. Aim for a daily correction of 8–10 mmol/l.

Management of SIADH can be difficult, particularly if a reversible underlying cause cannot be identified. Patients who do not respond to fluid restriction can be treated with demeclocycline at a dose of 600–1200 mg/day. This drug can cause photosensitivity and renal impairment. It works by inhibiting cAMP response to AVP in the kidney. Lithium carbonate is an alternative, but has a narrow therapeutic window, and a significant risk of side effects. Patients who are hypervolaemic and hyponatraemic require fluid restriction and sodium restriction (to less than 70 mmol/day), management of the underlying cause, and loop diuretic to promote both water and salt loss. Hypertonic (3%) saline contains 5 mmol sodium per 10 ml. An infusion of 25 ml/h corrects sodium by around 10 mmol in the first 24 hours.

Recent Developments

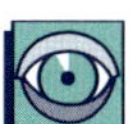

1. Osmotic demyelination syndrome is now well described.[3] It occurs when chronic hypo-osmolar states are corrected too rapidly. Central pontine myelinolysis occurs up to 10 days after acute fluid replacement. Dysarthria and dysphagia may be followed by flaccid quadriplegia, pseudobulbar palsy, seizures and coma; extrapontine myelinolysis occurs in about 10% of cases and presents with tremor, ataxia, parkinsonism and dystonia. Features are frequently not entirely reversible.

2. The effectiveness of diuretics in patients with heart failure is often limited by the side effects associated with hyponatraemia. Diuretic therapy increases sodium excretion out of proportion to water excretion. The V_2 receptor antagonist tolvaptan increases water excretion without affecting sodium excretion and thus increasing plasma sodium. The agent may prove very useful in patients with cardiac failure.[4] Combined V_1 and V_2 receptor antagonists, such as conivaptan, may be even more useful in cardiac failure as they combine effects on water excretion with haemodynamic benefits.

3. The mechanisms underlying hyponatraemia, which is a determinant of morbidity and mortality, in heart failure are complex.[4] When cardiac output and plasma volume decrease, there is activation of the sympathetic nervous system and the renin–angiotensin system, and AVP is released. The latter, along with diuretic therapy, is the major cause of hyponatraemia. There is increasing evidence for a beneficial effect

from AVP receptor blockers,[5] and these drugs may act synergistically with drugs that block the renin–angiotensin system.

4 Deaths occur in fewer than 1 in 50 000 participants in marathon runs. Usual causes are unrecognized cardiac disease, stroke and rhabdomyolysis. Hyponatraemia may occur in up to 30% of marathon participants and can reach dangerous levels. A recent study of participants in the Boston marathon reported significant hyponatraemia (<135 mmol/l) in 13% and serious hyponatraemia (<120 mmol/l) in 0.6%.[6] Risk factors were increased weight during the race, water intake every mile and race time greater than 4 hours. Most sports drinks are hypotonic.

Conclusions

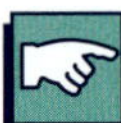

The patient has a history of smoking and has almost certainly developed a chest infection, and it is likely that he has SIADH as result of this. His clinical assessment should include estimation of the duration of his illness, whether he has symptoms attributable to the hyponatraemia, and his plasma volume status. If he is relatively asymptomatic, conservative management would be most suitable. He should have his fluid intake restricted and any diuretic therapy should be stopped if possible. Apart from his plasma electrolytes, measurement of plasma osmolality, and the osmolality and sodium concentration in urine would be helpful in establishing a precise diagnosis.

Further Reading

1 Hoorn EJ, Halperin ML, Zietse R. Diagnostic approach to a patient with hyponatraemia: traditional versus physiology-based approaches. *Q J Med* 2005; **98**: 529–40.

2 Reynolds RM, Seckl JR. Hyponatraemia for the clinical endocrinologist. *Clin Endocrinol* 2005; **63**: 366–74.

3 Abbott R, Silber E, Felber J, Ekpo E. Osmotic demyelination syndrome. *BMJ* 2005; **331**: 829–30.

4 Oren RM. Hyponatremia in congestive heart failure. *Am J Cardiol* 2005; **95**(suppl): 2B–7B.

5 Goldsmith SR. Current treatments and novel pharmacologic treatments for hyponatremia in congestive heart failure. *Am J Cardiol* 2005; **95**(suppl): 14B–23B.

6 Almond CSD, Shin AY, Fortescu EB, *et al.* Hyponatremia among runners in the Boston Marathon. *N Engl J Med* 2005; **352**: 1550–6.

PROBLEM

37 Hypokalaemia

Case History

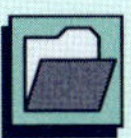

A 50-year-old woman complains of feeling generally unwell. She has recently had gastroenteritis. The bowel symptoms have now abated. She takes 20 mg of furosemide per day for peripheral oedema, but no other medications. You request plasma electrolytes and find that her potassium is decreased at 2.9 mmol/l (normal range 3.2–4.5 mmol/l).

Discuss the pathogenesis of her electrolyte abnormality.

What other conditions should be considered in a patient with hypokalaemia?

How would you correct the electrolyte abnormality?

Background

Potassium is the major intracellular cation. Hypokalaemia is common, both in outpatients and inpatients. A decrease in plasma potassium of 1 mmol/l usually indicates a deficit of 10–20% in total body potassium. Potassium is freely filtered by the glomerulus, 60–65% is reabsorbed in the proximal convoluted tubule, 25% is reabsorbed in the loop of Henle, and the ion is actively secreted under the influence of aldosterone in the distal convoluted tubule and collecting duct. Potassium balance is summarized in Figure 37.1.

Several factors are important in the regulation of plasma potassium level:

- *Extracellular pH*. Acidosis causes efflux of potassium from the cells (K^+–H^+ exchange—plasma potassium increases 0.6 mmol/l for every 0.1 decrease in pH. Conversely, alkalosis leads to decrease in extracellular potassium.
- *Insulin*. Increased potassium is a stimulus to insulin secretion, and insulin decreases circulating potassium by promoting entry into cells. States of insulin deficiency lead to hypokalaemia, and high levels of insulin, with glucose, lead to decreased circulating potassium.
- *Catecholamines*. Adrenaline and noradrenaline promote potassium entry into cells. β_2-agonists also promote potassium uptake and may, therefore, cause hypokalaemia. α-agonists inhibit uptake, and thus increase extracellular potassium.
- *Muscle activity*. In highly trained individuals, exercise promotes entry of potassium into muscle cells. Individuals who sustain muscle damage from high-intensity exercise may become hyperkalaemic because of potassium release from skeletal muscle.

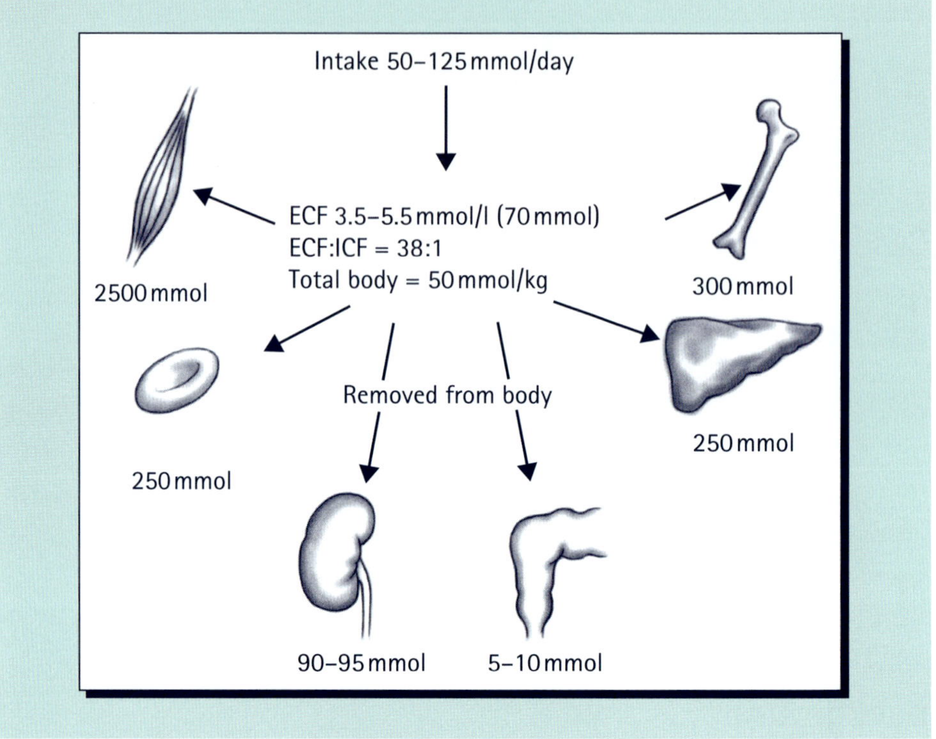

Fig. 37.1 Potassium balance. The majority of potassium is intracellular in the tissues shown (muscle, red blood cells, bone and liver). I/ECF = intra/extracellular fluid.

Symptoms from low plasma potassium are often non-specific. Patients with potassium in the range of 3.0–3.5 mmol/l are usually asymptomatic. Patients with lower levels of potassium complain of proximal muscle weakness. They often have diminished reflexes and may be areflexic. Decreased gastrointestinal motility can lead to constipation or ileus. Ventricular ectopic beats are common and, particularly in those with underlying heart disease, there is increased risk of arrhythmias. Electrocardiogram (ECG) changes are: increased amplitude of P wave, prolonged P-R interval, widening of the QRS complex, decreased T wave, increased U wave, and prolonged QU interval. Causes of hypokalaemia are summarized in Table 37.1.[1]

Eating disorders are present in up to 1% of young women. They often have anaemia (up to 40%), hyponatraemia (20%), hypokalaemia (20%) and elevated liver enzymes (20%). Familial periodic paralysis is an autosomal dominant condition, which also occurs in Asian men with thyrotoxicosis. Episodes of hypokalaemia and paralysis may occur following exercise, a high-carbohydrate meal, cold exposure, or after administration of insulin or adrenergic agents. Thyroid hormone may directly stimulate the Na-K-ATPase, potentiating catecholamine induced intracellular shift of potassium. β-blockers may inhibit this action and decrease risk of episodes of paralysis.[2]

Table 37.1 Causes of hypokalaemia

Without potassium deficit	Respiratory alkalosis Familial periodic paralysis Exercise (trained athlete) Treatment of megaloblastic anaemia β_2-adrenergic agents
With potassium deficit	
Decreased intake	Poor diet Alcoholics Anorexia nervosa (vomiting + purgatives also)
Increased gastrointestinal loss	Vomiting or diarrhoea Fistulas Villous adenoma Purgative abuse
Increased renal loss	Diuretics Mineralocorticoid excess (primary or secondary) Liquorice abuse Polyuria Low magnesium status Renal tubular acidosis Bartter's or Gitelman's syndrome Drugs (penicillamine, aminoglycosides)
Increased sweat loss	
Haemodialysis or peritoneal dialysis	

Several rare tubular disorders have been described and characterized in recent years.

- *Bartter's syndrome.* Mutations in the Na-K-2Cl co-transporter (*NKCC2*) gene in the thick ascending loop of Henle lead to increased urine excretion of potassium, calcium, sodium and chloride with metabolic alkalosis. The resultant dehydration leads to a high renin/high aldosterone state but blood pressure is usually normal or low. Children with Bartter's grow slowly, may be mentally retarded, have polyuria and dehydration. Symptoms are improved by drugs that help to retain potassium.
- *Gitelman's syndrome.* This is a variant of Bartter's but usually with milder clinical features. The spectrum of electrolyte and acid–base abnormalities is similar. Unlike in Bartter's, urine calcium is decreased and urine magnesium is increased. The disease is also inherited in an autosomal recessive fashion, and is due to mutations in the thiazide-sensitive Na-Cl co-transporter gene in the distal convoluted tubule. Both Bartter's and Gitelman's syndromes cause hypertrophy of the juxtaglomerular cells.
- *Liddle's syndrome.* This is an autosomal dominant disorder associated with severe hypertension and hypokalaemic metabolic alkalosis. The disorder is due to mutations in the renal sodium channel β subunit (SCNN1B) of γ subunit (SCNN1G) in the collecting duct. Increased sodium delivery leads to hypertension with low levels of renin and aldosterone. The potassium-sparing diuretics amiloride and triamterene may be useful in treating this condition.

- *Syndrome of apparent mineralocorticoid excess* (SAME). This is another rare genetic form of hypertension. Mutations in the renal form of the enzyme 11β-hydroxysteroid dehydrogenase (type 2) lead to decreased inactivation of cortisol in the kidney. The mineralocorticoid receptor binds cortisol with high affinity and the result is sodium retention with hypokalaemic alkalosis, but with low renin.

Treatment

Fluid and other electrolyte abnormalities need to be corrected concurrently. Patients with plasma potassium between 3.0 mmol/l and 3.5 mmol/l are usually asymptomatic and do not require urgent correction. In acute coronary syndromes, even mild hypokalaemia can predispose the patient to arrhythmias. In considering replacement, aim for a plasma level of 4.0 mmol/l. Since most of the deficit is intracellular, it will take some days to replace a deficit, even if the plasma level corrects quickly.

A 70 kg man with a plasma potassium of 2.5 mmol/l will have a total deficit of at least 350 mmol potassium. This should be corrected at a rate of 20–80 mmol/day in divided doses in the non-urgent situation. Non-effervescent tablets (Slow K) contain 8 mmol potassium. Two tablets three times daily would be a suitable dose for a patient with mild to moderate potassium deficiency. Effervescent tablets (Sando-K) contain 12 mmol potassium—one tablet four times daily is a suitable dose. Potassium syrup (1 mmol/ml) is also available.

For intravenous replacement, use ready-mixed solutions where possible. Alternatively, potassium chloride ampoules (1.5 g, 20 mmol) are available. Administering potassium with dextrose-containing solutions may further decrease the potassium. The rate of replacement depends on the degree of deficiency and the urgency of the situation. Up to 40 mmol (suitably diluted) can be given in 1 hour. Whether replacement is oral or intravenous, careful monitoring of plasma potassium is essential.

Recent Developments

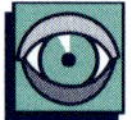

1 Hypokalaemia is a risk factor for morbidity and mortality in patients with cardiovascular disease.[3] This has traditionally been ascribed to the risk of arrhythmias in patients with low potassium. However, recent studies have also identified low potassium status as a predictive factor for morbidity from heart failure.

2 Both low potassium intake and high protein intake are risk factors for osteoporosis.[4] High intake of protein may lead to decreased bone density by increasing endogenous acid production, and intake of foods containing potassium salts may help to neutralize these acids.

3 Potassium-channel disorders in other tissues have also been associated with disease states including neonatal diabetes, hyperinsulinaemia, dilated cardiomyopathy, and Prinzmetal's angina.[5] The regulatory channel in the β cells of the pancreas is an octomeric complex of four Kir6 and four sulphonylurea receptor subunits. In high glucose states, the potassium channel is closed, the cell membrane depolarized, and the influx of calcium into the cytoplasm leads to increased insulin secretion. Disorders of this mechanism may contribute to type 2 diabetes.

4 Renal impairment is a well-recognized side effect of aminoglycoside antibiotics. Recently, Chou *et al.*[6] have reported four cases of Bartter-like syndrome following

gentamicin treatment. The syndrome caused renal wasting of sodium, potassium, chloride, calcium and magnesium, along with metabolic alkalosis. Gentamicin is a polyvalent cation, and the authors suggested that the disorder might be caused by gentamicin acting at the calcium-sensing receptor in the loop of Henle and distal convoluted tubule.

Conclusions

As with many hypokalaemic patients, the above patient has more than one cause for her low potassium. Diuretic prescriptions should be reviewed regularly and patients taking diuretics should be aware that if they develop vomiting, diarrhoea or any other illness, their electrolyte balance might be disturbed. Even mild potassium deficiency should be corrected, particularly in the light of recent evidence demonstrating effects of potassium status on multiple aspects of health. If this woman needs to carry on with her diuretic, she should be offered oral potassium supplementation, until her plasma potassium level is at least 4.0 mmol/l. If she does need to carry on taking diuretic, a milder (thiazide) preparation might be considered, or the concurrent use of a potassium-sparing diuretic.

Further Reading

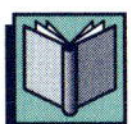

1 Schaefer TJ, Wolford RW. Disorders of potassium. *Emerg Med Clin North Am* 2005; **23**: 723–47.

2 Sinharay R. Hypokalaemic periodic paralysis in an Asian man in the United Kingdom. *Emerg Med J* 2004; **21**: 120–1.

3 Coca SG, Perazella MA, Buller GK. The cardiovascular implications of hypokalemia. *Am J Kidney Dis* 2005; **45**: 233–47.

4 Macdonald HM, New SA, Fraser WD, Campbell MK, Reid DM. Low dietary potassium intakes and high dietary estimates of net endogenous acid production are associated with low bone density in premenopausal women and increased markers of bone resorption in postmenopausal women. *Am J Clin Nutr* 2005; **81**: 923–33.

5 Ashcroft FM. ATP-sensitive potassium channelopathies: focus on insulin secretion. *J Clin Invest* 2005; **115**: 2047–58.

6 Chou CL, Chen YH, Chau T, Lin SH. Acquired Bartter-like syndrome associated with gentamicin administration. *Am J Med Sci* 2005; **329**: 144–9.

PROBLEM

38 Hypomagnesaemia

Case History

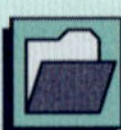

A 49-year-old man has had Crohn's disease for over 15 years. This was managed medically until he had a length of small bowel resected 4 years ago. The symptoms of Crohn's have improved since then but he still has frequent bowel habit with loose motions. On a routine clinical chemistry screen, you find his plasma magnesium level is low at 0.4 mmol/l (normal 0.9–1.2 mmol/l). His renal function and other electrolytes are otherwise normal.

What are the possible consequences of his low magnesium level?

Does it merit treatment?

What treatment should be considered and how would you monitor his condition?

Background

The fourth most abundant cation in the body and the second most abundant intracellular cation, magnesium is a co-factor for over 300 enzymes. The ion is also involved in regulation of muscular contraction, parathyroid hormone secretion and action, and acts as a calcium-channel blocker in neural and muscular tissues. Recent studies in acute asthma, myocardial infarction, diabetes, and pre-eclampsia have increased awareness of the clinical importance of magnesium and its deficiency.[1,2] Magnesium deficiency is present in up to 10% of patients admitted to hospital and in up to 60% admitted to critical care. It often coincides with deficiencies of other ions, particularly hypokalaemia (40% of cases), hyponatraemia, hypocalcaemia, and hypophosphataemia (each in 20% of cases).

Magnesium toxicity is hard to induce and is rare. The therapeutic target range for plasma magnesium in eclampsia is 2.0–3.5 mmol/l. Toxicity causes drowsiness and lethargy, and may progress to respiratory depression. Treatment consists of increasing excretion (diuresis) and intravenous calcium.

Causes of magnesium deficiency (Box 38.1) are listed in Table 38.1. As it is mainly an intracellular cation, total body magnesium deficiency can exist with normal plasma levels. In this instance, urinary excretion will be low. Also, over 70% of an intravenous dose

Box 38.1 Hypomagnesaemia

When plasma magnesium is below 0.7 mmol/l or where 24-hour urine magnesium is less than 1 mmol.

Table 38.1 Causes of magnesium deficiency

Poor intake and nutrition	Low dietary content – many countries relatively low, including the USA Vomiting or prolonged nasogastric suction Enteral or parenteral nutrition Alcoholism (also associated with increased renal and gastrointestinal loss) Burns (catabolic state + increased loss through skin)
Increased renal loss	Thiazide and loop diuretics Diuretic phase of acute renal failure Renal tubular acidosis Bartter's and Gitelman's syndromes (see Chapter 39)
Poor absorption or gastrointestinal loss	Malabsorption syndromes Short bowel or fistula Pancreatitis Diarrhoea Purgative abuse
Endocrine or electrolyte disorders	Hyperthyroidism Hyperparathyroidism Diabetes Hyperaldosteronism (Conn's or secondary) Catecholamine excess
Drugs	Aminoglycosides, carbenicillin, ticarcillin Digoxin Antineoplastic drugs – *cis*-platinum Ciclosporin

of magnesium (e.g. 30 mmol magnesium chloride) is usually excreted in the urine within 24 hours. Low urinary excretion following an intravenous magnesium load is indicative of deficiency.

A desirable daily intake of magnesium is in the region of 150–300 mg/day. Good dietary sources include wholegrain cereals, nuts, beans, seeds and food products made with yeast. Shellfish and green leafy vegetables are also good sources. The body contains 25 g of magnesium, and it is easy to see how deficiency can arise in the course of a few weeks of illness. The body has no sophisticated regulatory system for maintaining magnesium balance. Whole body magnesium balance is summarized in Figure 38.1. The clinical features of magnesium deficiency are shown in Box 38.2.

Treatment of magnesium deficiency depends on the degree of urgency. The usual parenteral replacement is magnesium sulphate available as a 50% solution (approximately 2 mmol/ml). Severe deficiency equates to a deficit of up to 160 mmol magnesium. As a rule of thumb, 0.15 mmol/kg is required for each 0.1 mmol/l below 0.7. In an emergency (fits or rhythm disturbances), 10 mmol can be given as a bolus. This is usually given intravenously. Intramuscular injection is painful. The bolus is followed by 20–60 mmol given over the next 24 hours, suitably diluted (20 mmol/l) in normal saline or 5% dextrose. Up to 5 days treatment is required for severe deficiency. Note that a large proportion of infused magnesium is excreted in the urine. Even when plasma magnesium is restored to normal, a total body deficit may persist. Be careful to treat any coexistent electrolyte abnormality, including hypokalaemia.

Box 38.2 Clinical features of magnesium deficiency

- Confusion, delirium, Wernicke's encephalopathy
- Mood changes, depression, hallucinations, psychosis
- Ataxia, tremor, involuntary movements
- Cramps, tetany

- Tachycardia
- Atrial and ventricular premature beats
- Torsades de pointes, ventricular dysrhythmias
- Electrocardiogram (ECG) changes – low amplitude P wave, low voltage and wide QRS, flattened T wave, prominent U wave, prolonged QT interval

- Increased tendon reflexes
- Positive Trousseau's and Chvostek's signs
- Plasma magnesium <0.7mmol/l
- Acidosis – lactic, ketoacidosis or renal tubular
- Low potassium, sodium, phosphate and calcium

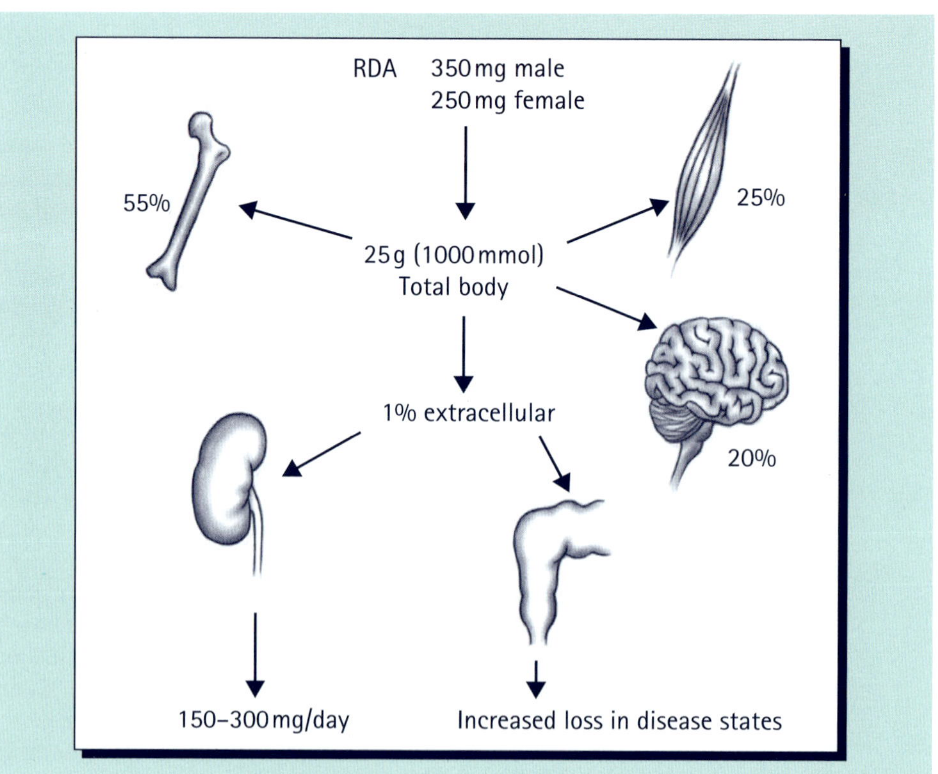

Fig. 38.1 Magnesium balance. RDA, recommended daily amount in diet.

Oral replacement at a dose of up to 24 mmol per day in divided doses is indicated in severe cases once intravenous loading is complete. This is best given as magnesium chloride—if a preparation is available. Other magnesium salts may precipitate hypochloraemic alkalosis. In some countries, a delayed release preparation (Slo-Mag) is available. This contains 64 mg magnesium chloride per tablet—use up to three tablets per day.

Recent Developments

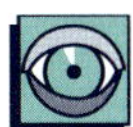

1. Recently, six trials have documented benefit of nebulized magnesium sulphate in patients with acute asthma.[3] Used with β_2-agonists, magnesium improves lung function and decreases the likelihood of hospital admission. The major benefit may result from muscle relaxation in respiratory smooth muscle.
2. There is increased interest in the use of magnesium in patients with severe illness. Its use is established as prophylaxis in women with severe pre-eclampsia. Given that up to 60% of patients admitted to intensive care areas may be magnesium deficient, the arguments for correcting the deficiency are now becoming persuasive.[4] Potential benefits include vasodilatation, protection against cardiac arrhythmias, neuroprotection including preventing fits and improved glucose tolerance.
3. Low magnesium status is a risk factor for insulin resistance, metabolic syndrome and type 2 diabetes. Data from the Nurses Health Study involving nearly 12 000 women show that magnesium status is inversely related to level of C-reactive protein.[5] Women in the highest quintile of plasma magnesium had a 27% lower risk of metabolic syndrome compared with those in the lowest quintile. There are now considerable data linking low magnesium status with diabetes risk.

Conclusions

Low magnesium is associated with a range of neurological and cardiovascular abnormalities. Magnesium replacement may decrease risk of cardiac arrhythmias, and might also protect the nervous system, and improve respiratory function and glucose intolerance in patients who are acutely unwell. Although magnesium status does not generally receive much attention in the management of an ill patient, there is an increasing tendency to measure magnesium and to correct deficiency. If the patient has fits or cardiac rhythm disturbances, treatment with intravenous magnesium is probably indicated. Otherwise, a more gradual approach with intravenous infusion or oral replacement is indicated. Patients with low magnesium have a high prevalence of other electrolyte disturbances which should also be corrected. Magnesium is predominantly an intracellular ion; correcting deficiency may take time and plasma levels are not a completely accurate guide to magnesium status.

Further Reading

1. Innerarity S. Hypomagnesaemia in acute and chronic illness. *Crit Care Nurs Q* 2000; **23**: 1–19.
2. Baker SB, Worthley LIG. The essentials of calcium, magnesium and phosphate metabolism: Pet II. Disorders. *Crit Care Resusc* 2002; **4**: 307–15.

3 Blitz M, Blitz S, Hughes R, *et al.* Aerosolised magnesium sulphate for acute asthma. A systematic review. *Chest* 2005; **128**: 337–44.

4 Tong GM, Rude RK. Magnesium deficiency in critical illness. *J Intensive Care Med* 2005; **20**: 3–17.

5 Song Y, Ridker PM, Manson JE, Cook NR, Buring JE, Liu S. Magnesium intake, C-reactive protein, and the prevalence of metabolic syndrome in middle aged and older US women. *Diabetes Care* 2005; **28**: 1438–44.

PROBLEM

39 Diabetes Insipidus

Case History

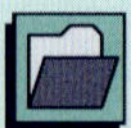

A 28-year-old psychiatric nurse presents with thirst and polyuria increasing over the past year. He describes passing copious amounts of dilute urine day and night. He may have to get up six or more times at night to pass urine. There is no history of note. He has never had a major head injury. He does not take any medications.

What is the differential diagnosis?

How should this situation be investigated?

What treatments are available?

How should this patient be followed up once on treatment?

Background

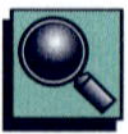

To maintain plasma osmolality in the critical, but narrow, physiological range three processes are important:[1] regulation of arginine vasopressin (AVP) release in response to increased plasma osmolality; renal response to AVP leading to increased reabsorption of water; and normal stimulation of thirst when plasma osmolality increases. Water intake in excess of requirements in patients with psychogenic or habitual polydipsia may overwhelm the normal physiological regulation of water balance and lead to polyuria in the face of low plasma osmolality. Water accounts for just under two-thirds of total body weight. Normal daily urine output varies widely from 0.5 l to 20 l according to fluid intake and a range of other physiological factors. Daily output in excess of 3 l should raise suspicion of a disorder of water balance.

AVP is synthesized in the neurones of the supraoptic and paraventricular nuclei of the hypothalamus. It is a nonapeptide with a six-member disulphide ring and a tripeptide tail, and is transported in axons within the pituitary stalk to the posterior pituitary, from where it is released into the circulation. The major stimulus to AVP release is decreased plasma osmolality detected by osmoreceptors in the anterior hypothalamus. Neuronal outputs from these cells alter in response to changes in cell volume, and this is responsive to changes in prevailing extracellular osmolality. Non-osmotic triggers to AVP release include hypovolaemia, hypotension, nausea, pain and acidosis. The hormone acts through the V_2 receptors in the renal collecting ducts to stimulate water reabsorption. Of the 13 or so isoforms of aquaporin, aquaporin-2 (AQP2) is mainly responsible for mediating the effects of AVP. Following occupancy of the V_2 receptor, increased cyclic AMP leads to activation of protein kinase A (PKA) and then phosphorylation and translocation of AQP2 to the cell membrane.

Cranial diabetes insipidus

The major symptoms of inadequate AVP secretion or defective action of the hormone are polyuria, frequency, nocturia, enuresis and thirst. At least 80% of secretory potential needs to be lost before clinical diabetes insipidus develops. Differential diagnosis of cranial diabetes insipidus is shown in Table 39.1. Up to 30% are idiopathic—no demonstrable cause, although autoantibodies to AVP-secreting neurones have been demonstrated in some cases. A triple response is recognized after brain injury where the patient has an initial diuresis due to impaired AVP release, followed by an antidiuretic phase as preformed AVP is released, then a further diuretic phase due to deficient AVP. The clinical course is extremely variable and patients may recover after any one of the phases. Familial cases are recognized and are due to mutations in the AVP gene located at chromosome 20p13. Wolfram's syndrome (Diabetes Insipidus, Diabetes Mellitus, Optic Atrophy and Deafness [DIDMOAD]) is caused by mutations in the gene for wolframin (*WFS1*) located at chromosome 4p16.1. The protein is an integral membrane glycoprotein localized to the endoplasmic reticulum.

Table 39.1 Differential diagnosis of cranial diabetes insipidus

Idiopathic	Some autoimmune
Head injury	See recent advances
Neurosurgery tumours	Pituitary, craniopharyngioma, hypothalamic metastases
Infection	Meningitis, encephalitis
Granulomatous	Sarcoid, histiocytosis
Vascular	Sheehan's syndrome, sickle cell disease, aneurysm, subarachnoid haemorrhage, stroke
Drugs	Alcohol, phenytoin, naloxone
Familial	Autosomal dominant DIDMOAD (Wolfram's syndrome)

Gestational diabetes insipidus

Symptoms of pre-existing diabetes insipidus may worsen during pregnancy or, in rare instances, the condition may arise *de novo* in late pregnancy. This is due to increased metabolic clearance of AVP by the placenta, perhaps because of increased activity of an vasopressinase enzyme. The syndrome responds to conventional doses of synthetic vasopressin (desmopressin) and usually disappears promptly after delivery.

Primary polydipsia

Primary polydipsia can arise in patients with psychological or psychiatric diagnoses but not invariably. It is unusual to find a structural lesion on computed tomography or magnetic resonance imaging. Dipsogenic polydipsia is a situation where the sensitivity of the thirst mechanism is altered so that thirst is stimulated at a lower than normal plasma osmolality. The vasopressin response to plasma osmolality is unaltered in this condition.

Nephrogenic diabetes insipidus

Nephrogenic diabetes insipidus occurs when the renal tubules are partially or completely resistant to the action of vasopressin. Causes may be divided into primary or secondary and reversible or irreversible (Table 39.2). Primary and irreversible causes are most commonly due to mutations that cause decreased expression or defective action of *AQP2*. These may be sporadic or, more commonly, familial. Autosomal recessive inheritance is much more common although autosomal dominant forms are recognized. Over 30 mutations of the *AQP2* gene leading to nephrogenic diabetes insipidus have now been described. Acquired nephrogenic diabetes insipidus is usually due to drugs or metabolic disturbances.[2] Lithium is the most common drug to cause nephrogenic diabetes insipidus.

Investigation

Diagnosis of diabetes insipidus is made using a water deprivation test. The patient is allowed fluid and food overnight and should be fully hydrated at the beginning of the

Table 39.2 Differential diagnosis of nephrogenic diabetes insipidus

Primary	
Mutations of *AQP2* gene	Autosomal recessive
	Autosomal dominant
Idiopathic	
Secondary	
Drugs	Lithium
	Antibiotics (demeclocycline, rifampicin)
	Antifungals (amphotericin B)
	Antiviral agents
	Antineoplastic (cyclophosphamide, methotrexate)
	Others (contrast agents, colchicine, mesalazine)
Metabolic	Hypercalcaemia
	Hypokalaemia
Vascular	Sickle cell disease
Renal	Chronic renal failure
	Post obstruction

test. Water deprivation is not necessary if the patient has high plasma sodium and osmolality with urine osmolality below 300 mOsm/kg at the beginning of the test. It should not be carried out in patients who are hypovolaemic, have renal failure or uncontrolled diabetes, or in those with untreated hypothyroidism or adrenal failure. The patient should be observed throughout the test. Urine and plasma osmolality, along with the patient's weight is checked every 2 hours. The test is abandoned if the patient loses more than 5% of their body weight. At the end of 8 hours of fluid deprivation, osmolalities are checked and the patient is given 2 μg of 1-desamino-8-D-arginine vasopressin (DDAVP) intramuscularly. Those with cranial diabetes insipidus will concentrate their urine, whereas those with nephrogenic diabetes insipidus will be resistant to the hormone. Investigation of patients with polyuria is summarized in Figure 39.1. An alternative to the dehydration test is to increase plasma osmolality using hypertonic saline: 5% saline is infused over 2 hours at a rate of 0.06 ml/kg per minute. Blood is withdrawn for measurement of plasma osmolality and AVP level every 30 minutes for 2–4 hours. AVP will increase with increased plasma osmolality in patients with nephrogenic diabetes insipidus and primary polydipsia, whereas there will be no increase in patients with cranial diabetes insipidus.

Treatment

Mild diabetes insipidus with urine output less than 4 l/day may require no other treatment than to ensure that there is adequate fluid intake. Chlorpropamide and carbamazepine have been used in partial cranial diabetes insipidus to sensitize the collecting ducts to AVP. For management of cranial diabetes insipidus, DDAVP is used since it has a longer duration of action and less pressor activity than either lysine or arginine vasopressin. This is most conveniently administered in oral form (300–600 μg/day in three divided doses). Given by nasal spray, the dose of DDAVP should be 10–40 μg/day—divided for larger doses. Fluid intake should be limited to 500 ml in the 8 hours after DDAVP administration. Dose regimen should be tailored to allow diuresis at some point each day and it is often useful to suggest that patients omit the treatment 1 day per week to avoid risk of water overload. Gestational diabetes insipidus, when it requires treatment, is also best treated with DDAVP.

In addition to being used in treatment of diabetes insipidus, vasopressin is also used in haemophilia A and von Willebrand's disease, in patients who are bleeding due to portal hypertension, and there is significant trial evidence supporting use of a single intravenous dose as a pressor agent in patients who have suffered a cardiac arrest. Nephrogenic diabetes insipidus is treated by removing the underlying cause if possible and with thiazide diuretics or amiloride if necessary.

Recent Developments

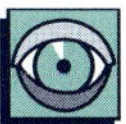

1 Two recent reports[3,4] have examined the incidence of diabetes insipidus after traumatic brain injury (TBI). The incidence of TBI is around 200 per 100 000 population per year, and diabetes insipidus occurs in less than 1%. Some degree of pituitary dysfunction occurs in up to 40% of patients after TBI. Increased prolactin, adrenocorticotrophic hormone and growth hormone, along with decreased gonadotropin and thyroid-stimulating hormone secretion are regarded as part of the adaptive response. Diabetes insipidus is present in up to 20% of patients admitted to neurosurgical units

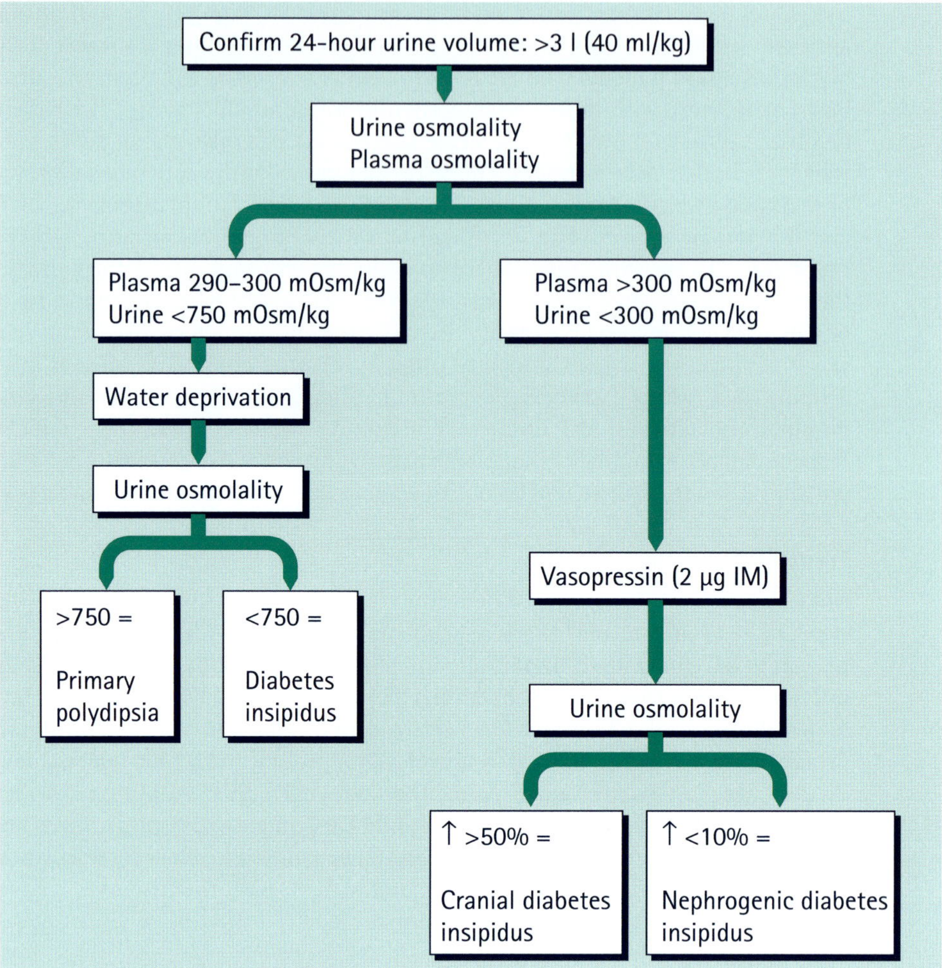

Fig. 39.1 Investigation of polyuria. IM, intramuscular.

with head injury, and in a third of patients who have damage in the region of the optic chiasm.

2 Kim *et al.*[5] have recently demonstrated that hydrochlorothiazide, used in an animal model of lithium-induced diabetes insipidus, partially reversed the downregulation of *AQP2* induced by lithium. Furthermore, the thiazide also increased expression of ENaC and the Na-Cl co-transporter.

3 Nocturia is an important symptom in elderly people. Its prevalence increases with age and is associated with increased risk of nocturnal falls and accidents, as well as with increased overall morbidity and mortality.[6] The fraction of total urine output excreted at night increases from 15% in young adults to around 30% in healthy elderly people. In extreme cases, this may be up to 85%. Around 3–4% of elderly people have little or no nocturnal AVP secretion.

Conclusions

The most important investigation in a patient with confirmed polyuria is usually a water deprivation test with a desmopressin test at the end of a period of water deprivation. This will distinguish diabetes insipidus from primary polydipsia and indicate whether the defect is in AVP secretion or action. DDAVP is used for treatment of cranial diabetes insipidus. The oral form is most convenient in the majority of cases although nasal spray is preferred by some patients. Measures should be instituted to replace fluid losses and to satisfy thirst. Patients who have had head injury and have impaired thirst mechanism present a particular problem. Care should be taken not to overdose patients with DDAVP and the regimen should allow for intermittent diuresis. Most patients with uncomplicated diabetes insipidus do not require frequent follow-up. They should be instructed about the importance of fluid balance and have electrolytes and osmolality checked if they feel unwell at any stage.

Further Reading

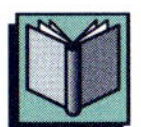

1 Lin M, Liu SJ, Lim IT. Disorders of water imbalance. *Emerg Med Clin North Am* 2005; **23**: 749–70.

2 Garofeanu CG, Weir M, Rosa-Arellano MP, Henson G, Garg AX, Clark WF. Causes of reversible nephrogenic diabetes insipidus: A systematic review. *Am J Kidney Dis* 2005; **45**: 626–37.

3 Aimaretti G, Ambrosio MR, Di Somma C, *et al.* Traumatic brain injury and subarachnoid haemorrhage are conditions at high risk of hypopituitarism: screening study at three months after brain injury. *Clin Endocrinol* 2004; **61**: 320–6.

4 Bondanelli M, Ambrosio MR, Zatelli MC, De Marinis L, degli Uberti EC. Hypopituitarism after traumatic brain injury. *Eur J Endocrinol* 2005; **152**: 679–91.

5 Kim GH, Lee JW, Oh YK, *et al.* Antidiuretic effect of hydrochlorothiazide in lithium-induced nephrogenic diabetes insipidus is associated with up regulation of aquaporin-2, Na-Cl co-transporter, and epithelial sodium channel. *J Am Soc Nephrol* 2004; **15**: 2836–43.

6 Asplin R. Nocturia in relation to sleep, health, and medical treatment in the elderly. *BJU Int* 2005; **96**(suppl): 15–21.

PROBLEM

40 Spontaneous Hypoglycaemia

Case History

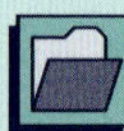

A 27-year-old woman who is separated from her husband and lives with her father attends complaining of recurrent attacks of feeling faint. She does not lose consciousness. The attacks typically occur mid-morning or mid-afternoon, and she finds the symptoms are better within 20 minutes if she eats something sweet. Her father has type 2 diabetes and has checked her blood sugar during an attack. On two occasions, he has noted the blood sugar to be around 2.0 mmol/l.

Do you think that she requires further investigations?

Is there a role for a prolonged glucose tolerance test?

What general advice should she receive?

Are there any drugs that might help?

Background

The vast majority of instances of hypoglycaemia are secondary to treatment of diabetes. Symptoms of hypoglycaemia vary widely from person to person, and are non-specific. Activation of the sympathetic nervous system occurs when glucose falls to between 2.5 mmol/l and 3.0 mmol/l. Adrenergic symptoms include sweating, tremor, hunger, nausea, agitation and headache. Patients with plasma glucose <2.5 mmol/l may experience neuroglycopenic symptoms. These include decreased concentration and coordination, diplopia or blurred vision, fatigue and disorientation or behavioural change. With more severe or prolonged hypoglycaemia, there may be clouding of consciousness, seizures or coma.[1]

Information about timing and frequency of symptoms is critical, and it may be useful to ask the patient to keep a symptom diary. Hypoglycaemia occurring more than 5 hours after a meal is termed fasting hypoglycaemia. That provoked by food and occurring between 2 and 5 hours is termed reactive. This latter term has proved to be controversial in recent years because of the inconsistent relation between symptoms and findings on the prolonged glucose tolerance test. There is not really universal agreement about the role of the 5-hour glucose tolerance test in patients who present with symptoms suggestive of functional reactive hypoglycaemia. In many cases, patients experience adrenergic symptoms without having low blood sugar. This has been termed adrenergic postprandial syndrome (APS). This and reactive hypoglycaemia may arise from a variety of physiological processes including increased insulin response (early responder), increased secretion of glucagon-like peptide-1 (GLP-1) and gastric insulotropic peptide, renal glycosuria, insulin resistance (late responder), and decreased glucagon secretion.

In practice, the most common initial questions are whether the patient truly has hypoglycaemia, and if it is likely to be reactive or whether there are grounds for considering insulinoma. Patients with access to blood glucose meters may also have access to insulin or oral hypoglycaemics, and the possibility of factitious hypoglycaemia should always be borne in mind. The provocative test for reactive hypoglycaemia is a prolonged glucose tolerance test or, perhaps more realistic, monitoring the glucose response over 5 hours following a mixed meal. For fasting hypoglycaemia, blood glucose (and insulin if hypoglycaemia is confirmed) following overnight fast or 30 minutes of exercise are useful as screening tests. Further investigation with 48–72 hours of fasting is required in some cases. For patients with fasting hypoglycaemia, the absence of ketones suggests that they are exposed to adequate insulin, or insulin-like activity. Plasma ketones >0.6 mmol/l or β-hydroxybutyrate >600 μmol/l suggests that the problem might be a failure to release stored glucose with consequent mobilization of fat. An algorithm for investigation of spontaneous hypoglycaemia is shown in Figure 40.1. Pituitary and adrenal disease should be excluded where appropriate.

Insulinoma is a relatively rare tumour, comprising around 25% of all functioning pancreatic endocrine tumours. The vast majority of insulinomas (>90%) are benign. They can occur at any age but the median age at diagnosis is around 50 years. They are slightly commoner in females (F:M = 3:2). The symptoms are those of hypoglycaemia, as described above, often provoked by exercise or fasting. Many patients experience increased appetite and weight gain. Diagnosis may require a prolonged fast of up to 72 hours. Fasting normally suppresses circulating insulin concentration to 3–5 μU/ml (18–30 pmol/l), and C-peptide to <0.6 ng/ml (<200 pmol/l). Abdominal ultrasound, computed tomography and magnetic resonance imaging all have a place in localizing these, often small, tumours. Endoscopic ultrasound improves the pick-up rate. In some cases, the tumours can only be localized at operation, either by palpation or by intra-operative ultrasound. ^{111}I-pentetreotide scanning is positive in about 50% of cases—many tumours lack the specific somatostatin receptors (particularly SSTR-2) required for this technique to be positive. Transhepatic portal venous, or intra-arterial sampling, with calcium infusion is used in specialist centres.

Medical treatment is generally only useful as part of preparation for surgery. Long-acting somatostatin analogues (octreotide, lanreotide) are useful in some cases. Diazoxide or verapamil are also used to decrease incidence of hypoglycaemic episodes. The preferred surgical approach depends on the ease with which the tumour can be localized, its size and position, and the experience of the surgeon. Many tumours can be selectively enucleated, while a partial pancreatectomy is required in some cases. In malignant insulinoma, removal or ablation of the metastases is considered worthwhile and not only improves prognosis but also alleviates the symptoms of hypoglycaemia.

Recent Developments

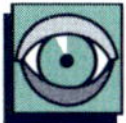

1 In spite of the controversy over whether reactive hypoglycaemia is a real clinical entity, it is common to find in hyperinsulinaemic women with polycystic ovarian syndrome (PCOS) that blood glucose is lower 3–4 hours after a glucose load than it was

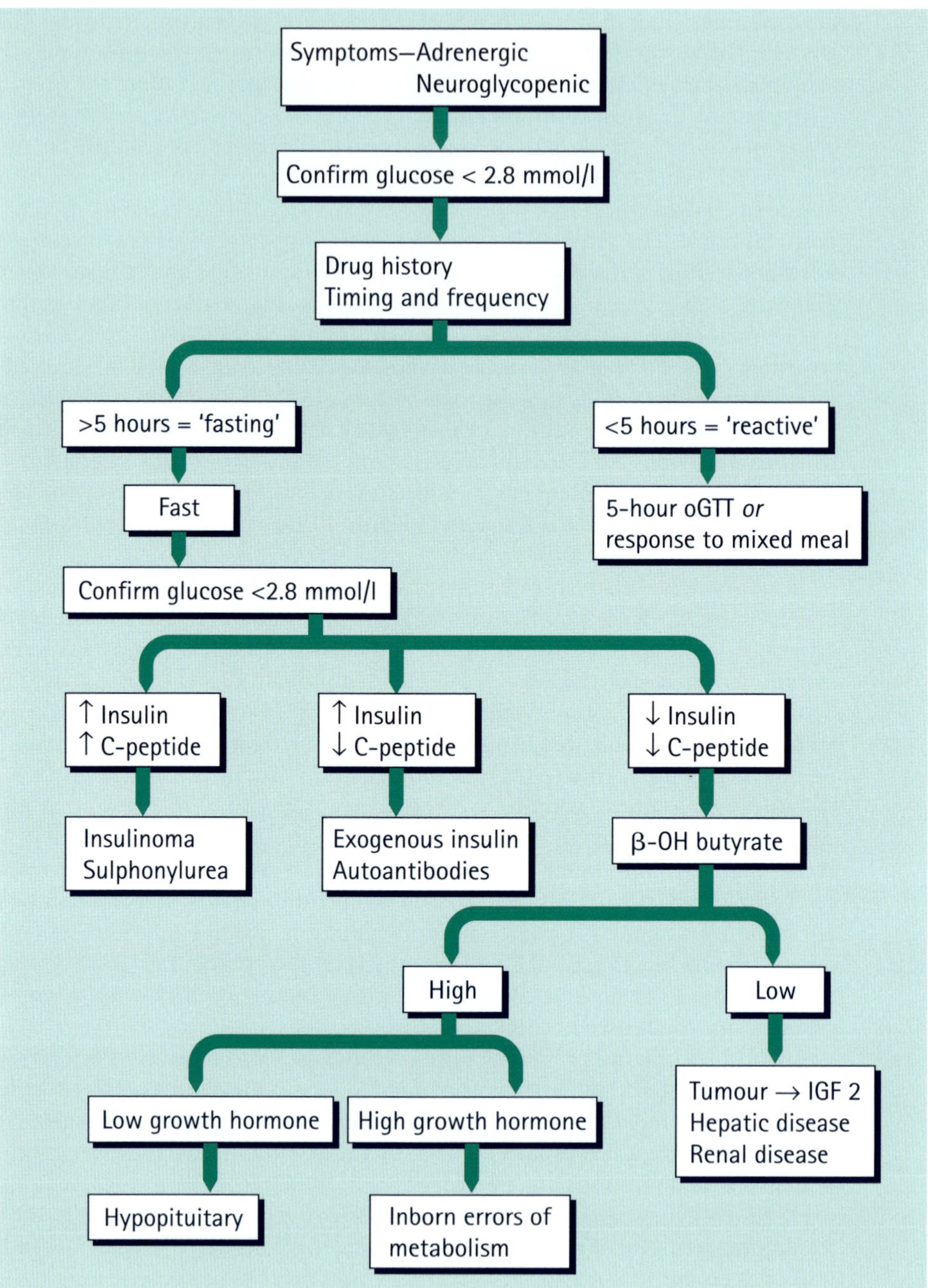

Fig. 40.1 Investigation of spontaneous hypoglycaemia. oGTT = oral glucose tolerance test.

at baseline. Even relative hypoglycaemia in these women may drive the hunger and carbohydrate cravings that many such women experience. In a recent study[2] of lean women with PCOS, reactive hypoglycaemia was reported to occur in 50%.

2 There has been considerable debate about whether 10% or 50% dextrose should be used in the management of acute hypoglycaemia. In children, very rapid increases in plasma glucose can cause cerebral oedema. Moore and Woollard[3] have conducted a randomized controlled trial of the two concentrations of glucose. Each was effective in reversing hypoglycaemia. Patients given 10% dextrose required less intravenous glucose and had lower post-treatment plasma glucose concentration.

3 Administration of GLP-1 to normal individuals can provoke hypoglycaemia, and the hormone has been implicated in the pathogenesis of late dumping syndrome following gastric surgery. Recently, hypoglycaemia was described in six patients following Roux-en-Y gastric bypass for severe obesity.[4] Increased delivery of nutrients to the small bowel through increased GLP-1 secretion was speculated to have produced nesidioblastosis.

Conclusions

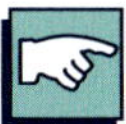

Hypoglycaemia should always be taken seriously, and should always be confirmed with a laboratory measurement of blood glucose. This may require admission for provocation tests. The role of the prolonged glucose tolerance test has become controversial as it can have false-positive and false-negative results. However, we believe the test to be useful, even if only to reassure the patient that their symptoms have been taken seriously and that some of the more worrying causes of hypoglycaemia have been excluded. Acarbose has been used to decrease the postprandial excursion in glucose and thus blunt the insulin response following a meal. Its routine use is not recommended, and the drug is associated with a high incidence of gastrointestinal side effects.

Further Reading

1 Gama R, Teale JD, Marks V. Best practice no. 173; Clinical and laboratory investigation of adult spontaneous hypoglycaemia. *J Clin Pathol* 2003; **56**: 641–6.

2 Altuntas Y, Bilir M, Ucak S, Gundogdu S. Reactive hypoglycemia in lean young women with PCOS and correlations with insulin sensitivity and with beta cell function. *Eur J Obstet Gynecol Reprod Biol* 2005; **119**: 198–205.

3 Moore C, Woollard M. Dextrose 10% or 50% in the treatment of hypoglycaemia out of hospital? *Emerg Med J* 2005; **22**: 512–15.

4 Service GJ, Thompson GB, Service FJ, Andrews JC, Collazo-Clavell ML, Lloyd RV. Hyperinsulinemic hypoglycemia with nedioblastosis after gastric-bypass surgery. *N Engl J Med* 2005; **353**: 249–54.

Therapeutic

PROBLEM

41 Corticosteroid and Mineralocorticoid Replacement

Case History

A 59-year-old woman has been known to have Addison's disease since her mid 20s. She has a family history of type 1 diabetes, and is presumed to have autoimmune adrenal failure. Although she has had no significant major illness in recent years she does not think that her health is as good as it might be. In particular she feels very tired in the middle of the day. She takes cortisone acetate 25 mg in the morning and 12.5 mg in the evening, as well as fludrocortisone 100 μg on alternate days.

What is the best form of glucocorticoid replacement?

How can you tell if her steroid replacement treatments are adequate?

Is it possible that she could develop side effects with standard replacement doses of glucocorticoid?

Background

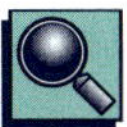

All patients with Addison's disease will require mineralocorticoid, as well as glucocorticoid, replacement, usually as fludrocortisone at 0.05–0.2 mg/day. The adequacy of replacement should be monitored by measuring erect and supine blood pressure, plasma electrolytes

Table 41.1 Relative potencies of steroid drugs

Steroid	Glucocorticoid potency (anti-inflammatory)	Glucocorticoid potency (glycogen deposition)	Mineralocorticoid potency (salt retention)	HPA axis suppression
Hydrocortisone (cortisol)	1			1
Cortisone	0.8	1	1	4
Prednisolone	3	3	0.75	4
Methylprednisolone	6.2	10	0.50	17
Dexamethasone	26	5	0	4
Triamcinolone	5	12	0	12
Fludrocortisone	12		125	

HPA = hypothalamic–pituitary–adrenal.

and plasma renin. The recent availability of assays for plasma renin concentration rather than for activity (i.e. an immunoassay) should lead to more widespread monitoring of mineralocorticoid replacement. Plasma renin concentration gives a good indication of under-replacement.[1] On the other hand, atrial natriuretic peptide may be a useful marker for over-replacement with mineralocorticoid. Clearly the latter may predispose to development of hypertension and cardiac failure in the longer term. Glucocorticoid replacement is usually given as hydrocortisone 15–25 mg/day. The dose is often prescribed as 10 mg on waking and 5 mg between 4 pm and 5 pm. An additional dose may be necessary at lunch time. Replacement with hydrocortisone may be monitored using a cortisol day curve. The dose of hydrocortisone should not be taken later than 6 pm as it may lead to greater suppression of morning adrenocorticotrophic hormone (ACTH) secretion. Cortisone acetate and prednisone are converted to cortisol and prednisolone, respectively, in the liver by the enzyme 11β-hydroxysteroid dehydrogenase type 1; it is therefore advisable to avoid these preparations. The dose equivalence of the different corticosteroid preparations used in clinical practice is given in Table 41.1.

Therapeutic doses of glucocorticoids which suppress the hypothalamic–pituitary–adrenal (HPA) axis can have a deleterious effect on a number of systems. In patients with Addison's disease, this should be avoided by offering the lowest possible dose as in this situation the aim is to use the lowest possible dose of replacement steroid, with appropriate increases during intercurrent illness. However, a number of clinical conditions require steroid therapy, and in these situations the steroid side effects are inevitable. The effects on bone can be prevented by the prophylactic use of bisphosphonates. Side effects of steroids are summarized in Box 41.1.

All patients on chronic corticosteroid therapy should carry a steroid card or warning bracelet and be advised to increase the dose of corticosteroid during intercurrent illness. In patients with Addison's disease on stable replacement doses of hydrocortisone, the dose of hydrocortisone may need to be increased to 100–150 mg/day. This may be given orally or parenterally if the patient is unable to take the drugs orally.

Box 41.1 Corticosteroid side effects

- Acute psychosis, euphoria, depression
- Osteoporosis
- Glucose intolerance, diabetes
- Peptic ulcer disease – perforation may be masked
- Hypertension
- Lack of a febrile response to infection
- Reactivation of latent tuberculosis

The complex physiology of hydrocortisone secretion and action makes it difficult to reproduce normal cortisol dynamics with two to three doses of hydrocortisone per day.[2] Recent estimates for cortisol production rates in man suggest normal values of around 10 nmol/ day, which is less than was previously thought. Many patients do not feel entirely well on such a low dose of replacement, but this is the physiological replacement dose that should be considered based on current evidence. Ninety per cent of circulating cortisol is bound to cortisol-binding globulin, with free cortisol levels ranging from up to 100 nmol/l at the diurnal peak to values as low as 1 nmol/l later in the day. Furthermore, the release of cortisol is pulsatile. It is not know whether this is of physiological significance, but it clearly cannot be reproduced with conventional oral replacement therapy. Circulating cortisol is inactivated to cortisone by the action of the enzyme 11β-hydroxysteroid dehydrogenase type 2 in the kidney. Cortisone circulates largely unbound and in concentrations that are, on average, higher than those of cortisol. Conversion of cortisone to cortisol occurs in target tissues through the action of 11β-hydroxysteroid dehydrogenase type 1. There is ample evidence from the literature that many patients with Addison's disease, hypopituitarism and other conditions requiring steroid replacement feel that their quality of life is impaired. Sometimes, it is justified to use higher doses to improve the patient's quality of life, knowing that they may then be exposed to slightly higher risk of steroid side effects.

Recent Developments

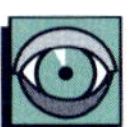

1. A recent study from Dublin examined glucocorticoid replacement in adult patients with partial ACTH deficiency.[3] Full dose hydrocortisone (10 mg twice daily) was compared with half dose (5 mg twice daily) and with no treatment in a crossover protocol. After each treatment, patients underwent a cortisol day curve, and results were compared with those of normal controls. The area under the cortisol day curve was greater for patients on full dose hydrocortisone compared with controls. There was no difference between controls and patients on half dose hydrocortisone or patients taking no treatment.

2. It is usual to start hydrocortisone replacement with a twice daily dose schedule, e.g. 20 mg in the morning and 10 mg in the evening. A three times daily schedule adding a dose at lunch time (e.g. 10 mg + 5 mg + 5 mg) is often used for patients who continue to experience symptoms suggestive of hypoadrenalism. These two regimens were compared by Alonso *et al.*[4] Although the three times daily regimen yielded a more

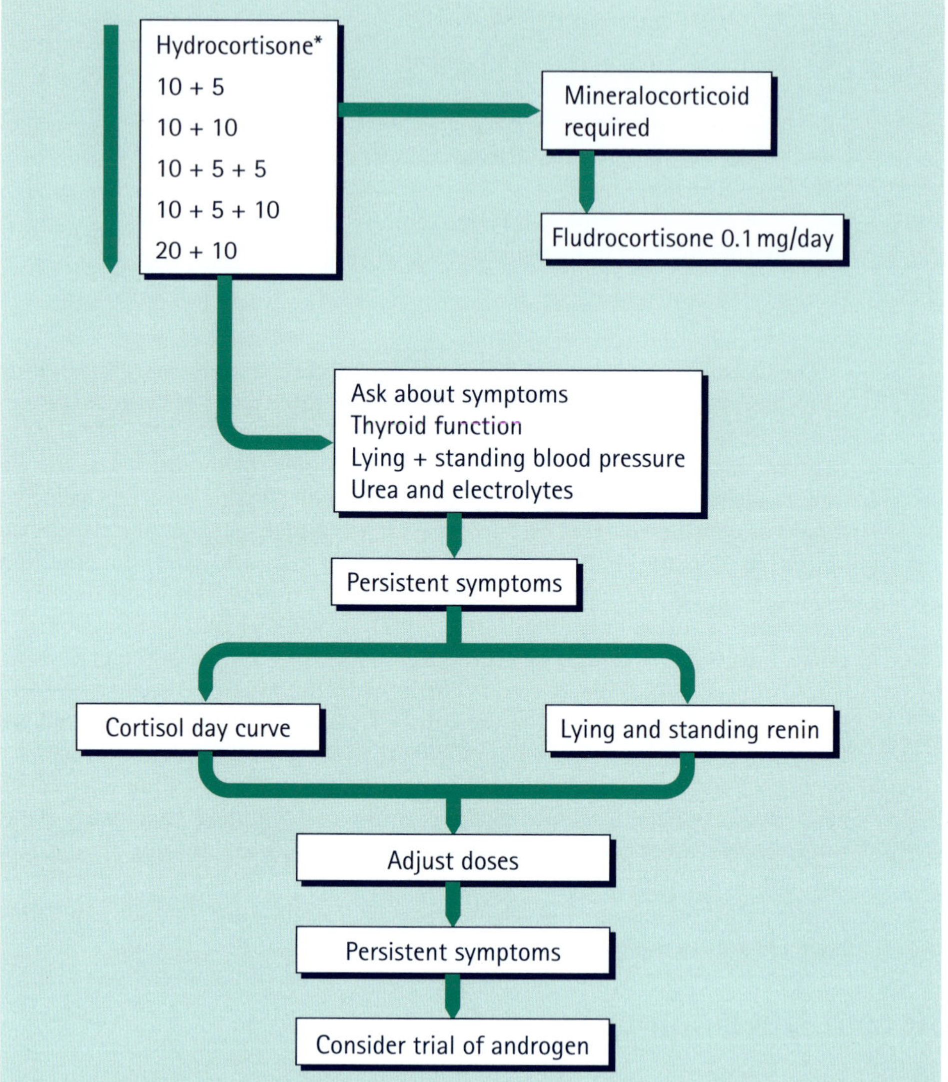

Fig. 41.1 Replacement therapy for hypoadrenalism. *Hydrocortisone dose (in mg) adjusted according to clinical response initially. Day curve will confirm absorption and physiological profile. Concomitant adrenocorticotrophic hormone measurements will exclude over-treatment.

physiological cortisol profile, there was no difference in health-related quality of life. Patients with Addison's disease in this study did rate their quality of life as being poorer compared with the general population.

3 Even though conventional doses of mineralocorticoid may be supraphysiological in terms of the cortisol day curve, the major question is whether they are harmful. There is no doubt that we should be treating patients with the lowest dose of replacement

that alleviates symptoms and minimizes risk of an adrenal crisis. Recent studies[5,6] have not shown increased risk of bone density loss in patients taking conventional replacement doses of hydrocortisone.

4 The role of androgen replacement in patients with hypoadrenalism remains controversial. A recent study[7] did not find any difference in lipid parameters, glucose levels, insulin sensitivity, or quality of life in Addison's patients given dehydro-3-epiandrosterone (DHEA) for four months. However, Addison's patients do have low androgen levels and do report symptoms suggestive of androgen deficiency.

Conclusions

There seems little doubt that hydrocortisone is the most appropriate glucocorticoid to use for replacement therapy in patients with adrenal failure. Fludrocortisone is the only mineralocorticoid widely available. A protocol for monitoring steroid replacement in patients with adrenal failure is suggested in Figure 41.1. It is often difficult to be sure that replacement doses are adequate when the patient continues to experience symptoms. It is clear from recent evidence that many patients are treated with doses of glucocorticoid that are greater than those they may produce physiologically. They may, therefore be exposed to risk of side effects of excess steroid. Caution should, however, be exercised in trying to minimize steroid doses as more patients seem to continue to experience hypoadrenal symptoms than develop serious steroid side effects.

Further Reading

1 Cohen N, Gilbert R, Wirth A, Casley D, Jerums G. Atrial natriuretic peptide and plasma renin levels in assessment of mineralocorticoid replacement in Addison's disease. *J Clin Endocrinol Metab* 1996; **81**: 1411–15.

2 Crown A, Lightman S. Why is the management of glucocorticoid deficiency still so controversial: a review of the literature. *Clin Endocrinol* 2005; **63**: 483–92.

3 Agha A, Liew A, Finunicane F, *et al.* Conventional glucocorticoid replacement over treats adult hypopituitary patients with partial ACTH deficiency. *Clin Endocrinol* 2004; **60**: 688–93.

4 Alonso N, Granada ML, Lucas A, *et al.* Evaluation of two replacement regimens in primary adrenal insufficiency patients. Effects on clinical symptoms, health-related quality of life and biochemical parameters. *J Endocrinol Invest* 2004; **27**: 449–54.

5 Jodar E, Vadlenpenas MPR, Martinez G, Jara A, Hawkins F. Long-term follow-up of bone mineral density in Addison's disease. *Clin Endocrinol* 2003; **58**: 617–20.

6 Chikada N, Imaki T, Hotta M, Sato K, Takano K. An assessment of bone mineral density in patients with Addisons disease and isolated ACTH deficiency treated with glucocorticoid. *Endocr J* 2004; **51**: 355–60.

7 Libe R, Barbetta L, Dall'Asta C, Salvaggio F, Gala C, Beck-Peccoz P. Effects of dehydroepiandrosterone (DHEA) supplementation on hormonal, metabolic, and behavioural status in patients with hypoadrenalism. *J Endocrinol Invest* 2004; **27**: 736–41.

PROBLEM

42 Neutropaenia on Carbimazole

Case History

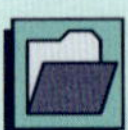

A 28-year-old woman was diagnosed as having thyrotoxicosis 4 months ago. She has a diffuse goitre and mild exophthalmos. She is not anticipating becoming pregnant in the foreseeable future. She presents with a sore throat and, on examination, has ulceration of her pharynx. She had been warned to report sore throat promptly and to discontinue the carbimazole. She has been taking 20 mg/day. Her white blood cell count is decreased at 0.4×10^9/l.

Was she correct to stop her carbimazole?

How should she be managed in the short term?

What approach would you now take to managing her Graves' disease?

Background

Antithyroid drugs are the commonest first line of treatment for thyrotoxicosis. The drugs are generally safe and well tolerated, and have been used since the 1940s. Minor side effects occur in up to 5% of patients and include urticaria or macular skin rash, nausea and vomiting, altered taste and arthralgia. Although usually relatively mild, the latter can signify onset of a more general drug reaction, and many would advise the drugs be discontinued if the patient develops arthralgia. A skin reaction severe enough to discontinue the drug occurs in 1 in every 100 to 200 patients. Side effects with carbimazole and methimazole (MMI) in particular are generally dose related, and there is about 50% crossover if the patient is changed to one of the other drugs.

Relative neutropaenia is not uncommon in patients with Graves' disease, especially in patients of African descent. Neutrophil dyscrasias (neutropaenia and agranulocytosis) are the most commonly reported serious side effects of thionamide drugs. Neutropaenia is defined as neutrophil count less than 1.5×10^9/l, and agranulocytosis is defined as neutrophil count less than 0.5×10^9/l. Agranulocytosis occurs in around one-third of 1% of patients taking antithyroid drugs. It usually occurs in the first 3 months of treatment. The drugs should be stopped immediately in all patients with granulocyte count less than 1×10^9/l. The complication may occur at any time in the course of antithyroid drug treatment, and may occur in patients who have previously taken a successful and uncomplicated course of thionamide drugs. Following agranulocytosis, treatment with any of the thionamide drugs is contraindicated. There should be a low threshold for checking full and differential blood counts in patients who are taking thionamides, but routine regular blood checks are not generally thought to be indicated.

Table 42.1 Fatal adverse reactions to carbimazole

Reaction	Total reported	Fatal (%)
Agranulocytosis	94	18 (19)
Neutropaenia	85	2 (2)
Aplastic anaemia	10	5 (50)
Thrombocytopaenia	17	3 (18)
Pancytopaenia	7	1 (14)
Hepatitis and jaundice	65	2 (3)
Vasculitis	2	0
Birth defects	59	3 (5)
Total reports	725	42 (6)

Data are from the UK,[1] where methimazole is not routinely used and propylthiouracil is generally only used as a second line drug. The table shows reports between 1963 and 2003.

Other serious side effects (apart from agranulocytosis, neutropaenia, thrombocytopaenia, pancytopaenia and aplastic anaemia) are hepatitis and vasculitis. Pearce[1] has reviewed adverse side effects with thionamides reported in the UK between 1963 and 2003. Fatal side effects were commoner in older subjects. Neutrophil dyscrasias were usually reported early in treatment, with a median time to reporting of only 30 days. The relative incidence of fatal side effects is shown in Table 42.1. There were 5.23 million prescriptions for thionamide drugs in the UK between 1981 and 2003. Reports of serious side effects (per million prescriptions) were 98.4 for carbimazole and 239.6 for propylthiouracil (PTU).

Antithyroid drugs are almost certainly the commonest cause of drug-induced agranulocytosis followed by sulphamethoxazole, sulfasalazine and clomipramine. The commonest presentations are fever and sore throat (due to pharyngitis or tonsillitis). Agranulocytosis is also associated with other infections including pneumonia and urinary tract infection. Positive blood cultures are common and may yield a range of organisms including *Pseudomonas aeruginosa*. The neutropaenia is thought to be of autoimmune origin with patients having a high frequency of antineutrophil cytoplasmic antibodies (ANCAs). A range of autoantigens has been described including proteinase 3 and myeloperoxidase. Management of agranulocytosis with antithyroid drugs is summarized in Figure 42.1. The drug should be withdrawn. Patients should be screened for infection and if febrile, or if there is evidence of infection, they should be commenced on broad-spectrum antibiotics, often with an antifungal agent. Use of granulocyte colony stimulating factor should be considered in severe cases.

Severe hepatotoxicity occurs in 0.1–0.25% of patients treated with PTU. It is difficult to diagnose as abnormalities in liver enzymes are common in patients with thyrotoxicosis at baseline. Furthermore, transient increases in liver enzymes (up to six times normal) also occur commonly in patients started on thionamide drugs. The commonest severe hepatic reaction to PTU is an allergic hepatitis with marked increases in transaminases. Like blood dyscrasias, the reaction is most common within the first few months of starting

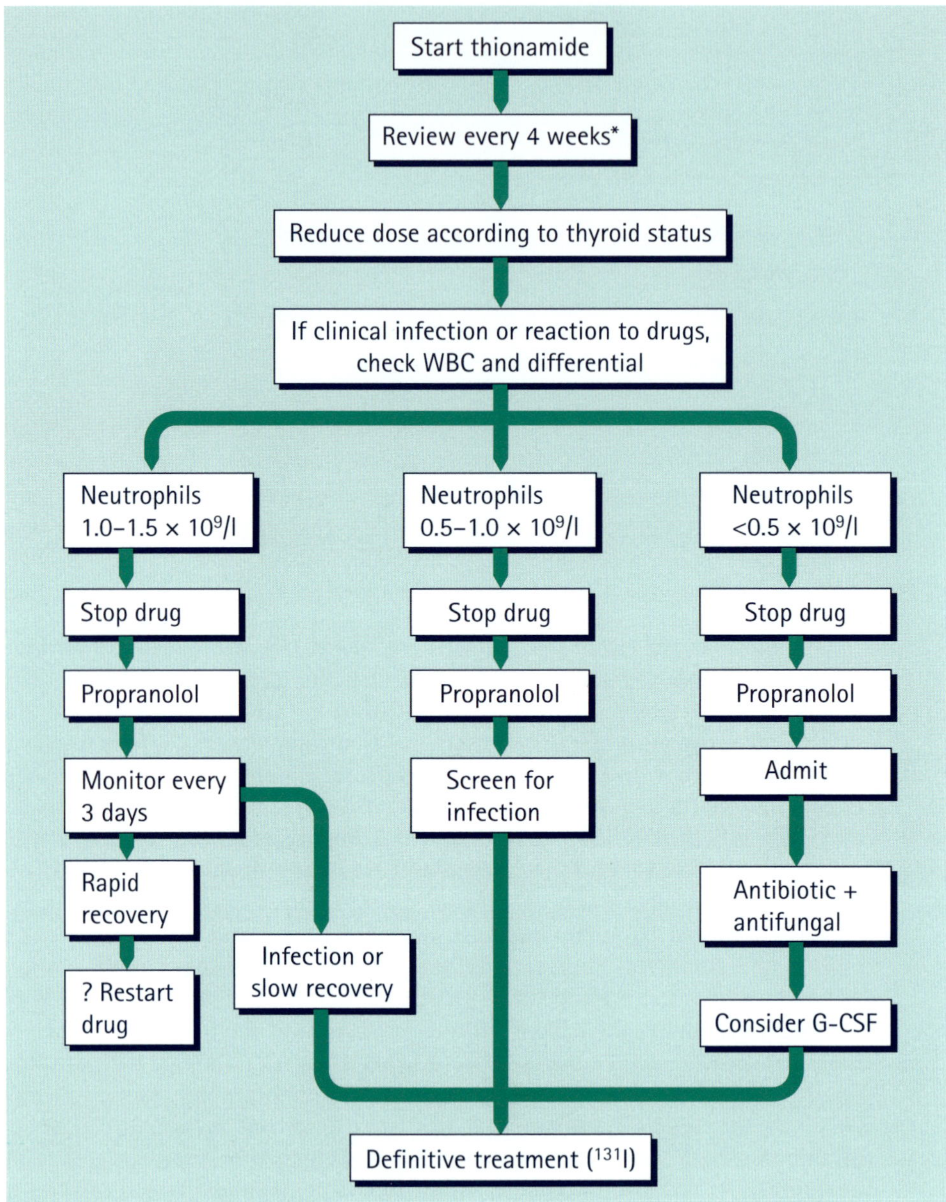

Fig. 42.1 Management of antithyroid drug-induced neutropaenia. *Until patient is clinically and biochemically euthyroid. G-CSF = granulocyte colony stimulating factor; WBC = white blood cell.

therapy. It may be fatal in up to 25% and can require liver transplantation. Hepatitis is less common with carbimazole and MMI, but these drugs can cause intrahepatic cholestasis, which usually resolves spontaneously on stopping the drug.

Vasculitis is also more common with PTU and may present with skin rash, arthritis, worsening renal function and respiratory symptoms including haemoptysis. ANCAs are positive in about 5% of patients with Graves' disease before treatment, in up to 15% taking carbimazole, and 30% taking PTU. Most patients with thionamide-induced vasculitis have perinuclear ANCAs with antibodies reacting against myeloperoxidase (perhaps not surprisingly due to cross-reactivity with thyroid peroxidase). Most cases resolve spontaneously on stopping the drug, but some require high-dose immunosuppressive therapy including corticosteroids and cyclophosphamide.

Recent Developments

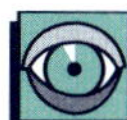

1. Harper and colleagues[2] screened a large number of patients with Graves' disease for ANCA. Results were compared with normal controls and with euthyroid patients with Hashimoto's thyroiditis. By indirect immunofluorescence, ANCA was positive in more patients with Graves' disease (19.9%) than euthyroid controls (4.6%; $P < 0.001$). ANCAs were also detected more frequently by enzyme-linked immunosorbent assay in Graves' sera. Anti-proteinase 3 and anti-myeloperoxidase were measured. The presence of ANCA was strongly associated with the use of antithyroid drugs, particularly PTU, rather than with the autoimmune state.
2. Low neutrophil count may occur in the presence of a normal total white blood cell count. Tajiri and Noguchi[3] noted white blood cell count of greater than 3.0×10^9/l in 18 out of 109 (16.5%) patients presenting with antithyroid drug-induced neutropaenia. Some of these patients had infections, and in some there was a further decrease in neutrophil count.
3. Only about a quarter of patients who become ANCA positive after PTU treatment is started develop clinical features of vasculitis. Yu *et al.*[4] measured antibodies to endothelial cells (AECAs) using an extract from human umbilical vein endothelial cells and an immunoblotting technique. Ten of 11 patients with ANCA-positive vasculitis were positive for AECAs in the active phase of their illness. Most of these became negative during the quiescent phase. AECAs were absent in patients who were ANCA positive after PTU but did not have vasculitis, and in normal controls.

Conclusions

The patient was correct to stop her carbimazole as she had severe neutropaenia. However, symptoms of sore throat and upper respiratory infection are common. It is preferable for patients to seek urgent advice and to have a full blood count and differential checked before stopping their drugs. Without antithyroid drug, the patient will require symptom control for thyrotoxicosis. We would use oral propranolol (80–240 mg/day) titrated to their resting pulse rate. If the patient is severely neutropaenic, severely thyrotoxic, or has clinical evidence of infection, they should be admitted to hospital and commenced on a suitable regimen of broad-spectrum antibiotics. Once the patient has recovered from the neutropaenia, the infections have been brought under control, and hyperthyroid symptoms are controlled, consideration should be given to definitive treatment with radioactive iodine. For those patients who prefer surgery, careful preoperative preparation with β-blockers and iodine is necessary.

Further Reading

1 Pearce SH. Spontaneous reporting of adverse reactions to carbimazole and propylthiouracil in the UK. *Clin Endocrinol* 2004; **61**: 589–94.

2 Harper L, Chin L, Daykin J, *et al*. Propylthiouracil and carbimazole associated-antineutrophil cytoplasmic antibodies (ANCA) in patients with Graves' disease. *Clin Endocrinol* 2004; **60**: 671–5.

3 Tajiri J, Noguchi S. Antithyroid drug-induced agranulocytosis: special reference to normal white blood cell count agranulocytosis. *Thyroid* 2004; **14**: 459–62.

4 Yu F, Zhao MH, Zhang YK, Zhang Y, Wang HY. Anti-endothelial cell antibodies (AECA) in patients with propylthiouracil (PTU)-induced ANCA positive vasculitis are associated with disease activity. *Clin Exp Immunol* 2005; **139**: 569–74.

PROBLEM

43 Lithium

Case History

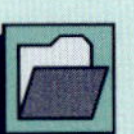

Mrs MH is a 57-year-old woman who has previously been very unwell with a bipolar disorder, necessitating admission to a psychiatric hospital. She has been well from the psychological point of view for the past 18 months and continues to take lithium carbonate. Her plasma levels are monitored regularly. She has noticed that she has to get up increasingly frequently at night to pass urine, and she is also passing urine fairly frequently during the day.

Are her urinary symptoms related to lithium, and what is the mechanism?

Should she stop taking the lithium?

Are there any treatments that might help with her urinary symptoms?

Should she be aware of any other long-term effects of lithium?

Background

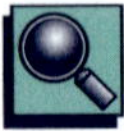

Although much less common than unipolar depression, bipolar illness may affect up to 1% of the population.[1] The disease is of variable severity, but can be life-threatening at its worst. The underlying cause is not known, although there is a strong genetic element with

Table 43.1 Side effects and toxic effects of lithium

Side effects	Toxic effects
Nausea	Blurred vision
Diarrhoea	Dysarthria
Dry mouth	Confusion
Oedema	Ataxia
Tremor	Coarse tremor
Weight gain	Drowsiness
Polyuria and polydipsia	Muscle weakness
Thyroid dysfunction	
Hypercalcaemia	

around half of sufferers having a family history. There is 10–20% concordance for the disease in dizygotic twins and a 40–80% concordance in monozygotic twins. Susceptibility loci for the disease have been identified on chromosomes 18 and 21.

Lithium has been used in management of bipolar illness for over 50 years. It is highly effective, and generally well tolerated, and may be used in the management of acute mania and as a mood stabilizer to prevent exacerbations of the disease. One of the problems with the drug is its narrow therapeutic window, making it necessary to monitor drug levels at regular intervals, usually every 3 months. The common side effects and toxic effects of lithium are listed in Table 43.1. Lithium may cause progressive nephropathy and a variety of endocrine abnormalities including hypothyroidism, hypercalcaemia and parathyroid adenoma, osteoporosis, nephrogenic diabetes insipidus, and weight gain with insulin resistance. These endocrine side effects are sufficiently common that an argument could be advanced for all patients taking lithium treatment to be seen regularly by an endocrinologist. A care pathway for patients treated with lithium is suggested in Figure 43.1.

Side effects may occur with drug levels in the therapeutic range (0.6–1.0 mmol/l), whereas some may appear only with prolonged exposure to the drug. Toxic effects would only usually be experienced when the levels of lithium are above the upper limit of the therapeutic range. Levels of lithium may be increased by a number of drugs including thiazides, non-steroidal anti-inflammatory agents, angiotensin-converting enzyme inhibitors, serotonin selective reuptake inhibitors and theophylline.

Renal abnormalities are common in patients taking lithium and they fall into three categories: nephrogenic diabetes insipidus; acute intoxication; chronic renal impairment. The renal impairment associated with acute intoxication is partially due to rehydration and is usually reversible with hydration and temporary discontinuation of the drug. The chronic renal impairment seen in a minority of patients on lithium is due partially to functional and partially to structural change. The distal tubules and collecting ducts are the main targets for damage. Lithium competes with magnesium which acts as a co-factor for many G proteins and enzymes within the kidney. The major changes are usually

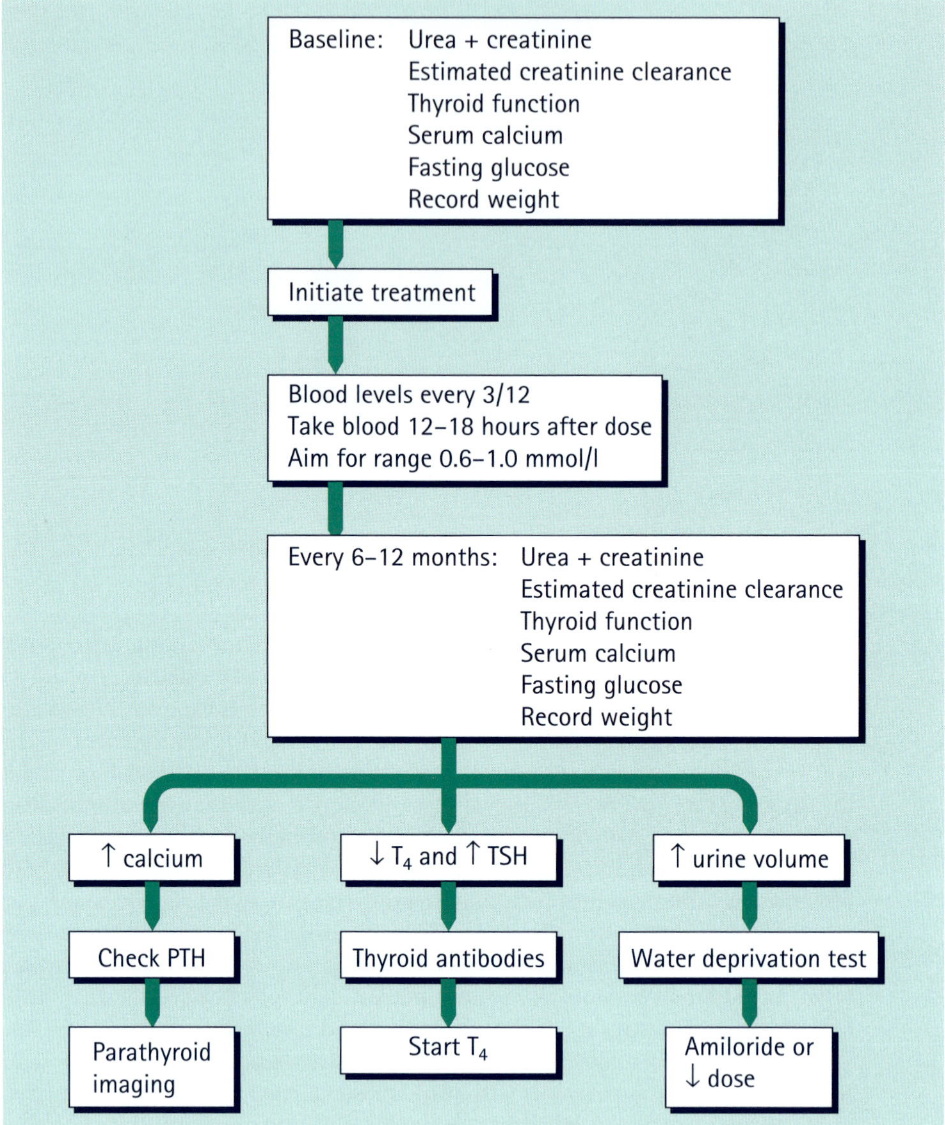

Fig. 43.1 Care pathway for patients taking lithium. PTH = parathyroid hormone; TSH = thyroid-stimulating hormone.

described as chronic tubulointerstitial nephropathy, which is associated with tubular atrophy and interstitial fibrosis. The result of these processes is steadily declining renal function and nephrotic protein loss in some (>3 g/day). Renal function often does not improve after discontinuing lithium.

Nephrogenic diabetes insipidus in patients taking lithium is due to downregulation of aquaporin (AQP2 and AQP3) in the collecting ducts. The aquaporins are membrane proteins that function as water channels. The changes range from mild inconvenience to severe hypernatraemia and dehydration with acute illness or when fluid intake is restricted.

Lithium therapy is the commonest drug-induced cause of nephrogenic diabetes insipidus. Up to 40% of patients taking lithium have increased urine volume, and nephrogenic diabetes insipidus is present in up to 12%. Age and duration of treatment are the major risk factors. The condition is said to be mild when plasma osmolality is normal, urine osmolality is <300 mOsm/kg, and urine output is between 2.5 l/day and 6 l/day. The most useful test is the water deprivation test. In nephrogenic diabetes insipidus, urine osmolality remains low (<300 mOsm/kg) after dehydration, and there is no response to vasopressin. Partial nephrogenic diabetes insipidus is said to be present when urinary osmolality is between 300 mOsm/kg and 750 mOsm/kg following dehydration, and does not rise above 750 mOsm/kg with vasopressin. Consideration should be given to stopping lithium therapy and substituting it with another antipsychotic drug. However, if this is not possible, the nephrogenic diabetes insipidus may be treated with amiloride which inhibits lithium entry into cells. Also, a decreased dose of lithium might be considered aiming at a therapeutic range of 0.5–0.8 mmol/l. Non-steroidal anti-inflammatory drugs such as indomethacin may be useful. Treatment of nephrogenic diabetes insipidus with a thiazide diuretic may reduce lithium excretion and precipitate lithium toxicity.

Lithium increases intrathyroidal iodine content, inhibits coupling of iodotyrosine residues to form T_4 and T_3 and it inhibits conversion of T_4 to T_3. The result is that up to 50% of lithium-treated patients are likely to develop goitre and many patients within this group have hypothyroidism. Hypothyroidism is usually subclinical (high thyroid-stimulating hormone [TSH] with normal T_4 and T_3) and occurs in up to 21% of patients. Overall, 3–5% of patients taking lithium have overt hypothyroidism. Lithium-induced goitre and hypothyroidism tend to appear within the first two years of lithium therapy in susceptible individuals. They are more likely to occur in women, and in those whose bipolar illness cycles rapidly. The role of autoimmunity in lithium-induced thyroid disorders has been controversial, but current evidence suggests that the disorders are not of autoimmune origin in most cases.

Long-term therapy is associated with mild increases in plasma calcium. In some cases this has been found to lead to primary hyperparathyroidism with associated parathyroid hyperplasia. This effect of lithium improves when the drug is stopped and the parathyroid gland returns to normal size in most cases. Of patients taking lithium, 10–15% develop hypercalcaemia, often mild and usually asymptomatic. A very small proportion develop parathyroid adenomas, and these can be multiple. Lithium also increases calcium turnover from bone and can contribute to development of osteoporosis. The mechanism underlying lithium-induced changes in calcium metabolism is not clear. Lithium inhibits calcium influx into cells, and may thus directly contribute to development of hypercalcaemia.

Recent Developments

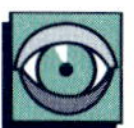

1 The cellular mechanism of lithium's actions is beginning to be understood.[1,2] The ion inhibits intracellular cyclic AMP generation by interfering with the interaction between G protein and intracellular adenylate cyclase. The enzyme inositol monophosphatase is inhibited by lithium. Some of the actions of the drug may be through intracellular inositol depletion, caused both by decreased recycling and decreased *de novo* synthesis. Lithium acts as a neuroprotective agent, and this action may be mediated in part through inhibition of the enzyme glycogen synthase kinase 3β.

2 A recent study from China confirms that the rate of development of hypothyroidism is markedly increased in patients who are prescribed lithium.[3] Similarly, in a review of prescribing for over 1.3 million patients in Ontario,[4] there was an increased rate of prescribing of thyroxine in patients who were concurrently prescribed lithium. The rate of development of hypothyroidism in lithium-treated patients was 5.65 per 100 patient-years. This was approximately twice that of the background population.

3 Growth regulatory effects on parathyroid tissue with increased expression of the transcription factor AP-1 have been noted.[5] However, it is not known whether the drug initiates growth of adenomas or whether it selects fast growing populations of cells from the parathyroid. A higher proportion of patients have adenomas of multiple glands than would be expected.

Conclusions

Urinary symptoms are common in patients taking lithium long term, occurring in up to 40% of patients. The symptoms are not generally severe enough to warrant stopping the drug. The condition should be explained to the patient, and the dangers of stopping lithium in a patient with severe bipolar illness should be recognized. Consideration could be given to lowering the dose to aim for the lower part of the therapeutic range. Alternatively, treatment with amiloride should be considered. Although very effective, the drug can lead to renal impairment, hypothyroidism, hypercalcaemia and weight gain.

Further Reading

1 Belmaker RH. Bipolar disorder. *N Engl J Med* 2004; **351**: 476–86.

2 Williams R, Ryves WJ, Dalton EC, Eickholt B, Shaltiel G, Agam G, Harwood AH. A molecular cell biology of lithium. *Biochem Soc Trans* 2004; **32**: 799–802.

3 Zhang ZJ, Li Q, Kang WH, *et al.* Differences in hypothyroidism between lithium-free and -treated patients with bipolar disorders. *Life Sci* 2006; **76**: 771–6.

4 Shulman KI, Sykora K, Gill SSS, Mamdani M, Anderson G, Marras C, Wodchis WP, Lee PE, Rochon P. New thyroxine treatment in older adults beginning lithium therapy. *Am J Geriatr Psychiatry* 2005; **13**: 299–304.

5 Awad SS, Miskulin J, Thompson N. Parathyroid adenomas versus four-gland hyperplasia as the cause of primary hyperparathyroidism in patients with prolonged lithium therapy. *World J Surg* 2003; **27**: 486–8.

PROBLEM

44 Calcium and Vitamin D

Case History

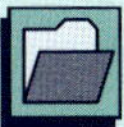

Mrs FS is a 48-year-old woman who has recently undergone subtotal thyroidectomy for a benign goitre. She has generally made a good recovery and is now taking thyroxine 150 μg/day. She is complaining of tingling around her mouth and in her fingers. On questioning, she recalls that she required intravenous calcium after her operation. Her serum calcium is 1.80 mmol/l (normal 2.2–2.6 mmol/l).

How would you approach management of her low serum calcium?

Is she likely to require replacement long term?

How would you manage severe hypocalcaemia?

Background

The complication rate from subtotal thyroidectomy will depend on the expertise of the surgeon, and it is therefore difficult to generalize its frequency. Transient hypoparathyroidism after surgery results from the inadvertent removal of some parathyroids and ischaemia in the remaining. The symptoms of hypocalcaemia develop within a week of surgery but the rapidity of onset will depend on the severity of the injury. Permanent hypoparathyroidism occurs in up to 3.6% of cases. In mild hypocalcaemia oral calcium carbonate is necessary. In more severe and prolonged hypocalcaemia, calcium and vitamin D or one of its analogues will be required long term.

Vitamin D exists in two forms: vitamin D_2 (ergocalciferol) and vitamin D_3 (cholecalciferol). Vitamin D_2 is the principal form available in diet and pharmaceutical agents. Vitamin D_3 is produced endogenously from 7-dehydrocholesterol. The metabolism of vitamin D is summarized in Figure 44.1. 1α-hydroxylase is stimulated by parathyroid hormone (PTH), hypocalcaemia and hypophosphataemia. 1α-hydroxylase activity is present in epidermis, placenta, bone, macrophages and prostate in addition to the kidney. Extra-renal production of $1,25(OH)_2$ D is not controlled by calcium or PTH. Cytokines such as γ-interferon are responsible for increased 1α-hydroxylase activity in macrophages in sarcoidosis or other lymphoproliferative diseases. $1,25(OH)_2$ D production in such cases is independent of PTH action. Renal disease reduces 1α-hydroxylase activity and $1,25(OH)_2$ D levels drop. Levels of $1,25(OH)_2$ D begin to decrease when the glomerular filtration rate approaches 40 ml/min.

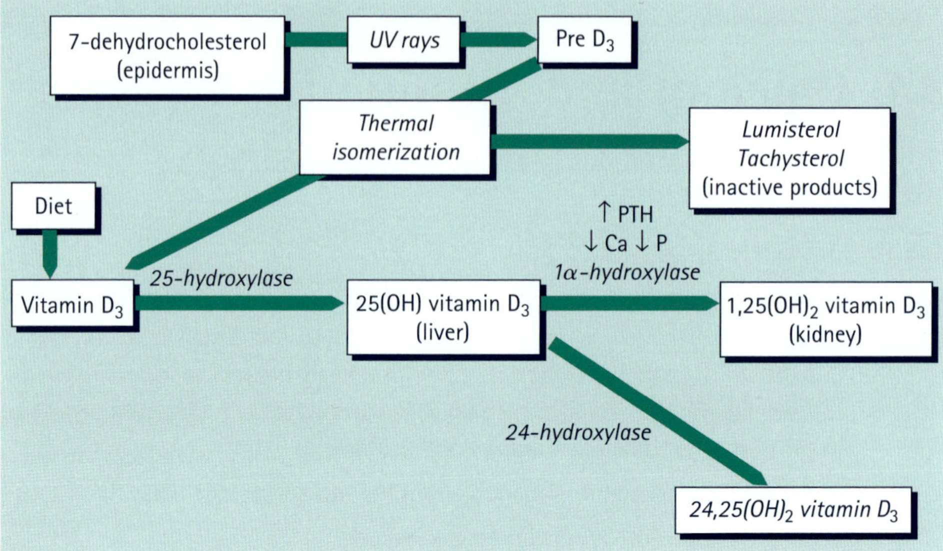

Fig. 44.1 Metabolism of vitamin D. PTH = parathyroid hormone.

Table 44.1 Causes of vitamin D deficiency

Defective intake or production	Low dietary intake Lack of exposure to sunlight Malabsorption
Defective 25-hydroxylation	Liver disease
Defective 1α-hydroxylation	Renal failure Ketoconazole X-linked hypophosphataemic rickets Vitamin D dependent rickets type 1
Increased metabolism	Phenytoin Rifampicin Glutethimide
Target organ resistance	Vitamin D dependent rickets type 2

Causes of vitamin D deficiency

These are summarized in Table 44.1. Daily vitamin D requirement for children and adults up to the age of 50 is 200 U, for adults aged 51–70 it is 400 U, and the daily requirement for subjects aged 71 or older is 600 U. Vitamin D dependent rickets type 1 is an autosomal recessive disease due to mutations in the gene for the 1α-hydroxylase enzyme located at chromosome 12q14. The condition should be treated with forms of vitamin D that are 1α-hydroxylated. Vitamin D dependent rickets type 2 is also an autosomal recessive condition, this time due to defects in the gene for the vitamin D receptor. Levels of vitamin D and its 25-hydroxylated derivative are normal while 1,25-dihydroxyvitamin D levels are markedly increased.

Calcium supplementation

This is not necessarily required in patients who have vitamin D deficiency, although many vitamin D preparations contain calcium. Per unit weight, different calcium salts yield varying amounts of elemental calcium. Calcium phosphate, citrate and gluconate have a relatively low yield. Calcium carbonate is cheap, and is the most widely used salt. It needs acidification to be absorbed and is therefore best taken with food or can be taken with a citrus fruit drink. Absorption can be a problem in elderly people with achlorhydria. In the emergency situation 10 ml of 10% calcium gluconate (2.25 mmol) can be administered slowly intravenously followed by 40 ml (9 mmol) over the next 24 hours.

Vitamin D replacement

A wide range of preparations are available, and the choice depends on the underlying diagnosis. The available forms of vitamin D are: ergocalciferol (calciferol, vitamin D_2); cholecalciferol (vitamin D_3); dihydrotachysterol (a synthetic analogue of vitamin D_3); alfacalcidol (1α-hydroxycholecalciferol); calcitriol (1,25-dihydroxycholecalciferol); and paricalcitol (analogue use to prevent secondary hyperparathyroidism in renal failure).

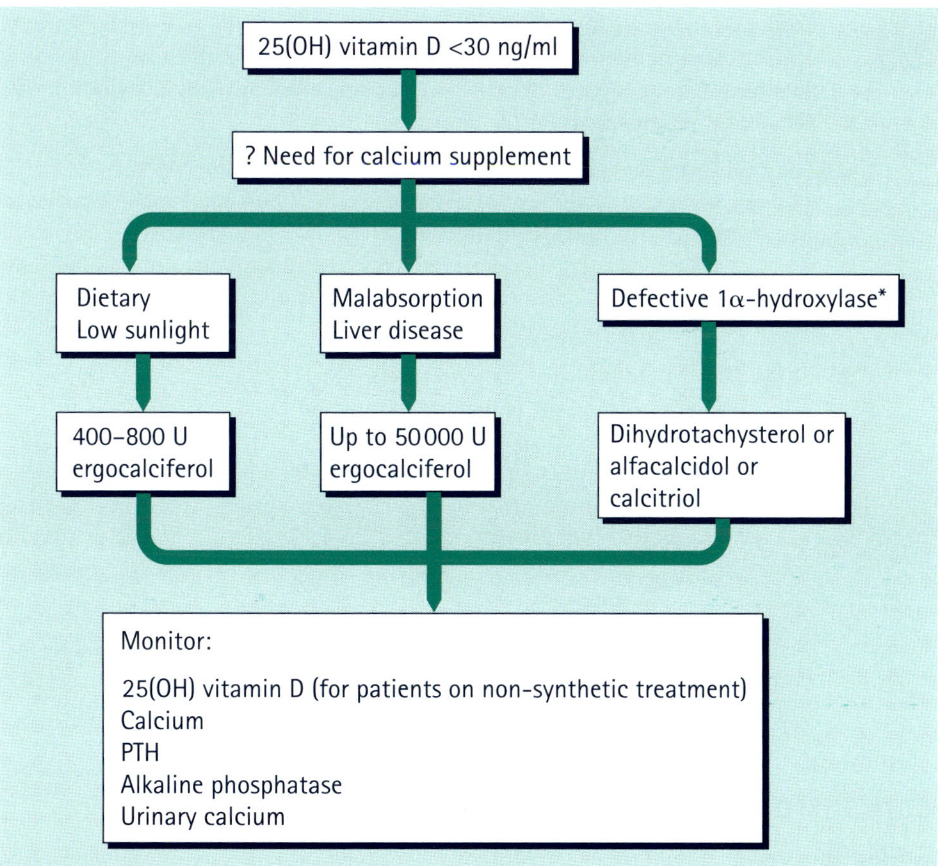

Fig. 44.2 Calcium and vitamin D replacement. *Defective 1α-hydroxylation occurs in renal failure, hypoparathyroidism, parathyroid hormone (PTH) resistance and in type 1 vitamin D dependent rickets.

For simple vitamin D supplementation 400–800 U (10–20 μg) ergocalciferol per day is suitable. This may be given with up to 1500 mg calcium, depending on dietary intake. More severe forms of vitamin D deficiency should be treated with doses of up to 50 000 U/day for up to 3 weeks before starting the patient on maintenance therapy. Patients with malabsorption or liver disease require pharmacological doses of up to 40 000 U (1 mg) ergocalciferol per day. Hypoparathyroidism requires treatment with high doses of ergocalciferol (if this is the chosen or available treatment) of up to 100 000 U (2.5 mg)/day. 1α-hydroxylation is impaired in patients with renal failure, hypoparathyroidism, parathyroid hormone resistance, and vitamin D dependent rickets. In these conditions, use dihydrotachysterol, calcitriol, or alfacalcidol.

In monitoring vitamin D replacement, ensure that hypocalcaemia is corrected. PTH should be suppressed into the normal range, and urine calcium excretion should be greater than 100 mg per 24 hours. Alkaline phosphatase may remain elevated for some months after starting treatment but should ultimately return to normal. A treatment flow chart for vitamin D replacement is shown in Figure 44.2.

Recent Developments

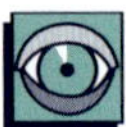

1. In the recent study by Diamond *et al.*,[1] a single injection of 600 000 U cholecalciferol (15 mg) maintained adequate vitamin D status during the 12 months of follow-up. Furthermore, adequate vitamin D status was confirmed by the finding of decreased levels of PTH during the study period.
2. Vitamin D status is probably the major factor in governing levels of PTH in the general population.[2] Part of the importance of vitamin D status as a determinant of bone health may be through regulating secretion of PTH. Increased PTH has also been associated with increased tendency to hypertension and insulin resistance. It may well be that measures of PTH and urinary calcium excretion should be taken into account when assessing vitamin D status routinely.
3. Up to 80% of elderly patients with osteoporosis are at least somewhat vitamin deficient. However, even in the younger and more ambulant population, the prevalence of low levels of vitamin D may be up to 10%.[3] This is now thought to be a major determinant of a number of aspects of health including risk of osteoporosis, type 1 diabetes and rheumatoid arthritis, hypertension, heart disease and some cancers. It has been suggested that measurement of 25(OH) vitamin D levels should be part of routine medical assessment.
4. The prevalence of low vitamin D status is high, even in women who do not have evidence of osteoporosis.[4] A recent study in community-dwelling elderly women has confirmed that supplementation with 400–800 U/day vitamin D corrected vitamin D status in a large proportion of subjects within 3 months.[5] At baseline, low vitamin D status was associated with decreased physical activity and slower gait.

Conclusions

This patient should receive urgent intravenous calcium as a bolus followed by an infusion of calcium. If hypocalcaemia appears to be relatively resistant to treatment, intravenous magnesium should also be given if the patient is, or may be, magnesium deficient. If she does prove to have hypoparathyroidism, she will require life-long calcium and vitamin D. In cases of nutritional vitamin D deficiency this may be stopped once the hypocalcaemia has been corrected.

Further Reading

1 Diamond TH, Ho KW, Rohl PG, Meerkin M. Annual intramuscular injection of a megadose of cholecalciferol for treatment of vitamin D deficiency: efficacy and safety data. *Med J Aust* 2005; **183**: 10–12.

2 Pepe J, Romagnoli E, Nofroni I, *et al.* Vitamin D status as the major factor determining the circulating levels of parathyroid hormone: a study in normal subjects. *Osteoporos Int* 2005; **16**: 805–12.

3 Holick MF. The vitamin D epidemic and its health consequences. *J Nutr* 2005; **135**: 2739S–48S.

4 Gaugris S, Heaney RP, Boonen S, Kurht H, Bentkover JD, Sen SS. Vitamin D inadequacy among post-menopausal women: a systematic review. *Q J Med* 2005; **98**: 667–76.

5 Greenspan SL, Resnick NM, Parker RA. Vitamin D supplementation in older women. *J Gerontol* 2005; **60A**: 754–9.

PROBLEM

45 Oestrogen and Progesterone

Case History

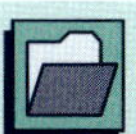

A 52-year-old woman consults you wanting advice on hormone replacement therapy (HRT). Her periods have stopped recently. She has noted hot flushes over the past 6 months and thinks that she is lacking in energy. She also complains of a marked decrease in her libido.

What are the major considerations regarding whether she should take HRT or not?

How would you help her choose the route of treatment and the preparation?

Is there a role for androgen replacement after the menopause?

Background

Menopause is the time when menstrual function and ovarian activity cease. Average age at menopause is 51 years. It cannot be definitively diagnosed until 1 year after the last period. A transition phase of up to 4 years often precedes the final period. During this time, women may experience symptoms and signs of developing oestrogen deficiency. These include: altered menstrual function with shortening, lengthening or irregularity of periods and change in the amount of bleeding; hot flushes and night sweats; sleep and mood disturbances; urinary and vaginal symptoms (stress incontinence), recurrent urinary tract infections, soreness and dryness, dyspareunia; thin skin and hair, brittle nails; impaired wellbeing.

Eighty per cent of women experience symptoms before, during or after the menopause, and these are severe in up to half. Serum follicle-stimulating hormone (FSH) is the most useful test: levels of greater than 30 U/l are consistent with menopause, although levels fluctuate widely in pre-menopausal women and FSH should therefore be measured on more than one occasion several weeks apart. Declining ovarian function is associated with increased FSH levels in early follicular phase. FSH >10 U/l on days 2–3 after the onset of bleeding is suggestive of incipient ovarian failure. Weight gain is common after the menopause and the prevalence of urogenital problems, osteoporosis, cardiovascular disease and stroke all increase. Oestrogen replacement therapy combined with progestogen is provided to women who have an intact uterus.

Since menopausal symptoms are self-limiting in most cases, HRT or other pharmacological treatment should only be started where necessary, and only after due consideration of potential benefits and risks. Lifestyle management such as looser clothes, cooler environment, avoiding triggers for vasomotor symptoms (alcohol, spicy foods etc.) should be discussed. Oestrogen replacement is the most effective treatment for vasomotor symptoms. Tibolone, a compound with oestrogenic, androgenic and progestogenic activity is effective, as is progestogen-only HRT. The antidepressant drugs paroxetine (20 mg/day) or venlafaxine (75 mg/day) may be helpful in some cases, and clonidine (25–50 mg/day) is sometimes helpful. Loss of libido can be treated with tibolone or, in specialist hands, small doses of testosterone. Vaginal symptoms often respond to low-dose vaginal oestrogen.

The increased risk of breast cancer is very small with short-term use of HRT. It is slightly higher with combined therapy, but increased risk does not become apparent until 4 years of treatment, and declines to normal population levels 5 years after stopping HRT. Unopposed oestrogen in women with intact uterus increases endometrial hyperplasia, and thus the risk of endometrial carcinoma. Use of progestogen for at least 12 days of the cycle is recommended. HRT also increases risk of ischaemic stroke and venous thromboembolism. It should no longer be used as first line for prevention or treatment of osteoporosis, and should not be prescribed for cardiovascular prevention. Evidence that HRT prevents tooth loss or cognitive decline with ageing is not sufficiently strong to justify routine use for these purposes.

The oestrogen dose in standard HRT preparations is not sufficient to act as a contraceptive. Women with menopause before the age of 50 should be advised to continue to use contraception for 2 years after their last period. One year is sufficient for women who go through menopause after the age of 50.

In women with intact uterus, monthly cyclical regimens are usually preferred. Oestrogen should be given in the lowest dose that will control symptoms. Three-monthly cyclical regimens are usually reserved for women who experience side effects with the progestogen component. Up to a third of women have to stop or change the first preparation prescribed because of side effects. Low dose oestrogens (e.g. 0.3 mg conjugated oestrogen or 0.5 mg oestradiol) may be sufficient to control symptoms in some women.

Higher doses (0.625 mg conjugated oestrogen or 2 mg ostradiol) are associated with bone protection. Oestrogen replacement is not generally used for long enough to make a material long-term difference to risk of osteoporosis. Oral preparations are cheaper, but more likely to cause nausea and are best avoided in women taking drugs that induce liver enzymes. Other side effects related to oestrogen include dyspepsia, fluid retention, breast enlargement, bloating, migraine and cramps. Weight gain is not thought to occur. When these side effects occur consider a change of dose, route or preparation.

Progestogen can be given orally or by patch, and may be administered for 12–14 days of each cycle or continuously. Women on combined regimens who experience irregular or no bleeding may require a change of progestogen type or dose or duration of treatment. Side effects of progestogen include mood changes/depression, fluid retention/breast tenderness, headache/migraine, acne, and back pain. Side effects are more common with the more androgenic progestogens (norethisterone, norgestrel, levonorgestrel) compared with the less androgenic compounds (medroxyprogesterone or dydrogesterone). Some progestogens are anti-androgenic, particularly cyproterone. Newer agents, including Nestorone and trimegestone, are very potent progestogens with little or no effect on the other steroid axes. A suggested scheme for initiating HRT is shown in Figure 45.1.

Recent Developments

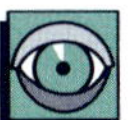

1 The Women's Health Initiative (WHI) enrolled 10 739 women aged 50–79 years who were post-menopausal and had prior hysterectomy. Women were randomized to receive either 0.625 mg conjugated equine oestrogen (CEE) or placebo. This wing of WHI was stopped prematurely in 2003 after 7 years. Use of CEE was associated with possible decreased breast cancer risk in this group (relative risk [RR] 0.77; 95% confidence interval [CI] 0.59 to 1.01) and decreased risk of hip fracture (RR 0.61; 95% CI 0.41 to 0.91). Risk of stroke was increased (RR 1.39; 95% CI 1.10 to 1.77). There was no effect on the risk of heart disease or colon cancer.

2 Selective oestrogen receptor modulators have oestrogen antagonist effects on breast and uterus but agonist effects on other tissues, including bone. In the Multiple Outcomes of Raloxifene Evaluation (MORE) trial, use of the drug appeared to be associated with increased risk of new diabetes or worsening of pre-existing diabetes. Lasco *et al.*[1] have studied a small group of women before and after raloxifene using the euglycaemic hyperinsulinaemic clamp. Although there were no changes in glucose tolerance, insulin sensitivity did decrease in women treated with the drug.

3 Newer oestrogen modulators with improved selectivity are being developed. Bazedoxifene has been tested in animal models.[2] This compound has low potency on the uterus but maintains a high action in bone, decreasing resorption. One possible advantage of the drug is its low effect in contributing to vasomotor phenomena.

4 There is now considerable evidence to support use of androgen replacement in some women. However, there is debate about which androgen, the optimal dose, and the preferred route of administration. Oral testosterone can cause changes in liver enzymes and adverse effects on lipid profile. The hormone can also be administered as subcutaneous implants and by the transdermal route. Testosterone gel is easy to administer and can restore circulating testosterone to the normal pre-menopausal level with a minimal risk of side effects.[3]

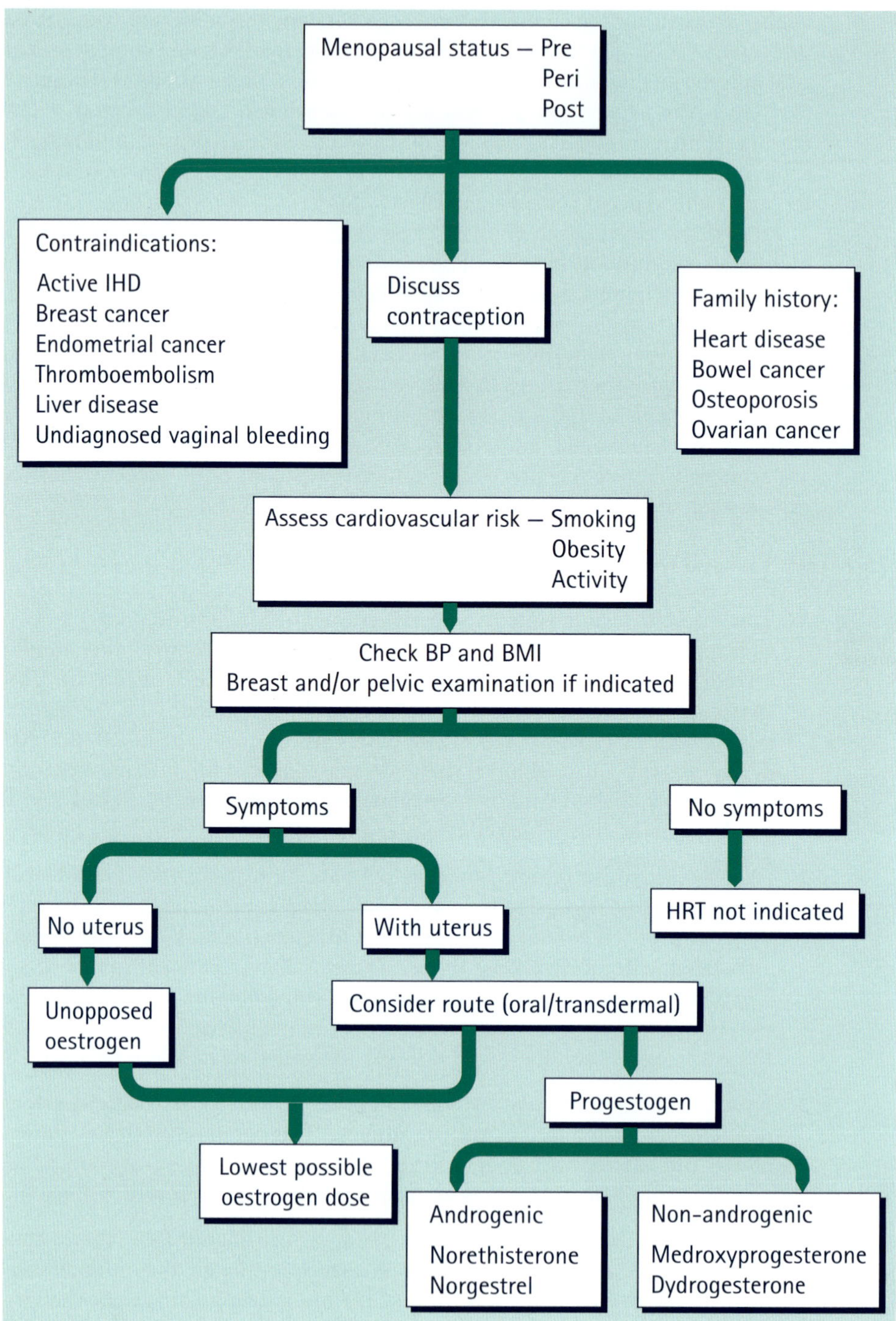

Fig. 45.1 Initiating hormone replacement therapy. *All women, whether on HRT or not, should have an annual medical check. BMI = body mass index; BP = blood pressure; IHD = ischaemic heart disease.

5 Adrenal androgen status also decreases in later life, and some of the effects of ageing have been ascribed to the decline in dehydroepiandrosterone (DHEA) levels with ageing. Administration of DHEA to post-menopausal women not only restores levels of this hormone, but also those of other androgens (testosterone and androstenedione).[4] The result is improved muscle mass and function, improved sexual function, and better self-reported quality of life.

Conclusions

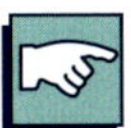

Current evidence favours use of HRT for relief of menopausal symptoms only. Its use should be reviewed regularly and it should only be continued for as long as it is useful in relieving symptoms, but for no more than 5 years. Monthly cyclical treatment is the approach of choice for women with an intact uterus. The lowest dose of oestrogen that can control symptoms should be used. Many of the side effects attributed to HRT arise from the progestogen component. Agents with higher androgenic activity may improve libido and wellbeing but are more likely to give rise to side effects. Monthly cyclical treatment can be by oral or transdermal routes, or by a combination of the two. The route of administration largely depends on the patient's personal preference.

Further Reading

1 Lasco A, Gaudio A, Morabito N, *et al.* Effects of a long-term treatment with raloxifene on insulin sensitivity in postmenopausal women. *Diabetologia* 2004; **47**: 571–4.

2 Komm BS, Kharode YP, Bodine PVN, Harris HA, Miller CP, Lyttle CR. Bazedoxifene acetate: a selective estrogen receptor modulator with improved selectivity. *Endocrinology* 2005; **146**: 3999–4008.

3 Nathorst-Boos J, Jarkander-Rolff M, Carlstrom K, Floter A, Von Schoultz B. Percutaneous administration of testosterone gel in postmenopausal women—a pharmacological study. *Menopause* 2005; **20**: 243–8.

4 Dayal M, Sammel MD, Zhao J, Hummel AC, Vandenbourne K, Barnhart KT. Supplementation with DHEA: effect on muscle size, strength, quality of life, and lipids. *J Women's Health* 2005; **14**: 391–400.

PROBLEM

46 Thyroid Hormone Replacement

Case History

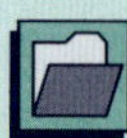

Mr HF is a 50-year-old executive who enjoys good general health. He was diagnosed as having hypothyroidism 4 years ago. His previous general practitioner has tried very hard to find a dose of thyroxine that suits him, but the patient continues to complain that his energy and mental functioning are not what they should be. He has read that thyroid extract is available and wonders whether this may be of benefit to him. He currently takes 150 μg thyroxine per day – free T_4 is 20 pmol/l (normal 12–25 pmol/l) and his thyroid-stimulating hormone (TSH) is 2.1 mIU/l (normal 0.35–3.5 mIU/l).

How would you approach his thyroid replacement therapy?

Is there a role for thyroid extract?

Should he consider combined replacement with thyroxine and triiodothyronine?

Background

Hypothyroidism affects over 5% of the female population and 5% of the population over 60 years. Many patients continue to complain of symptoms despite what appears to be adequate replacement therapy. It remains controversial whether such patients benefit from combined treatment with thyroxine (T_4) and triiodothyronine (T_3).[1] About 20% of hormone produced by the thyroid is T_3, and this is the active hormone. Experiments in rats show that replacement with both hormones is necessary to restore tissue levels of T_3 and T_4, and that the optimal ratio is around 14:1 which equates for a human to 100 μg T_4 and 6 μg T_3 per day. T_4 has a plasma half-life of 6 days and can be administered in a single daily dose. Levels of T_3 peak 2–4 hours after administration, and the half-life is less than 24 hours. It needs to be given in multiple daily doses. To date, only one clinical study has shown improved mood, quality of life and psychometric performance with combined therapy. The balance of opinion at present is, therefore, that routine use of combined replacement therapy is not justified.

The first controlled clinical trial of combined therapy was published in 1970 by Smith and colleagues (discussed in reference 1). In their double-blind, crossover study, patients were treated with 100 μg T_4 or 80 μg T_4 + 20 μg T_3. Those on combined therapy experienced frequent palpitations, tremor and anxiety. No benefit from the combined therapy was documented. In fact, prior to the advent of modern thyroid tests offering high sensitivity measurement of TSH and free thyroid hormones, many patients with hypothyroidism were over-treated. Impaired quality of life, cognitive performance, and other symptoms can result from both under- and over-treatment. The study by Bunevicius published in 1999,[2] supported the use of combined replacement: 33 hypothyroid patients took part in a crossover study with each phase lasting 5 weeks. During one of the two phases 50 μg of their thyroxine replacement was replaced by 12.5 μg T_3. The authors used 17 tests of cognition and mood. With combined treatment, T_4 level decreased, T_3 increased, and there was no change in TSH. Combined therapy was associated with improved mood, neuropsychological functioning and self-assessed physical status. Five further clinical trials published in 2003 and 2004 (reviewed in reference 1) did not show any difference between thyroxine alone and thyroxine combined with triiodothyronine. Some of these involved only small numbers of subjects, and may not have been suitably powered to detect relatively subtle differences in neuropsychological functions. In a recent large study of 697 patients, Saravanan *et al.*[3] substituted 10 μg of T_3 for 50 μg of usual T_4 replacement. Although there were temporary improvements in some cases, no specific benefit was seen with the combined therapy over 12 months.

Although there does not appear to be strong evidence for combined T_3 and T_4 replacement in hypothyroid patients, the fact is that many patients experience persistent hypothyroid symptoms while biochemical tests appear satisfactory. Many of the studies reported have been small and short term. Also, they have not focused on patients who are experiencing symptoms. Further, it is surprisingly difficult to compare two thyroid replacement regimens: TSH concentration indicates pituitary status but different tissues may respond in different ways to varying thyroid hormone concentrations. Saravanan and colleagues[4] surveyed 961 patients taking thyroxine from five general practices. They used the short form of the General Health Questionnaire (GHQ-12) and a twelve-item thyroid symptom questionnaire. In spite of having TSH in the normal range, patients reported dissatisfaction with their state of health. The differences were still apparent when observations were corrected for presence of other chronic diseases and use of other drugs in a multivariate analysis.

Recent Developments

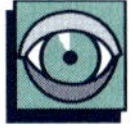

1 Two very recent trials[4,5] again did not demonstrate objective benefit of combined therapy, but reported a marked patient preference for the combination. Appelhof *et al.*[6] divided patients into three groups—those taking their usual replacement, those taking T_4 and T_3 in a ratio of 10:1, and those taking the hormones in a ratio of 5:1. Plasma TSH in the three groups was 0.64, 0.35 and 0.07 mIU/l, respectively. Weight change was +0.1, −0.5, and −1.7 kg, respectively. Although patients reported a preference for the combined treatment, there was no evidence for improved neuropsychological functioning.

2 Bianchi *et al.*[7] used the Short Form-36 (SF-36) and the Nottingham Health Profile questionnaires in a large series of patients with thyroid disorders. Physical and emotional function was decreased, as was general health and social function. Mood disturbances are common in patients with hypothyroidism and may, of course, contribute to cognitive and social impairment.

3 Decreased functioning of the nuclear retinoid and thyroid hormone pathways in the nucleus has been implicated in the cognitive decline that occurs with ageing. A recent

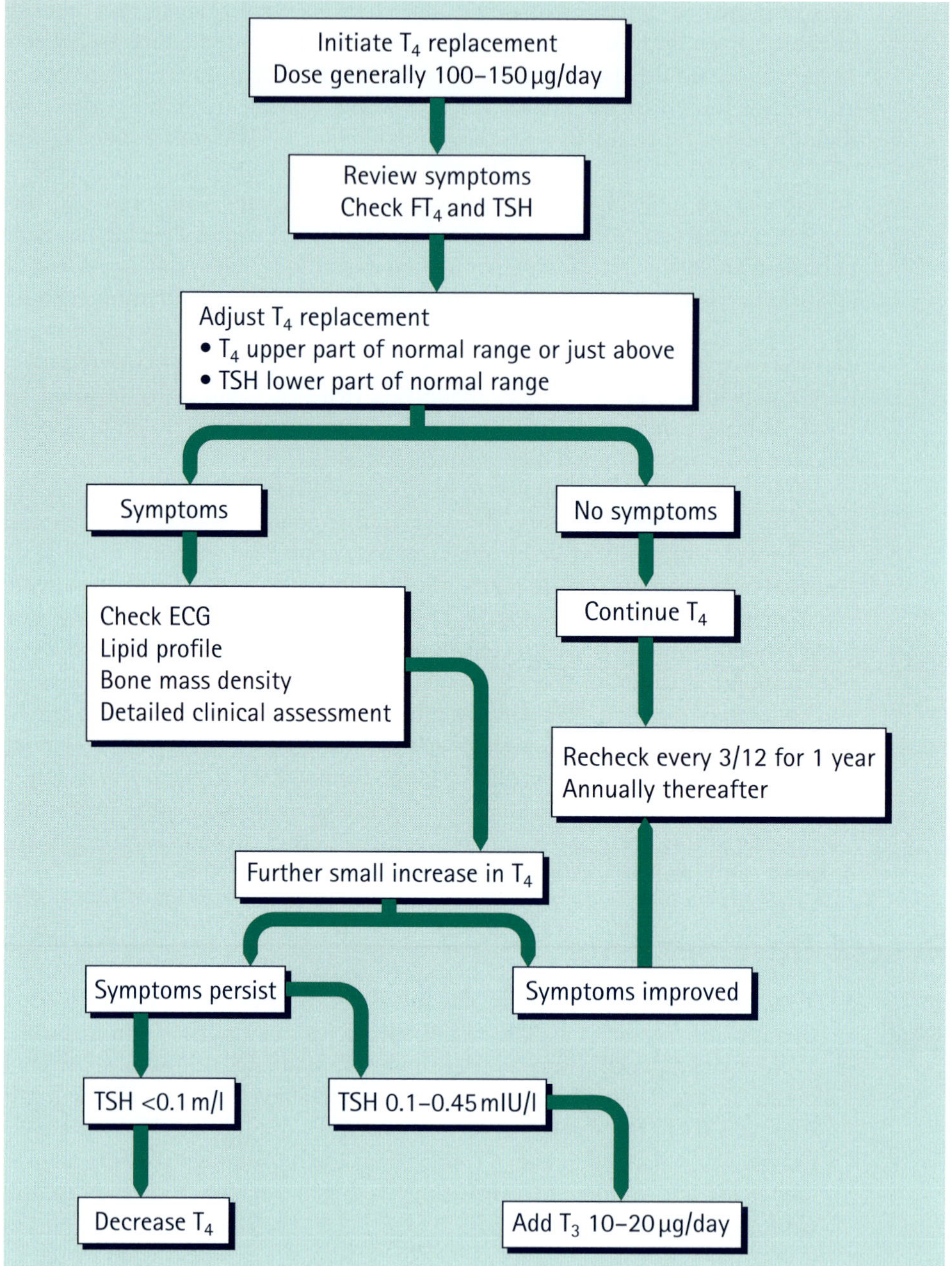

Fig. 46.1 Optimization of thyroid replacement. ECG = electrocardiogram; TSH = thyroid-stimulating hormone.

study[8] has demonstrated decreased receptor expression in the brains of ageing subjects. It is not clear at present whether increased doses of thyroid hormone are required, justified, or effective in overcoming this effect of ageing.

Conclusions

It is very common for patients to feel that their thyroid hormone replacement is inadequate. This issue often does not receive due attention. The balance of evidence does not suggest a particular benefit from combined replacement with T_3 and T_4. However, patients often feel better on the combination. There is no justification for the use of thyroid extract. It is always easier for the patient, and for monitoring therapy, if treatment with one agent (thyroxine) is suitable. Every effort should be made to optimize monotherapy and to obtain a realistic assessment of the patient's symptoms before considering dual therapy. Some patients do benefit from combination therapy. Our approach to this is summarized in Figure 46.1. A patient and measured approach is required since both TSH levels and symptoms take weeks, if not months, to alter following a change of treatment.

Further Reading

1 Escobar-Morreale HF, Botella-Carretero JI, Escobar del Rey F, Morrealle de Escobar G. Treatment of hypothyroidism with combinations of levothyroxine plus liothyronine. *J Clin Endocrinol Metab* 2005; **90**: 4946–54.

2 Bunevicius R, Kazanavicius G, Zalinkevicius R, Prange AJ. Effects of thyroxine as compared with thyroxine plus triiodothyronine in patients with hypothyroidism. *N Engl J Med* 1999; **340**: 424–9.

3 Saravanan P, Simmons DJ, Greenwood R, Peters TJ, Dayan CM. Partial substitution of thyroxine (T4) with tri-iodothyronine in patients on T4 replacement therapy: results of a large community-based randomized controlled trial. *J Clin Endocrinol Metab* 2005; **90**: 805–12.

4 Saravanan P, Chau WF, Roberts N, Vedhara K, Greenwood R, Dayan CM. Psychological well-being in patients on 'adequate' doses of l-thyroxine: results of a large, controlled community-based questionnaire study. *Clin Endocrinol* 2002; **57**: 577–85.

5 Escobar-Morreale HF, Botella-Carretero JI, Gómez-Bueno M, Galán JM, Barrios V, Sancho J. Thyroid hormone replacement therapy in primary hypothyroidism: a randomized trial comparing L-thyroxine plus liothyronine with L-thyroxine alone. *Ann Int Med* 2005; **142**: 412–24.

6 Appelhof BC, Fliers E, Wekking EM, *et al.* Combined therapy with levothyroxine and liothyronine in two ratios, compared with levothyroxine monotherapy in primary hypothyroidism: a double-blind, randomized, controlled clinical trial. *J Clin Endocrinol Metab* 2005; **90**: 2666–74.

7 Bianchi GP, Zaccheroni V, Solaroli E, *et al.* Health-related quality of life in patients with thyroid disorders. *Qual Life Res* 2004; **13**: 45–54.

8 Feart C, Pallet V, Boucheron C, *et al.* Aging affects the retinoic acid and the triiodothyronine nuclear receptor mRNA expression in human peripheral blood mononuclear cells. *Eur J Endocrinol* 2005; **152**: 449–58.

Index

H

N

O

P

Q

R

U

V

W

X

Y

Z

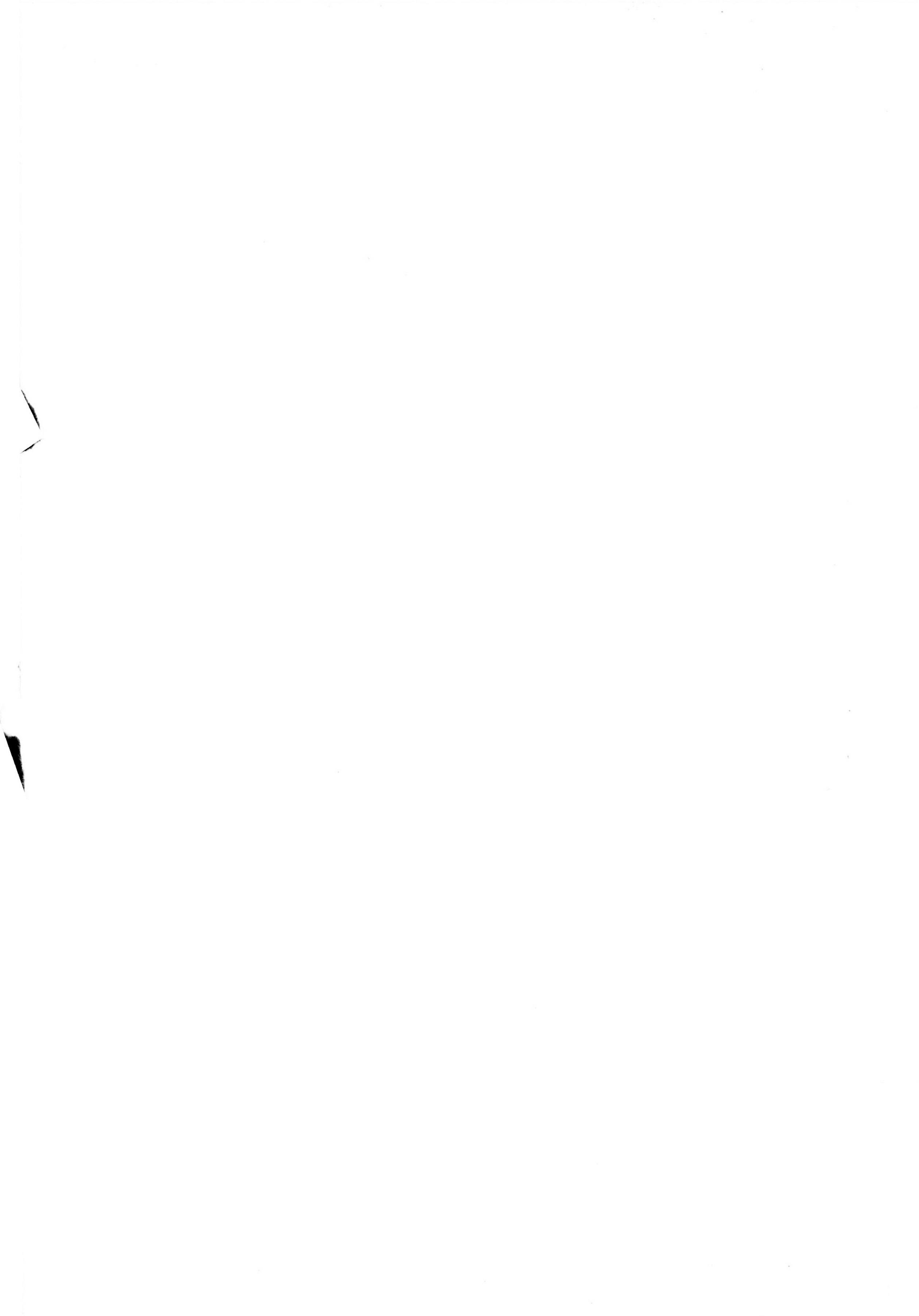